P9-DZA-118

Community as Partner

THEORY AND PRACTICE IN NURSING

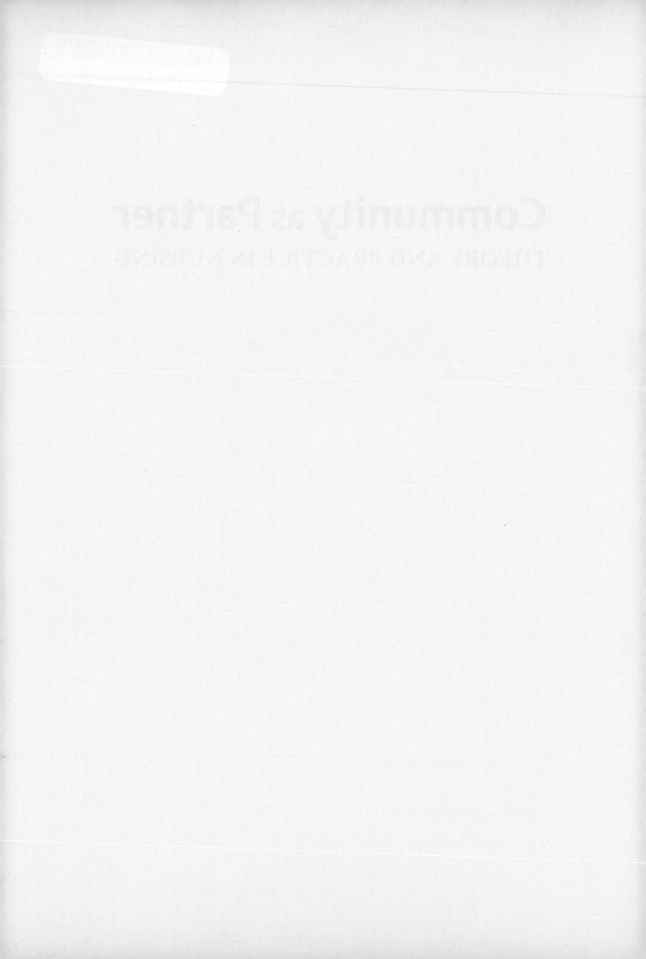

Community as Partner

THEORY AND PRACTICE IN NURSING

7th Edition

Elizabeth T. Anderson, DrPH, RN, FAAN

Professor Emerita
The University of Texas Medical Branch
School of Nursing
Galveston, Texas

Honorary Member
Pan American Nursing and Midwifery Collaborating Centers
Global Network of World Health Organization
Collaborating Centers for Nursing and Midwifery

Judith McFarlane, DrPH, RN, FAAN

Parry Chair in Health Promotion and Disease Prevention
Texas Woman's University
College of Nursing
Houston, Texas

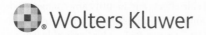
Wolters Kluwer

Philadelphia • Baltimore • New York • London
Buenos Aires • Hong Kong • Sydney • Tokyo

Acquisitions Editor: Chris Richardson
Product Development Editor: Meredith L. Brittain
Editorial Assistant: Zachary Shapiro
Design Coordinator: Holly Reid McLaughlin
Marketing Manager: Nicole Dunlap
Production Project Manager: Cynthia Rudy
Manufacturing Coordinator: Karin Duffield
Prepress Vendor: S4Carlisle Publishing Services

7th edition

Copyright © 2015 Wolters Kluwer.

Copyright © 2011 Wolters Kluwer Health | Lippincott Williams & Wilkins. Copyright © 2008 by Lippincott Williams & Wilkins, a Wolters Kluwer business. Copyright © 2004, 2000 by Lippincott Williams & Wilkins. Copyright © 1996 by Lippincott-Raven. Copyright © 1988 by J.B. Lippincott Company. All rights reserved. This book is protected by copyright. No part of this book may be reproduced or transmitted in any form or by any means, including as photocopies or scanned-in or other electronic copies, or utilized by any information storage and retrieval system without written permission from the copyright owner, except for brief quotations embodied in critical articles and reviews. Materials appearing in this book prepared by individuals as part of their official duties as U.S. government employees are not covered by the above-mentioned copyright. To request permission, please contact Wolters Kluwer at Two Commerce Square, 2001 Market Street, Philadelphia, PA 19103, via email at permissions@lww.com, or via our website at lww.com (products and services).

9 8 7 6 5 4 3 2

Printed in China

Library of Congress Cataloging-in-Publication Data
Anderson, Elizabeth T., author.
  Community as partner : theory and practice in nursing / Elizabeth T. Anderson, Judith McFarlane. — Seventh edition.
    p. ; cm.
  Includes bibliographical references and index.
  ISBN 978-1-4511-9093-9
  I. McFarlane, Judith M., author.   II. Title.
  [DNLM: 1. Community Health Nursing.   2. Health Promotion.   3. Nurse's Role.   4. Nursing Theory.   WY 106]
  RT98
  610.73'43—dc23
                                                                                        2014018428

This work is provided "as is," and the publisher disclaims any and all warranties, express or implied, including any warranties as to accuracy, comprehensiveness, or currency of the content of this work.

   This work is no substitute for individual patient assessment based upon healthcare professionals' examination of each patient and consideration of, among other things, age, weight, gender, current or prior medical conditions, medication history, laboratory data and other factors unique to the patient. The publisher does not provide medical advice or guidance and this work is merely a reference tool. Healthcare professionals, and not the publisher, are solely responsible for the use of this work including all medical judgments and for any resulting diagnosis and treatments.

   Given continuous, rapid advances in medical science and health information, independent professional verification of medical diagnoses, indications, appropriate pharmaceutical selections and dosages, and treatment options should be made and healthcare professionals should consult a variety of sources. When prescribing medication, healthcare professionals are advised to consult the product information sheet (the manufacturer's package insert) accompanying each drug to verify, among other things, conditions of use, warnings and side effects and identify any changes in dosage schedule or contradictions, particularly if the medication to be administered is new, infrequently used or has a narrow therapeutic range. To the maximum extent permitted under applicable law, no responsibility is assumed by the publisher for any injury and/or damage to persons or property, as a matter of products liability, negligence law or otherwise, or from any reference to or use by any person of this work.

LWW.com

CCS0915

Dedication

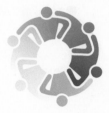

To the memory of public health mentors, colleagues, and friends

Edith Wright
Shirley Hutchinson

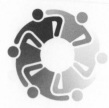

Contributors to the 7th Edition

Elizabeth T. Anderson, DrPH, RN, FAAN
Professor Emerita
The University of Texas Medical Branch
School of Nursing
Galveston, Texas
Honorary Member
Pan American Nursing and Midwifery
    Collaborating Centers
Global Network of World Health Organization
    Collaborating Centers for Nursing and
    Midwifery

Judith C. Drew, PhD, RN
Professor Emeritus
The University of Texas Medical Branch
Galveston, Texas

Nina M. Fredland, PhD, RN, FNP
Associate Professor
Texas Woman's University
Houston, Texas

Heidi Gilroy, MSN, APHN-BC
Senior Project Manager
Texas Woman's University
Houston, Texas

Julia Henderson Gist, PhD, RN, CNE
Division Chair of Health Sciences/
    Director of Nursing
Arkansas State University Mountain Home
Mountain Home, Arkansas

Deanna E. Grimes, DrPH, RN, FAAN
Professor
The University of Texas Health Science Center at
    Houston
Houston, Texas

David Hartley, PhD, MHA
Research Professor
University of Southern Maine
Portland, Maine

**Bruce Leonard, PhD, RN, APRN, FNP-BC,
NP-C**
Associate Professor
University of Nevada
Las Vegas, Nevada

Teresa L. Maharaj, RN, MS
Assistant Clinical Professor
Texas Woman's University
Houston, Texas

Ann T. Malecha, PhD, RN
Professor and Research Liaison
Texas Woman's University
Houston, Texas

Judith McFarlane, DrPH, RN, FAAN
Parry Chair in Health Promotion and Disease
    Prevention
Texas Woman's University
College of Nursing
Houston, Texas

Robert W. McFarlane, PhD
Consulting Ecologist
Houston, Texas

Elnora P. Mendias, PhD, RN, APRN, FNP-BC
Professor, ret.
The University of Texas Medical Branch School
    of Nursing
Galveston, Texas

Susan Scoville Walker, EdD, RN, FAAN
Professor Emeritus
University of Nebraska Medical Center
Omaha, Nebraska

Lynda Law Wilson, PhD, RN, FAAN
Professor
The University of Alabama
Birmingham, Alabama

Teresa J. Walsh, PhD, RNC, MS
Associate Clinical Professor
Texas Woman's University
Houston, Texas

For a list of the contributors to the Student and Instructor Resources accompanying this book, please visit http://thepoint.lww.com/Anderson7e.

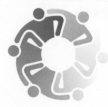

Contributors to the 6th Edition

Judith C. Drew, PhD, RN
Professor Emerita
The University of Texas Medical Branch
School of Nursing
Galveston, Texas

Nina M. Fredland, PhD, RN
Assistant Professor
University of Texas at Austin
School of Nursing
Austin, Texas

Julia Henderson Gist, PhD, RN
Visiting Assistant Professor
Arkansas Tech University
Russellville, Arkansas

Deanna E. Grimes, DrPH, RN, FAAN
Professor
The University of Texas Health Science
    Center-Houston
School of Nursing
Houston, Texas

David Hartley, MHA, PhD
Director
Maine Rural Health Research Center
Portland, Maine

Shirley F. Hutchinson, DrPH, RN
Associate Professor
Texas Woman's University
Houston, Texas

Bruce Leonard, PhD, RN, FNP, NP-C, BC
Associate Professor
The University of Texas Medical Branch
School of Nursing
Galveston, Texas

Ann T. Malecha, PhD, RN
Professor
Texas Woman's University
Houston, Texas

Robert W. McFarlane, PhD
Consulting Ecologist
Houston, Texas

Elnora P. Mendias, PhD, RN
Associate Professor
The University of Texas Medical Branch
School of Nursing
Galveston, Texas

Susan Scoville Walker, PhD, RN
Professor Emerita of Nursing
Texas A&M International University
Laredo, Texas

Teresa J. Walsh, PhD, RNC
Associate Clinical Professor
Texas Woman's University
Houston, Texas

Lynda Law Wilson, PhD, RN, FAAN
Professor, Assistant Dean for
    International Affairs
Deputy Director, WHO/PAHO Collaborating
    Center on International Nursing
University of Alabama at Birmingham
Birmingham, Alabama

Nancy Zamboras, RN, CCM, COHN-S
Occupational Health Associate
Chevron Phillips Chemical Company
The Woodlands, Texas

Reviewers

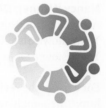

Debborah Bolian, MSN
Assistant Professor
Mississippi College School of Nursing
Clinton, Mississippi

Angeline Bushy, PhD
Professor
University of Central Florida
Daytona Beach, Florida

Barbara Cheyney, BSN, MS
Adjunct Professor
Seattle Pacific University
Seattle, Washington

Susan Coyle, PhD
Assistant Professor
West Virginia University School of Nursing
Morgantown, West Virginia

Michelle Dang, PhD, RN, APHN-BC
Assistant Professor
California State University
Sacramento, California

Rhonda Goodman, PhD, ARNP, FNP-BC,
NCSN, AHN-BC
Assistant Professor
Florida Atlantic University
Boca Raton, Florida

J. Mari Beth Linder, PhD, MSN, BSN
Professor of Nursing
Missouri Southern State University
Joplin, Missouri

Kalay Naidoo, MSN
Assistant Professor
Bon Secours Memorial College of Nursing
Richmond, Virginia

Barbara Poremba, EdD, MPH, MS, RNCS,
ANP, CNE
Professor
Salem State University
Salem, Massachusetts

Collette Renstrom, DNP, APRN, FNP-C
Assistant Professor
Weber State University
Ogden, Utah

Sheila Stroman, MSN, PhD
Assistant Professor
University of Central Arkansas
Conway, Arkansas

Candace Tavormina, MSN, CNE
Associate Professor
Mercy College of Ohio
Toledo, Ohio

Roseann Vivanco, RN, MSN
Clinical Instructor
The University of Texas Health Science Center
San Antonio, Texas

Della Wagner, MSN
Assistant Professor
The University of Texas Health Science Center
San Antonio, Texas

Nancy Wagner, DNP
Associate Professor
Youngstown State University
Youngstown, Ohio

Dolores Wright, PhD
Professor
Loma Linda University
Loma Linda, California

For a list of the reviewers of the Test Generator accompanying this book, please visit http://thepoint.lww.com/Anderson7e.

Preface

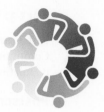

This user-friendly text is presented as a handbook for students and practicing nurses who work with communities to promote health. *Community as Partner* focuses on the essentials of practice with the community. Students will find this text helpful for the many examples of working with the community as partner. For over 20 years and seven editions, this textbook has served undergraduate, RN to BS and RN to MS students, and graduate students alike as a framework for professional nursing practice in the community. Our intention is to keep the text basic and accessible to all who practice in the community. Using this text with distance education and virtual learning with internet resources will enrich practice in any community.

Organizational Philosophy

This seventh edition continues the philosophy of the authors by strengthening the theoretical base with updated chapters on globalization and rural health. All other chapters have been revised and updated from the sixth edition. We continue with a series of chapters that takes the reader through the entire nursing process by using a real-life community as our example. The urban example is enhanced and expanded throughout the remainder of the book by selected aggregates that serve as exemplars of working with the community as partner as well.

Part 1: Essential Elements for Healthy Partnerships

Part 1 of the book describes content areas basic to the practice of community health nursing. The areas encompassed include globalization, essentials of practice, theoretical foundations, epidemiology, environmental health, ethics, empowerment, cultural competence, health policy, informatics, and infectious diseases and disasters. Emphasis is on theory-based practice, with those theories critical to community as partner described and explicated.

Part 2: The Process of Working With the Community

Part 2 covers the process of working with the community. The assessment chapter (Chapter 11) includes an introduction to the community-as-partner model, which then serves as a framework for the remaining chapters in this section. One sample community is used to illustrate each step of the nursing process for community health nursing practice. The chapters guide the reader through processes of community assessment; data analysis; formulation of a community nursing diagnosis; and the planning, implementation, and evaluation of a community health program. Emphasis throughout is on understanding the community as a dynamic system that is more than the sum of its parts and in continual interaction with the environment.

Part 3: Practicing With Diverse Communities

Part 3 provides examples in which nurses play a major role as partners in health promotion. Communities and aggregates in this section include marginalized groups, the workplace, rural populations, schools, faith communities, and the elderly.

Postscript

An editorial describing some of the roots of public health nursing is reproduced at the end of the book as both a reminder of our past and a challenge for the future.

Special Features

- **Learning Objectives** at the beginning of each chapter focus readers' attention on important chapter content.
- **Take Note** boxes highlight key concepts for readers as they go through the steps of the nursing process for a community.
- **Critical Thinking Questions** at the end of each chapter enable students to review and apply chapter content.
- **Further Readings** offer additional references on the chapter subject matter.

Additional Resources

Community as Partner includes additional resources for both instructors and students that are available on the book's companion website at http://thepoint.lww.com/Anderson7e.

Instructors

Approved adopting instructors will be given access to the following additional resources:

- Brownstone test generator with more than 400 multiple choice questions
- PowerPoint presentations, including multiple choice questions for use with interactive clicker technology
- An image bank, containing images from the text in formats suitable for printing, projecting, and incorporating into websites

Students

Students who have purchased *Community as Partner* have access to the following additional resources:

- Adams County interactive case studies engine
- Learning objectives

Acknowledgments

Our colleagues who contributed to this edition have enriched both the book and our lives. Along with our families and friends, they have sustained this process and helped us to feel proud of our profession.

Community as Partner: Theory and Practice in Nursing could not have been written without the thoughts, critiques, and examples provided by our students and colleagues in public health.

The fine folks at Wolters Kluwer Health have facilitated the process of doing this seventh edition so that it was an enjoyable experience.

We thank each of you.

Elizabeth T. Anderson
Judith McFarlane

Contents

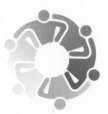

PART

3

Practicing With Diverse Communities   279

Essential Elements for Healthy Partnerships

CHAPTER 1

The World as Community: Globalization and Health

Lynda Law Wilson

LEARNING OBJECTIVES

This chapter provides a global perspective to community health nursing, introducing the concepts of globalization, major global health challenges, and the role of the nurse in contributing to the goals of promoting global health equity and reducing health disparities.

After studying this chapter, you should be able to:

1. Discuss the concepts of global health and globalization.

2. Analyze the relationship between globalization and health.

3. Discuss major global health challenges.

4. Describe the contributions of the Millennium Development Goals (MDGs) campaign to promoting global health.

5. Analyze the implications of health diplomacy for nurses.

6. Explore ways that nurses can contribute to reducing global health challenges and promoting the goal of Health for All.

Introduction

The world is indeed a global community, and this is an exciting time to be a nurse. There are unlimited opportunities to truly make a difference in promoting social justice and global health equity and in reducing health disparities for all of the world's peoples. Nurses provide 60% to 80% of the world's health care, although in some rural areas in Africa, nearly 85% of the health care is provided by nurses (World Health Organization [WHO] Department of Human Resources for Health, 2008, p. 83). Thus, it is critical that nurses have an awareness of key global health challenges, and the roles that they might play in addressing these challenges. Wilson et al. (2012) recently surveyed nursing faculty in the United States, Canada, Latin America, and the Caribbean to identify global health competencies for nurses.

The 593 respondents to this survey supported the importance of addressing the 30 competencies that were included in the survey in undergraduate nursing curricula.

One of the greatest challenges to global health that leads to health disparities is poverty and the associated problems related to lack of access to adequate food, water, shelter, and health care. The World Bank estimates that in 2008 about 1.2 billion people (or 22% of the world's population) lived below the international poverty line of $1.25 a day (World Bank, 2013a). Although the percentage of the world's population living in poverty has declined from 52% in 1981 to 22% in 2008, there are significant disparities in the poverty rates among countries. In East Asia, the poverty rate has decreased from 84% in 1981 to 13% in 2008. In contrast, in sub-Saharan Africa, the poverty rate has decreased only 4% from 52% in 1981 to 48% in 2008 (World Bank, 2013b). In addition to poverty, there are many other factors that contribute to health disparities, including racial/ethnic status, presence of physical or mental disabilities, stigma associated with certain health problems such as mental illness or HIV/AIDS, and inequitable distribution of global resources, including funding for research to address global health problems. The term "10/90 gap" has been used to characterize this imbalance, referring to the concept that only 10% of the world's research resources are used to address the health problems that affect 90% of the world's population (Kilama, 2009). Although the gap has narrowed in recent years, there remain significant disparities in spending for health and for health research between the rich and poor countries of the world.

 Take Note

"Health disparities are systematic, plausibly avoidable health differences according to race/ethnicity, skin color, religion, or nationality; socioeconomic resources or position (reflected by, e.g., income, wealth, education, or occupation); gender, sexual orientation, gender identity; age, geography, disability, illness, political or other affiliation; or other characteristics associated with discrimination or marginalization." (Braveman et al., 2011, p. S150)

GLOBAL HEALTH AND GLOBALIZATION

In 1997, the Institute of Medicine in the United States published a landmark report that highlighted America's vital interest in global health. In this report, global health was defined as "health issues that transcend national boundaries, and may best be addressed by cooperative actions" (Institute of Medicine, 1997). *Globalization* is a term used to refer to the increasing economic, political, social, technological, and intellectual interconnectedness of the world. Changes in the economy in one part of the world quickly influence the markets in other countries. Similarly, emerging infectious diseases can quickly spread across the globe. Globalization is not a new phenomenon; however, the current phase of globalization is different from earlier phases because of the speed with which new technologies promote the sharing of information, resources, and people (Bauman & Blythe, 2008). The process of globalization has also been influenced by global trade policies and deregulation that facilitate the movement of products and people across national borders. These trade policies can have significant impacts on public health when products that are imported from countries with lax safety and monitoring standards are exported internationally. One example was the discovery of a problem in the food supply chain in China when many exported products were found to be contaminated with banned drugs or toxic chemicals (Ramzy & Yang, 2008).

With the growing strength of organizations such as the World Trade Organization (WTO) and trade pacts such as the North American Free Trade Agreement (NAFTA), with their emphasis on free trade, free financial markets, and economic profits, governments—especially those of resource-poor nations—find themselves losing the ability to define and control their own futures. Political scientists and sociologists warn of the declining strength of the "nation state" and the questionable future of international organizations such as the United Nations (UN) and its related units such as the World Health Organization (WHO). If many countries are weakening in relation to powerful international forces, what does this mean for the development of our local communities? How are they affected by the emphasis on profit—usually for a few privileged individuals and companies?

Globalization has both positive and negative effects on health. The positive effects include diffusion of ideas, technologies, and other innovations that lead to improvements in many areas such as availability of safe water, medications, and treatments for both acute and chronic health problems. Expansion of trade has resulted in increased living standards for many, especially for women (Abbot & Coenen, 2008). Another positive effect noted in the 2008 World Health Report is the emerging "global stewardship" that has been influenced by more international and global exchanges, leading to growing recognition of common threats as well as opportunities, and a sense of growing solidarity and commitment to collaboration to promote global social justice and equity (WHO, 2008c). Negative effects include increased crowding in urban areas, increased health problems (such as obesity and chronic disease) associated with adoption of unhealthy Western lifestyles, and faster transmission of infectious diseases associated with increased global travel and "so-called 'microbial hitchhikers'" (Abbot & Coenen, 2008). Examples include the 2003 outbreak of the severe acute respiratory syndrome (SARS) (Murphy, 2006) and the 2007 incident in which a US citizen with extensively drug-resistant tuberculosis (XDR TB) failed to comply with medical orders and traveled on a commercial airplane to Paris, Athens, and then Rome for his honeymoon. The travel exposed more than 600 fellow passengers, requiring follow-up and tracking for testing and treatment as needed (Hitti, 2007).

Other negative effects of globalization are the "brain drain" that results from migration from lower-resource countries to higher-resource countries (WHO Department of Human Resources for Health, 2008) and growing disparities between the "haves" and the "have-nots." Birdsall noted that globalization has resulted in benefits for those who are already ahead—the high-resource countries, and among low- and middle-resource countries (those who are at the higher end of the socioeconomic spectrum) (Birdsall, 2006). Abbott and Coenen noted that although increased access to information that is associated with globalization and advances in information and communication technology (ICT) has resulted in many benefits to health as well as education and social development, some societies find this open exchange of information threatening to their ideologies and social structures (Abbot & Coenen, 2008). These authors also noted that many groups who could most benefit from increased access to ICT are unable to enjoy these benefits because of challenges with limited access to ICT due to untrained personnel and lack of infrastructure and resources. Grootjans and Newman suggested that in today's globalized world, nurses need to consider environmental determinants of health and illness, and "look beyond local influences on the well-being of clients towards national and global events that have direct impact on people's lives" (Grootjans & Newman, 2013, p. 83).

MAJOR GLOBAL HEALTH PROBLEMS

Although there continue to be significant disparities in the global burden of disease, there has been considerable progress in leading health indicators over the past 30 years. The 2008 World Health Report noted that although 9.5 million children died in 2006, a total of 16.2 million children would have died that year if the child mortality rates remained the same as they were in 1978. Despite these improvements, there remain significant inequities in the global burden of disease, and many of these inequities are directly related to the effects of poverty and the unequal distribution of the world's resources (WHO, 2008b). The global burden of disease is defined as "the disability-adjusted life year (DALY), [which is a] time-based measure combin[ing] years of life lost due to premature mortality and years of life lost due to time lived in states of less than full health" (WHO, 2008a). In 2012, *The Lancet* published a series of papers describing findings from the 2010 Global Burden of Disease Study, which was the "first systematic and comprehensive assessment of data on disease, injuries, and risk since 1990" (Horton, 2013, p. 2053). The results showed that life expectancies were increasing across the globe, and that rates of HIV, malaria, TB, and other infectious diseases were decreasing. Deaths due to cancer and road accidents have increased, and nearly 25% of all deaths are due to heart disease. The greatest disease risks were high blood pressure, followed by the use of tobacco and alcohol, and poor diet (Horton, 2013). Box 1.1 illustrates the top 12 causes of death across all regions of the world, and Box 1.2 summarizes key facts about the state of global health.

These global data provide important guidance for nurses and other health workers in identifying priorities for programs to address the most pressing health needs, but it is also important for nurses to be familiar with the specific problems in the communities where they practice. Nurses also need to be aware of new and emerging health problems associated with infectious diseases, climate change, and other factors such as potential threats to public health security resulting from industrial accidents, natural disasters, bioterrorism, or other health emergencies.

Infectious Diseases

The HIV/AIDS pandemic has had a devastating effect in many countries since it was first identified in the 1980s. In 2011, there were 34 million people living with HIV, and 0.8% of those between ages 15 and 49 were infected with HIV. There continue to be wide variations in the HIV infection rate globally. In sub-Saharan Africa nearly 5% of adults are infected with HIV, and this region accounts for 69% of adults living with HIV and 90% of children infected with HIV worldwide (Joint United Nations Programme on HIV/AIDS [UN-AIDS], 2012). Other emerging infections include those caused by newly evolved strains of

---

Box 1.1 Top 12 Causes of Death in the World, in Order of Prevalence

1. Ischemic heart disease
2. Cerebrovascular disease
3. Chronic obstructive pulmonary disease
4. Lower respiratory infections
5. Lung cancer
6. HIV/AIDS
7. Diarrheal diseases
8. Road injury
9. Diabetes mellitus
10. Tuberculosis
11. Malaria
12. Cirrhosis

Source: Institute for Health Metrics and Evaluation. (2013). *The global burden of disease: Generating evidence, guiding policy* (p. 12). Seattle, WA: University of Washington. Retrieved from http://www.healthmetricsandevaluation.org/gbd/publications/policy-report/global-burden-disease-generating-evidence-guiding-policy

---

Box 1.2   10 Facts About the State of Global Health

1. **Around 7 million children under the age of five die each year**. Almost all of these children could survive with access to simple and affordable interventions. WHO is working with governments and partners worldwide to deliver integrated, effective care and strengthen health systems, both of which are crucial to reduce child deaths.

2. **Cardiovascular diseases are the leading causes of death in the world**. Cardiovascular diseases are diseases of the heart and blood vessels that can cause heart attacks and stroke. At least 80% of premature deaths from cardiovascular heart disease and strokes could be prevented through a healthy diet, regular physical activity and avoiding the use of tobacco.

3. **HIV/AIDS is the leading cause of adult death in Africa**. The annual number of people dying from AIDS-related causes worldwide is steadily decreasing from a peak of 2.2 million in 2005 to an estimated 1.8 million in 2010. HIV testing and counseling uptake has improved, access to antiretroviral therapy has increased, however many people living with HIV in low- and middle-income countries still do not know their HIV status.

4. **Population ageing is contributing to the rise in cancer and heart disease**. The increasing proportion of older people in the global population is contributing to the increase of age-associated chronic diseases, particularly in developing countries. Care-givers, health systems and societies need to be ready to cope with the growing needs of the elderly in every part of the world.

5. **Lung cancer is the most common cause of death from cancer**. Tobacco use is responsible for 70% of all lung cancers – it is the single largest preventable cause of cancer in the world.

6. **Complications of pregnancy account for almost 15% of deaths in women of reproductive age worldwide**. Every day, about 800 women die due to complications of pregnancy and child birth. The risk of a woman in a developing country dying from a pregnancy-related cause during her lifetime is about 25 times higher compared to a woman living in a developed country. WHO works to improve maternal health by assisting countries to improve care before, during and after childbirth.

7. **Mental disorders such as depression are among the 20 leading causes of disability worldwide**. Depression affects around 350 million people worldwide and this number is projected to increase. Fewer than half of those affected have access to adequate treatment and health care.

8. **Hearing loss, vision problems and mental disorders are the most common causes of disability**. These disorders can affect people's lives and livelihoods, but many are easily treatable (e.g. hearing loss and cataracts). Statistics vary between higher- and lower-income countries but high overall rates of these disorders underline the need for wider access to interventions that help people live productively.

9. **Nearly 3500 people die from road traffic crashes every day**. Road traffic injuries are projected to increase as rising income levels in developing countries lead to increased vehicle ownership. Strong action to improve road use policies and enforce road laws will be needed to avert this increase.

10. **Under-nutrition is the underlying cause of death for at least one-third of all children under age five**. Inadequate breastfeeding, inappropriate food and a lack of access to highly nutritious foods contribute to the problem. Common childhood diseases affect a child's ability to eat or absorb the necessary nutrients from food.

Source: World Health Organization. (2013). *10 facts on the state of global health*. Retrieved June 23, 2013, from http://www.who.int/features/factfiles/global_burden/facts/en/index.html

---

pathogens (e.g., multiple-drug-resistant tuberculosis, some *Staphylococcus aureus* infection, or chloroquine-resistant malaria) and newly recognized infections such as SARS (Jones et al., 2008; Murphy, 2006). In a recent analysis of the emergence of 335 global infectious diseases that were reported from 1940 to 2004, Jones et al. (2008) reported that 22.8% of these diseases were vectorborne, and that the incidence of these diseases corresponds to climate anomalies that occurred during the 1990s, lending support to the hypothesis that global warming and climate change may lead to the emergence of these types of diseases.

Climate Change

Although the specific health effects of climate change and global warming continue to be debated, it is likely that there will be shifts in patterns of disease in the coming decades that are attributable at least in part to the effects of climate change. There are several ways in which climate change might influence health outcomes, including (a) changes in intensity of extreme heat waves, floods, and droughts; (b) changes in air pollutants and allergens; (c) alterations in ecosystems, water, and food supplies that in turn influence the incidence of infectious diseases as well as nutritional status; and (d) population displacement due to rising sea levels (Patz, Campbell-Lendrum, Gibbs, & Woodruff, 2008). Luber and Hess (2007), from the United States Centers for Disease Control, identified the following potential health effects of climate change: (a) the elderly and other vulnerable groups will be at greatest risk for exposure to catastrophic weather events such as hurricanes and extreme heat; (b) increased flooding will result in possible food and water shortages and may lead to mass migration, "environmental refugees, and regional tension and conflict"; (c) persons affected by disasters and economic problems due to ecosystem and climate changes will be vulnerable to mental health stresses; and (d) many vectorborne diseases may become more frequent and widespread. Kjellstrom and McMicheal (2013) reported that the average global temperature may increase by 3 to 4°C by 2011, and called for urgent action to reduce the potential devastating impact of global warming.

Threats to Global Public Health Security and Health Diplomacy

In today's world, it is essential that countries work together to minimize risks from disease outbreaks or health hazards related to factors such as natural disasters, infectious disease outbreaks, bioterrorism incidents, or other emergencies. Recognizing the importance of such global cooperation, the 2007 World Health Report was devoted entirely to the issue of global public health security in the 21st century (WHO, 2007). The Healthy People 2020 document included a global health goal to improve public health and strengthen U.S. national security through global disease detection, response, prevention, and control strategies (United States Department of Health and Human Services, 2013). It is important that every nurse be familiar with plans in his/her local community for dealing with potential threats to public health security, since nurses will be key first responders to any such threats. Global health diplomacy has emerged as an increasingly important strategy for addressing global health security threats. Global health diplomacy is "a political change activity that meets the dual goals of improving global health while maintaining and strengthening international relations abroad, particularly in conflict areas and resource-poor environments" (Novotny & Adams, 2007, p. 1). Hunter et al. (2013) recently reviewed the literature related to global health diplomacy and the implications of this emerging field for nurses. These authors recommended that nurses make important contributions to health diplomacy, but identified the need for nurses to engage in "critical dialogue about the ethical and moral conflicts inherent in this concept—providing health care as a humanitarian responsibility versus using health care as an instrument of political activity" (Hunter et al., 2013, p. 90).

MILLENNIUM DEVELOPMENT GOALS

In a historic meeting in New York in September 2000, representatives of 189 UN member states met and endorsed a plan called the Millennium Declaration, which has been described as "a new vision for humanity." The Millennium Declaration is a set of eight goals and specific targets under each goal designed to reduce poverty, reduce global inequities, and promote health and social welfare of the world's citizens (United Nations Department of Economic and Social Affairs, 2012). This plan, named the UN Millennium Development Goals (MDGs), outlined eight broad goals and specific targets for each goal, which were to be achieved by the year 2015. The eight goals, which are listed in Box 1.3, have served as guiding principles for both public and private organizations that focus on addressing global health and social welfare issues.

Each year the United Nations issues a MDG report to summarize the progress in addressing the eight goals. The 2012 report summarized the progress made on each of the eight goals at the midpoint of the 15-year target period. In the introduction to this report, Ban Ki-Moon, the Secretary General of the United Nations, noted that

This year's report on progress towards the Millennium Development Goals (MDGs) highlights several milestones. The target of reducing extreme poverty by half has been reached five years ahead of the 2015 deadline, as has the target of halving the proportion of people who lack dependable access to improved sources of drinking water. Conditions for more than 200 million people living in slums have been ameliorated—double the 2020 target. Primary school enrolment of girls equaled that of boys, and

---

Box 1.3 Millennium Development Goals

1. **Eradicate extreme poverty and hunger.**
   a. Target 1: Halve, between 1990 and 2015, the proportion of people whose income is less than $1 a day.
   b. Target 2: Halve, between 1990 and 2015, the proportion of people who suffer from hunger.
2. **Achieve universal primary education.**
   a. Target 1: Ensure that, by 2015, children everywhere, boys and girls alike, will be able to complete a full course of primary schooling.
3. **Promote gender equality and empower women.**
   a. Target 1: Eliminate gender disparity in primary and secondary education preferably by 2005 and in all levels of education no later than 2015.
4. **Reduce child mortality.**
   a. Target 1: Reduce by two-thirds, between 1990 and 2015, the under-five mortality rate.
5. **Improve maternal health.**
   a. Target 1: Reduce by three-quarters, between 1990 and 2015, the maternal mortality ratio.
6. **Combat HIV/AIDS, malaria, and other diseases.**
   a. Target 1: Have halted by 2015 and begun to reverse the spread of HIV/AIDS.
   b. Target 2: Have halted by 2015 and begun to reverse the incidence of malaria and other major diseases.
7. **Ensure environmental sustainability.**
   a. Target 1: Integrate the principles of sustainable development into country policies and programmes and reverse the loss of environmental resources.
   b. Target 2: Halve, by 2015, the proportion of the population without sustainable access to safe drinking water and basic sanitation.
   c. Target 3: To improve the lives of at least 100 million slum dwellers by 2020.
8. **Develop a global partnership for development.**
   a. Target 1: Address the special needs of the least developed countries, landlocked countries, and small island developing states.
   b. Target 2: Develop further an open, rule-based, predictable, nondiscriminatory trading and financial system.
   c. Target 3: In cooperation with developing countries, develop and implement strategies for decent and productive work for youth.
   d. Target 4: In cooperation with the private sector, make available the benefits of new technologies, especially information and communications.

Source: United Nations Department of Economic and Social Affairs. (2012). *Millenium Development Goals Report 2012.* New York, NY: Author.

we have seen accelerating progress in reducing child and maternal mortality . . . These results represent a tremendous reduction in human suffering and are a clear validation of the approach embodied in the MDGs. But, they are not a reason to relax. Projections indicate that in 2015 more than 600 million people worldwide will still be using unimproved water sources, almost one billion will be living on an income of less than $1.25 per day, mothers will continue to die needlessly in childbirth, and children will suffer and die from preventable diseases. Hunger remains a global challenge, and ensuring that all children are able to complete primary education remains a fundamental, but unfulfilled, target that has an impact on all the other Goals. Lack of safe sanitation is hampering progress in health and nutrition, biodiversity loss continues apace, and greenhouse gas emissions continue to pose a major threat to people and ecosystems. (United Nations Department of Economic and Social Affairs, 2012, p. 3)

This section highlights some of the key indicators of progress that were noted in the 2012 MDG Report, and also describes the use of microfinance as a key strategy that has been used in many low-resource countries to reduce poverty and thereby enhance health and well-being.

Goal 1: Eradicate Extreme Poverty and Hunger

The 2012 MDG Report indicated that the goal of reducing the percentage of people living on less than $1.25 per day to one half of what it was in 1990 will be achieved before the 2015 deadline. Even though the overall global poverty rate has been reduced, there are still significant disparities, with the highest rates in sub-Saharan Africa. One strategy that has shown much promise in reducing poverty, and thereby contributing to improvements in health status, has been the use of microfinance programs to provide the poor with access to financial services, including savings plans and opportunities for low-interest loans to stimulate income-generating businesses. Pronyk, Hargreaves, and Morduch (2007) reported that the repayment rates across these programs are often greater than 95%, and that programs generally recover most of their administrative costs through user fees and interest rates. Leatherwood, Metcalf, Geisslar, and Dunford (2012) reviewed the literature on microfinance programs and noted that there are more than 3,500 microfinance institutions providing financial services and microcredit to over 150 million households globally. These authors concluded that microfinance is not only effective in reducing poverty but may also contribute to improved health outcomes by increasing knowledge as well as access to health care. In 2006, Muhammad Yumus and the Grameen Foundation won the Nobel Peace Prize in recognition of their use of microfinance as a means to reduce poverty, improve health, and stimulate social change. Poor village women in Bangladesh who received microloans were able to purchase cell phones and become village phone operators (VPOs), selling calls to their neighbors and increasing access to the outside world. This access in turn stimulated local businesses and had other community benefits as the VPOs earned enough money to invest in the education, health, and nutrition of their children and families (Grameen Foundation, 2013). Abbott and Coenen (2008) noted that the VPO model has been implemented in much of Africa and is viewed as a tool to promote sustainable development, as "wealth has impacted health.".

Goal 2: Achieve Universal Primary Education

Although enrollment in primary education increased in developing countries from 82% to 90% between 1999 and 2010, the rate of increase has slowed since 2004, and there is still much to be done in order to achieve the second MDG goal by 2015. More than half of the world's children who are not attending primary school are in sub-Saharan Africa, where only 76% of children attend primary school (United Nations Department of Economic and Social Affairs, 2012). Given the strong correlation between education and health, there is a need to strengthen programs to ensure that all children have access to quality educational programs.

Goal 3: Promote Gender Equality and Empower Women

The 2012 MDG Report included some encouraging statistics to indicate that gender parity in education is improving, although in many nations women still lag behind men in accessing tertiary education. Equal job access for men and women has increased globally from 35% to 40% between 1990 and 2010. There has also been a global increase in the percentage of parliamentary positions held by women from 14% in 2000 to 20% in 2012 (United Nations Department of Economic and Social Affairs, 2012). Because women are often the major family caregivers and assume primary responsibility for healthcare decisions, there is a clear relationship between health and the goal of promoting gender equity and women's empowerment.

Goal 4: Reduce Child Mortality

Although the target of a two-thirds reduction in mortality rates of children under age 5 has not yet been met, the rate in developing nations has decreased from 97/1,000 in 1990 to 63/1,000 in 2010. The rates are highest in sub-Saharan Africa, and there has been less progress in neonatal mortality (United Nations Department of Economic and Social Affairs, 2012). Child mortality is closely related to poverty, AIDS, malaria, and to wars and conflicts.

Goal 5: Improve Maternal Health

The 2012 MDG Report noted that the maternal mortality rate has decreased from 440/100,000 live births in 1990 to 240/100,000 live births in 2010. Only two-thirds of deliveries in the developing world are now attended by skilled personnel, however (United Nations Department of Economic and Social Affairs, 2012). Key strategies to improve maternal health include increased access to prenatal care and skilled birth attendants and prevention of teen and unplanned pregnancies.

Goal 6: Combat HIV/AIDS, Malaria, and Other Diseases

The 2012 MDG Report indicated that there were 21% fewer new HIV infections than the peak reported in 1997, although there are still disparities across the globe, with highest rates in sub-Saharan Africa and the Caribbean. The report estimated that only 48% of those needing HIV treatment are receiving it. The President's Emergency Program for AIDS Relief (PEPFAR), an initiative of the U.S. government that was launched in 2004, has provided significant funding for medications, care, and treatment of patients with HIV, targeting 15 countries with the highest rates of HIV (see http://www.pepfar.gov/). Gender imbalances continue to contribute to increasing numbers of women, including married women, becoming infected. Clearly there is a need to strengthen programs for prevention, treatment, and support to address the HIV pandemic. Malaria remains a significant cause of morbidity and mortality throughout the world, although there have been substantial improvements in malaria control programs since 1990. In 2012, 43 of 99 countries with malaria reported a 50% reduction of new cases (United Nations Department of Economic and Social Affairs, 2012). One of the most effective prevention strategies is the use of insecticide-treated bed nets, since the mosquitoes that cause malaria typically bite only between dusk and dawn. Unfortunately, the use of bednets is still limited in many areas. In sub-Saharan Africa, it is estimated that the percentage of children under the age of 5 who sleep under these bednets has increased from 2% in 2000 to 39% in 2010. There is also an urgent need to increase access to appropriate medicines to treat malaria, and to address the problem of resistance to many of the traditional antimalarial medications (United Nations Department of Economic and Social Affairs, 2012).

Other infectious diseases also present considerable threats in many countries. Such diseases include tuberculosis, cholera, measles, typhoid, polio, guinea worm, diarrheal diseases, and upper respiratory infections. The 2012 MDG Report also noted that the number of new cases of tuberculosis has started to decline, and predicted that, "If this trend is sustained, the world will achieve the target of halting the spread and beginning to reverse the incidence of the disease" (United Nations Department of Economic and Social Affairs, 2012, p. 44).

Goal 7: Ensure Environmental Sustainability

The 2012 MDG Report noted some encouraging data related to the seventh goal, as the international community has increased the amount of protected land and expanded the development and use of cleaner energy technologies such as biofuels and hydroelectric power. The goal of reducing the percentage of people without access to clean water by one half has been met, with the percentage falling from 24% to 11%. However, the report noted that only 56% of the world's population has access to basic sanitation, short of the 75% target set for 2015 (United Nations Department of Economic and Social Affairs, 2012).

Goal 8: Develop a Global Partnership for Development

It is clear that achieving the MDGs will require global partnership and collaboration and increased commitment to international aid by high-resource countries. The 2012 MDG Report noted that the amount of global development aid decreased for the first time in a decade because of global economic problems. One of the targets associated with the eighth MDG was to make available the benefits of increased technology and communication. The 2012 MDG Report noted that access to technology has increased, particularly for mobile cell phones, with mobile cell phone service available to 87% of the world's population (including 79% of those living in developing regions). Internet access is also increasing, with 35% of the world having internet access (and 67% of internet users being in developing countries) (United Nations Department of Economic and Social Affairs, 2012).

Abbott and Coenen (2008) provided an excellent review of the relationships between globalization, health, and the use of ICT, identifying numerous opportunities for nursing to contribute "in this flattening and increasingly interconnected world" (p. 238). Such opportunities include using ICT to (a) provide educational and collaborative learning programs, (b) deliver nursing and health care using telenursing or telehealth services, (c) help to develop interoperable Electronic Health Record Systems (EHRS) to facilitate sharing data and to improve clinical decision-making, (d) facilitate knowledge management and utilization to promote evidence-based practice, and (e) develop collaborative partnerships and communities of practice (CoPs) involving nurses throughout the world.

One such CoP is the Global Alliance for Nursing & Midwifery (GANM), which was initiated by the WHO Department of Human Resources for Health, the WHO Office for Nursing & Midwifery, and the Johns Hopkins University School of Nursing Collaborating Center for Nursing Knowledge & Information Management. Membership in the GANM is free and open to nurses and midwives throughout the world. There are currently more than 3,192 members from 123 countries who share knowledge and best practices, participate in continuing education, and have access to library resources (Global Alliance for Nursing and Midwifery Communities of Practice, 2013). Other examples of CoPs are the Global Health Delivery Online Nursing and Midwifery Community, which currently has 1708 members (Global Health Delivery Online: Global Health Nursing and Midwifery, 2013), and the Network for Nurses in Child Health (Red Internacional de Enfermeria en Salud Infantil, Red ENSI). This network is one of more than 15 specialty nursing networks that has been promoted by the Pan American Health Organization (PAHO) (Harrison et al., 2008). This network has coordinators from every country in Latin America and from Spain and the United States. Participants hold virtual meetings using internet technology, facilitated by the PAHO/WHO Collaborating Center on International Nursing at the University of Alabama at Birmingham, and also share information via email correspondence and a website (http://www.enfermeriainfantil.org/R-ENSI/).

Another example of using ICT for global networking is the Nightingale Initiative for Global Health (NIGH) (Dossey, Beck, & Rushton, 2008). The NIGH was established in 2003 and has two goals: (a) to globally unite 10 million nurses through the internet and through developing regional groups around the world to promote a healthier world by 2020 and (b) to demonstrate the significance of nursing's contribution to global health. A key strategy to achieving these goals is the creation of the web-based Nightingale Global Alliance Campaign for a Healthy World (www.NightingaleDeclaration.net). A final example of how ICT can facilitate information management and sharing, even when access to internet and other technologies is limited, is the eGranary Digital Library, a collection of digital resources (such as web pages, articles, clinical practice guidelines, and other media), that can be accessed in areas where internet connectivity is limited. The eGranary project is coordinated by the Widernet project, with support from many global partners, including the WHO, universities, and private corporations (Widernet, 2013). The nursing collection has been developed with input and recommendations from nurses all over the world.

OTHER OPPORTUNITIES FOR NURSES TO CONTRIBUTE TO GLOBAL HEALTH AND THE GOAL OF *HEALTH FOR ALL*

In addition to using ICT to facilitate global partnerships and collaboration as described in the previous section, there are many other ways in which nurses can make significant contributions to global health at the local, national, and international levels. This final section will highlight four additional opportunities for nurses to make a difference in global health: (a) supporting primary health care initiatives; (b) helping to address challenges associated with the global nursing shortage and international nurse migration; (c) promoting global health equity through leadership and involvement in health policy development; and (d) participating in international exchanges and collaborations.

Primary Health Care

The year 2008 marked the 60th anniversary of the WHO and the 30th anniversary of a famous declaration supporting the essential role of primary health care in achieving the goal of global health equity, the Alma-Ata Declaration (WHO, 2008c). The Alma-Ata Declaration was the result of a meeting of delegates from 134 nations of the world, plus representatives from non-governmental organizations (NGOs) officially accredited by WHO, in what was then known as Alma-Ata, USSR (now Almaty, Kazakhstan). In that historic meeting, the nations of the world committed themselves and their resources to the achievement of Health for All by the year 2000 through primary health care. The 2008 WHO Report (Primary Health Care: Now More than Ever) reflected the ongoing commitment to the Alma-Ata Declaration and identified four reforms necessary to achieving the Health for All goal: (a) universal access to social health protection; (b) service delivery reforms to reorganize health services around people's needs and expectations; (c) public policy reforms; and (d) leadership reforms to promote more inclusive and participatory leadership. The eight elements essential to the primary health care approach reflect the priorities identified in 1978 at Alma-Ata (Box 1.4). Nurses are the backbone for provision of primary health care services. Although applied differently around the world, these elements remain valid for all countries, at all levels of socioeconomic development.

Box 1.4 **Eight Essential Elements of Primary Health Care**

The 1978 Report of the Alma-Ata Conference on Primary Health Care identified eight essential elements of primary health care. These remain relevant today.

1. Education for the identification and prevention/control of prevailing health problems
2. Proper food supplies and nutrition
3. Adequate supply of safe water and basic sanitation
4. Maternal and child care, including family planning
5. Immunization against the major infectious diseases, prevention and control of locally endemic diseases
6. Appropriate treatment of common diseases using appropriate technology
7. Promotion of mental health
8. Provision of essential drugs

Source: World Health Organization and United Nations Children's Fund. (1978). *Alma-Ata, 1978: Primary health care: Report of the International Conference on Primary Health Care.* Retrieved from http://www.unicef.org/about/history/files/Alma_Ata_conference_1978_report.pdf

---

Addressing Challenges Associated With the Global Nursing Shortage and International Nurse Migration

Numerous professional and governmental organizations have identified the critical shortage of nurses in countries around the globe as a major challenge to providing adequate health care services. The American Academy of Nursing's Expert Panel on Global Health published a White Paper in 2007 (Rosenkoetter & Nardi, 2007), addressing many of these challenges and reviewing the factors that contribute to the shortage and to the unequal global distribution of nurses. The average number of nurses per 100,000 people ranges from 10 to 1,000, with the ratios in Europe nearly 10 times higher than the ratios in many countries in Africa and Southeast Asia. Factors that contribute to the shortage in low-resource countries include challenges related to HIV/AIDS, high-stress work environments, gender-based discrimination and violence, and international migration of nurses. Many high-resource countries, faced with their own nursing shortages, contribute to this problem by recruiting nurses from lower-resource countries, further compounding the problem (Dovlo, 2005; Simpson, 2004).

Wilson and Fowler (2012, p. 52) recommended the following specific actions for nurses that could help to address the global nursing shortage:

1. *Advocate for strengthening nursing and midwifery leadership at all levels of the WHO and in state, local, and national governmental organizations responsible for health policy;*
2. *Support policies for the ethical recruitment and retention of nurses/midwives;*
3. *Implement policies to promote safe and just working environments for nurses;*
4. *Strengthen professional nursing organizations and inter-organizational communication and collaboration to promote policies and funding priorities to support critical global health workforce needs;*
5. *Partner with health-related nongovernmental organizations to address global healthcare and nursing workforce needs; and*
6. *Promote policies and standards to ensure that nursing educational curricula incorporate concerns for global citizenship and political participation in a substantive way.*

It is critical that nurses promote international efforts to promote ethical practices in international nurse recruitment. During the World Health Assembly in 2004, the WHO adopted a resolution (WHA57.19) addressing "International Migration of Health Personnel: A Challenge for Health Systems in Developing Countries" (World Health Organizaton, 2004). This resolution included a series of recommendations, including international collaboration to collect information to monitor migration patterns and identify effects of such migration, strengthening mechanisms to train sufficient numbers of health care workers, and developing a code of practice on international recruitment of health personnel. In 2010, the World Health Assembly passed WHA 63.16, a voluntary code of practice to manage recruitment of nurses to the United States and to support the WHO and the Ethical Globalization initiative (WHO, 2010).

Promoting Global Health Equity Through Leadership and Policy Development

The first step in making a contribution to global health equity involves developing a global perspective and awareness of important global health issues, and then finding ways to make a personal contribution to address these issues. Smith identified several questions that could help guide nurses in finding ways that they could make such contributions, and suggested that some of the strategies outlined in the Academy of Nursing White Paper on Global Nursing and Health could provide a useful road map (Smith, 2006). Such strategies include promoting ethical models of nurse recruitment, incorporating more global health content into nursing curricula, supporting appropriate-technology distance-learning initiatives, and supporting legislation that supports *global* health research. Walker and Elberson (2005) suggested that organizational leaders have a responsibility to facilitate changes that will promote collaboration among organizational members, and suggested that the use of technology can facilitate these leadership initiatives.

Participating in International Exchanges and Collaborations

We all have much to learn from one another, and participation in international exchanges and collaborative projects can facilitate this learning. There are many ways to facilitate these types of exchanges. Spry described the goal of the International Networking Committee of the Association of periOperative Registered Nurses (AORN) to welcome and engage international attendees at the AORN annual conference (Spry, 2008). Leite de Silva (2008) identified the need for "emancipating education" for nurses, which would prepare them to know about local and global reality and develop culturally competent practice. McAuliffe and Cohen (2005) reviewed 79 articles that were published in English describing international educational or research exchanges, and concluded that although such exchanges provide valuable opportunities for learning and for knowledge development, there is a need for further development of theoretical models to guide such exchanges. These authors also suggested that faculty and student exchanges are most useful when they address priorities identified by the host country and when they ensure that the projects increase the capacity of nurses in the host countries. Baumann and Blythe (2008) noted that the trend toward globalization of higher education in nursing brings both benefits and challenges. One of the challenges is the need for mechanisms to compare different educational qualifications of nurses against global standards. These authors noted several initiatives that have begun to address this challenge, including the Code of Good Practice in the Provision of Transnational Education adopted by the European Union in 2001 and Guidelines on Quality Provision in Cross-Border Education developed by the United Nations Educational, Scientific, and Cultural Organization (UNESCO).

Summary

Nurses today have multiple and exciting opportunities to truly make a difference in addressing health disparities and promoting the goal of Health for All. The world is indeed a community, and each nurse is a global citizen. We can begin by embracing the Nightingale Declaration of Commitment for a Healthy World by 2020:

> We, the nurses and concerned citizens of the global community, hereby dedicate ourselves to achieve a healthy world by 2020.
>
> We declare our willingness to unite in a program of action, to share information and solution and to improve health conditions for all humanity—locally, nationally and globally.
>
> We further resolve to adopt personal practices and to implement public policies in our communities and nations—making this goal achievable and inevitable by the year 2020, beginning today in our own lives, and in the life of our nations and in the world at large. (© NIGH, 2007. The Nightingale Initiative for Global Health. Available from http://www.nightingaledeclaration.net/the-declaration.)

Critical Thinking Questions

1. Describe the relevance of one of the MDGs to the community in which you live. How would you promote that goal to your own community? What types of data would you need to present your "case"?

2. Climate change affects everyone worldwide. Describe one major "natural disaster" that may be connected to climate change that had an impact on your community recently. What were the effects? Who was affected? How were nurses involved in the aftermath of that disaster?

3. Consider the recommendations of this chapter about how you can be involved in making a difference in global health. What does being a "global citizen" mean to you? Where can you go to find international opportunities for nurses?

4. Explore the websites listed at the end of this chapter. How can you use the information about global issues in your own practice?

REFERENCES

Abbot, P. A., & Coenen, A. (2008). Globalization and advances in information and communication technologies: The impact on nursing and health. *Nursing Outlook, 56*(5), 238–246.

Bauman, A., & Blythe, J. (2008). Globalization of higher education in nursing. *OJIN: Online Journal of Issues in Nursing, 13*(2). Retrieved from http://www.nursingworld.org/MainMenuCategories/ANAMarketplace/ANAPeriodicals/OJIN/TableofContents/vol132008/No2May08/GlobalizationofHigherEducation.html

Birdsall, N. (2006). *The world is not flat: Inequality and injustice in our global economy* (WIDER Annual Lecture 9). Helsinki, Finland: United Nations University World Institute for Development Economics Research.

Braveman, P. A., Kumanyika, S., Fielding, J., LaVeist, T., Borrell, L. N., Manderscheid, R., & Troutman, A. (2011). Health disparities and health equity: The issue is justice. *American Journal of Public Health, 101*(Suppl. 1), S149–S155. doi:10.2105/AJPH.2010.300062

Dossey, B. M., Beck, D., & Rushton, C. H. (2008). 21st-century nightingales and global health. *Dean's Notes, 29*(3), 4.

Dovlo, D. (2005). Taking more than a fair share? The migration of health professionals from poor to rich countries. *PLoS Medicine, 2*(5), 376–379.

Global Alliance for Nursing and Midwifery Communities of Practice. (2013). *Global alliance for nursing and midwifery communities of practice.* Retrieved June 24, 2013, from http://knowledge-gateway.org/ganm

Global Health Delivery Online: Global Health Nursing and Midwifery. (2013). *Community at a glance.* Retrieved June 22, 2013, from http://www.ghdonline.org/nursing/members/

Grameen Foundation. (2013). *Village phone: Connecting technology and innovation.* Retrieved June 23, 2013, from http://www.grameenfoundation.org/who-we-are

Grootjans, J., & Newman, S. (2013). The relevance of globalization to nursing: A concept analysis. *International Nursing Review*, *60*(1), 78–85. doi:10.1111/j.1466-7657.2012.01022.x

Harrison, L., Montenegro, G., Malvares, S., Astudillo, M., Behn, V., Bertolozzi, M. R., . . . Verissimo, M. D. O. (2008). The network for nursing in child health. *Pediatric Nursing*, *34*(2), 113–116, 138–139.

Hitti, M. (2007). Officials seeking more than 600 passengers on patient's flight; patient feeling well in hospital. *WebMD Health News*. Retrieved June 23, 2013, from www.medicinenet.com/script/main/art.asp?articlekey=81465

Horton, R. (2013). GBD 2010: Understanding disease, injury, and risk. *Lancet*, *380*(9859), 2053–2054. doi:10.1016/S0140-6736(12)62133-3

Hunter, A., Stanhope, M., Wilson, L., Hatcher, B., Hattar, M., Messias, D. K. H., & Powell, D. (2013). Global health diplomacy: An integrative review of the literature and implications for nursing. *Nursing Outlook*, *61*, 85–92. doi:10.1016/j.outlook.2012.07.013

Institute of Medicine. (1997). *America's vital interest in global health*. Washington, DC: National Academy Press.

Joint United Nations Programme on HIV/AIDS (UNAIDS). (2012). *UNAIDS report on the global AIDS epidemic*. Retrieved from http://www.unaids.org/en/resources/publications/2012/name,76121,en.asp

Jones, K. E., Patel, N. G., Levy, M. A., Storeygard, A., Balk, D., Gittleman, J. L., & Daszak, P. (2008). Global trends in emerging infectious diseases. *Nature*, *451*, 990–994.

Kilama, W. L. (2009). The 10/90 gap in sub-Saharan Africa: Resolving inequities in health research. *Acta Tropica*, *112*(Suppl. 1), S8–S15. doi:http://dx.doi.org/10.1016/j.actatropica.2009.08.015

Kjellstrom, T., & McMichael, A. J. (2013). Climate change threats to population health and well-being: The imperative of protective solutions that will last. *Global Health Action*, *6*, 20816. doi:10.3402/gha.v6i0.20816

Leatherman, S., Metcalfe, M., Geissler, K., & Dunford, C. (2012). Integrating microfinance and health strategies: Examining the evidence to inform policy and practice. *Health Policy Plan*, *27*(2), 85–101. doi:10.1093/heapol/czr014

Leite de Silva, A. (2008). Nursing in the era of globalisation: Challenges for the 21st century. *Revista Latino-Americana de Enfermagem*, *16*(4), 787–790.

Luber, G., & Hess, J. (2007). Climate change and human health in the United States. *Journal of Environmental Health*, *70*(5), 43–46.

McAuliffe, M. S., & Cohen, M. Z. (2005). International nursing research and educational exchanges: A review of the literature. *Nursing Outlook*, *53*(1), 21–25.

Murphy, C. (2006). The 2003 SARS outbreak: Global challenges and innovative infection control measures. *OJIN: The Online Journal of Issues in Nursing*, *11*(1). Retrieved from http://www.nursingworld.org/MainMenu Categories/ANAMarketplace/ANAPeriodicals/OJIN/TableofContents/Volume112006/No1Jan06/tpc29_516064.html

Novotny, T. E., & Adams, V. (2007). *Global health diplomacy: A global health sciences working paper*. San Francisco: University of California San Francisco Global Health Sciences. Retrieved from http://igcc.ucsd.edu/assets/001/500883.pdf

Patz, J., Campbell-Lendrum, D., Gibbs, H., & Woodruff, R. (2008). Health impact assessment of global climate change: Expanding on comparative risk assessment approaches for policy making. *Annual Review of Public Health*, *29*, 27–39.

Pronyk, P. M., Hargreaves, J. R., & Morduch, J. (2007). Microfinance programs and better health: Prospects for sub-Saharan Africa. *JAMA*, *298*(16), 1925–1927. doi:10.1001/jama.298.16.1925

Ramzy, A., & Yang, L. (2008). *Tainted-baby-milk scandal in China*. Retrieved December 18, 2008, from www.time.com/time/world/article/0,8599,1841535,000.html

Rosenkoetter, M. M., & Nardi, D. A. (2007). American Academy of Nursing Expert Panel on global nursing and health: White Paper on global nursing and health: Academia Americana de Enfermeria, Panel de Expertos en Enfermeria Global y Salud: Documento de Opinion en Enfermeria Global y Salud. *Journal of Transcultural Nursing*, *18*(4), 305–315. doi:10.1177/1043659607305188

Simpson, R. L. (2004). Global informing. Impact and implications of technology in a global marketplace. *Nursing Administration Quarterly*, *28*(2), 144–149.

Smith, B. A. (2006). The role of nursing leaders in global health issues and global health policy. *Nursing Outlook*, *54*(6), 309–310.

Spry, C. (2008). Global perspectives. International sharing: What's in it for us? *AORN Journal*, *88*(3), 443.

United Nations Department of Economic and Social Affairs. (2012). *Millenium Development Goals Report 2012*. New York, NY: Author.

United States Department of Health and Human Services. (2013). *2020 topics and objectives: Global health*. Retrieved June 21, 2013, from http://www.healthypeople.gov/2020/topicsobjectives2020/overview.aspx?topicid=16

Walker, P. H., & Elberson, K. L. (2005). Collaboration: Leadership in a global technological environment. *OJIN: Online Journal of Issues in Nursing*, *10*(1). Retrieved from http://www.nursingworld.org/MainMenuCategories/ANAMarketplace/ANAPeriodicals/OJIN/TableofContents/Volume102005/No1Jan05/tpc26_516012.html

Widernet. (2013). *eGranary digital library*. Retrieved June 24, 2013, from http://www.widernet.org/egranary/

Wilson, L., & Fowler, M. (2012). Leadership needed to address the global nursing and midwifery shortage. *Nursing Outlook*, *60*(1), 51–53.

Wilson, L., Harper, D. C., Tami, I., Zarate, R., Salas, S., Farley, J., . . . Ventura, C. (2012). Global health competencies for nurses in the Americas. *Journal of Professional Nurses*, *28*(4), 213–222.

World Bank. (2013a). *Poverty and equity data*. Retrieved June 1, 2013, from http://povertydata.worldbank.org/poverty/home/

World Bank. (2013b). *World Bank atlas of global development*. London: HarperCollins.

World Health Organizaton. (2004). *WHA57.19 International migration of health personnel: A challenge for health systems in developing countries*. Geneva, Switzerland: Author.

World Health Organization. (2007). *The World Health Report 2007—A safer future: Global public health security in the 21st century*. Geneva, Switzerland: Author.

World Health Organization. (2008a). *Global burden of disease (definition)*. Retrieved December 19, 2008, from http://www.who.int/topics/global_burden_of_disease/en/

World Health Organization. (2008b). *Global burden of disease, 2004 update*. Geneva, Switzerland: Author.

World Health Organization. (2008c). *World Health Report 2008: Primary health care now more than ever*. Geneva, Switzerland: Author.

World Health Organization. (2010). *WHA 63.16: Global code of practice on international recruitment of health personnel*. Geneva, Switzerland: Author.

World Health Organization Department of Human Resources for Health. (2008). *Report of the global consultation on an implementation framework for scaling up nursing and midwifery capacity*. Geneva, Switzerland: World Health Organization.

CHAPTER 2

Community Health Nursing: Essentials of Practice

Elizabeth T. Anderson

LEARNING OBJECTIVES

This chapter continues the conceptual basis of community as partner. As such, it introduces the key concepts of community health nursing and public health nursing.

After studying this chapter, you should be able to:

1. Describe the historical development of community health nursing.

2. Define community health nursing in the 21st century.

3. Identify the domains of community health nursing competency.

4. Describe nursing roles in the community.

Introduction

The second decade of the 21st century is bustling with phenomenal opportunities and challenges for health care delivery and community health nursing. There is no better time to be a community health nurse. The discussion that follows represents some reflections on what we believe will characterize the practice of community health nursing in the 21st century. We use the term *community health nursing* to denote the practice of nursing by professional nurses who have been educated in the processes of population-based nursing and whose principal client is the aggregate community.

In the past, population-based nursing was referred to as public health nursing. Public health nurses usually worked in health departments. This chapter uses the term *community health nurse,* which was adopted in recent years and intended to be more inclusive of population-based nursing practiced in a variety of community settings, including schools, worksites, shelters, health departments, and a multitude of others, some of which will be discussed in Part 3 of this book. You will encounter both terms, *public health nursing* and *community health nursing,* during your education and practice. Titles and practice settings are not as relevant as the nature of the practice itself. This chapter discusses the essence and diversity of that practice.

Until now the majority of your nursing education has focused on individual behavior. The theoretical basis for your nursing care has included knowledge about chemistry, physiology, pharmacology, and so on. Community health nursing, too, relies on that basic knowledge, but is also based on theories about populations. Hence, you will discover in subsequent chapters the concepts of epidemiology, demography, empowerment, ethics, environment, culture, and policy. To understand why these theories are important to the community health nurse, let's begin with a bit of history.

REFLECTIONS ON THE PAST

Reflecting on the historical contributions of community health nurses is both instructive and inspirational. Examining our roots allows us to take the best from the past in order to shape the future. Community health nurses can gain motivation and direction from the work of Lillian Wald, Lavinia Dock, and Margaret Sanger, who "make up nursing's 'distinguished history of concern . . . for social justice'" (Bekemeier & Butterfield, 2005, p. 153) and who, more than 100 years ago, ". . . grew indignant from witnessing the destructive health outcomes of institutionalized poverty and of gender and ethnic inequalities" (Bekemeier & Butterfield, 2005, p. 153). Observing rapid industrialization, large concentrations of people moving into cities, unsanitary environmental conditions, poor housing, poverty, misuse of child labor, infectious diseases, and short life expectancy, Lillian Wald and Mary Brewster were moved to action. Together, they founded the Henry Street Settlement House in New York City. There they lived and worked among the people, teaching hygiene practices, visiting the sick in homes, and crusading for better health care in all aspects of the community. Lillian Wald recognized the intertwining of health status, environmental sanitation, and social and political forces. Her work targeted the root causes of ill health, which meant that she had to take on institutions, politics, and social policy to effect change for the improvement of the community's health. Lillian Wald had an exceptional ability to inform and convince people of the need for social change (Backer, 1993). Wald first coined the term *public health nurse* and is regarded as the "mother of public health nursing" in the United States. Her contributions include establishing nursing schools, advocating better housing, working to change child labor laws, teaching preventive practices, advocating occupational health nursing, and improving the education of public health nurses, to name a few (Coss, 1989; Feld, 2008).

With the discovery of antibiotics in the 1940s and vaccines for mass immunizations in conjunction with tremendous improvements in environmental sanitation, the United States experienced a considerable decline in morbidity and mortality due to communicable diseases. According to the Centers for Disease Control and Prevention (CDC), public health is credited with adding 25 years to the life expectancy of people in the United States. In addition, the CDC has identified 10 great achievements of public health in the 20th century that have contributed to this increase in longevity (CDC, 1999). These achievements are listed in Box 2.1. Public health nurses were at the forefront of ensuring that these great achievements were carried out in the community.

Beginning in the 1960s, as communicable diseases declined, attention turned to the prevention of chronic diseases and related risk factors such as cigarette smoking and dietary fat. Community health nurses working in health departments focused attention on screening, case finding, home visiting to individual clients, and health education activities related to disease prevention. This trend continued into the early 1980s, when the focus of health shifted somewhat to health promotion, prompted by the Health for All era established by the World Health Organization (WHO, 1978). However, the 1990s were marked by considerable emphasis on clinical care and high-tech medicine as ways to increase life span in the United States. Health departments began to emphasize clinical care, such as prenatal care, family planning, treatment

---

Box 2.1 Ten Great Public Health Achievements in the 20th Century

1. Immunizations
2. Improvements in motor vehicle safety
3. Workplace safety
4. Control of infectious diseases
5. Decline in deaths from heart disease and stroke
6. Safer and healthier foods
7. Healthier mothers and babies
8. Family planning
9. Fluoridation of drinking water
10. Tobacco as a health hazard

Source: Centers for Disease Control and Prevention. (1999). Ten great public achievements—United States, 1900–1999. *Morbidity and Mortality Weekly Report, 48*(12), 241–243.

---

of communicable diseases, and immunizations, particularly for citizens without access to basic preventive services. The 1990s can also be characterized as the era in which the high cost of health care in the United States became a major concern of policymakers.

In recent years, official agencies have become more involved in direct clinical care, and community health nursing has focused on clinical and illness care or "clinic" roles and functions, assigning less importance to family- and community-focused roles and functions. This shift was primarily in response to clinical services that could be reimbursed. Now public health is shifting back to its "roots" by focusing more on disease prevention, health promotion, and assurance that care is provided, rather than providing one-on-one care. To respond to the challenges facing community health nursing in the future, we must understand the changes occurring in health care delivery, including directions for population-based health.

COMMUNITY HEALTH NURSING IN THE UNITED STATES: THE CONTEXT

Past debates about health care reform largely ignored the contributions of population-based community health, concentrating almost entirely on clinical care, with the exception of immunizations. Mechanisms to deliver and pay for illness care are driving current health care system changes. The debate really ought to be about what can be done to make our population the healthiest, rather than how we can best pay for illness. Some elected officials have been reluctant to fund health-promotion services at the levels needed, but it takes excellent health promotion to minimize the cost of illness care. Health promotion results in wellness. Community health in the 21st century must offer integrated services and activities that focus on minimizing threats to health, promoting wellness, and then focusing on illness management.

To improve the health of communities, community health nurses need to focus on the 10 essential public health services (Table 2.1). The essential public health services provide a fundamental framework by describing the public health activities that should be undertaken in all communities. The essential services provide a working definition of public health and a guiding framework for the responsibilities of local public health systems. Table 2.1 includes both the essential services as well as selected nursing activities for each. These essential services comprise an impressive list, and each service can be used to direct community health nursing practice in diverse settings.

TABLE 2.1 Essential Public Health Services and Selected Nursing Activities

Essential Public Health Services	Selected Nursing Activities/Competencies
Monitor health status to identify community health problems.	Participate in community assessment; identify potential environmental hazards.
Diagnose and investigate health problems and hazards in the community.	Understand and identify determinants of health and disease.
Inform, educate, and empower people about health issues.	Develop and implement community-based health education.
Mobilize community partnerships to identify and solve health problems.	Explain the significance of health issues to the public and participate in developing plans of action.
Develop policies and plans that support individual and community health efforts.	Develop programs and services to meet the needs of high-risk populations as well as members of the broader community.
Enforce laws and regulations that protect health and ensure safety.	Regulate and support safe care and treatment for dependent populations such as children and the frail elderly.
Link people to needed personal health services, and ensure the provision of health care when otherwise unavailable.	Establish programs and services to meet special needs.
Ensure a competent public health and personal health care workforce.	Participate in continuing education and preparation to ensure competence.
Evaluate effectiveness, accessibility, and quality of personal and population-based health services.	Identify unserved and underserved populations in communities.
Research new insights and innovative solutions to health problems.	Participate in early identification of factors detrimental to the community's health.

Sources: Centers for Disease Control and Prevention. (n.d.). *Public health system and the 10 essential public health services*. Retrieved July 6, 2013, from http://www.cdc.gov/nphpsp/essentialServices.html. Quad Council of Public Health Nursing Organizations. (2011). *Core competencies for public health nurses*. Washington, DC: Author.

In addition to the services, community health practice is focused on prevention rather than illness care. The levels of prevention—primary, secondary, and tertiary—are described in Chapter 3.

COMMUNITY HEALTH NURSING PRACTICE

The focus of this text is on populations and systems, as you will see from our selected model as well as the exemplars described in Part 3. As the basis for your practice, as with any professional role, you are expected to be familiar with the scope and standards of practice. Developing the statements has been an iterative process with input from the Quad Council as well as numerous nurses in practice, education, and research. The American Nurses Association (ANA) published the scope and standards using the term public health nursing (ANA, 2007) (Box 2.2).

Box 2.2 Public Health Nursing Perspectives

Public health nursing practice and roles are defined from "the perspective, knowledge base, and the focus of care, rather than by the site in which these nurses practice. Even though they are frequently employed by agencies in which direct care is provided to individuals and families, these nurses view individual and family care from the perspective of the community and/or the population" (ACHNE, 2003, p. 10).

The four organizations of the Quad Council (the ANA, Council of Community, Primary, and Long-Term Care; American Public Health Association [APHA]—Public Health Nursing Section; Association of Community Health Nurse Educators; and Association of State and Territorial Directors of Nursing) met over time to describe community health nursing more clearly. Their definition of public health nursing is as follows:

> *Public health nursing is the practice of promoting and protecting the health of populations using knowledge from nursing, social, and public health sciences* (American Public Health Association, Public Health Nursing Section, 1996). *The practice is population-focused with the goals of promoting health and preventing disease and disability for all people through the creation of conditions in which people can be healthy.*
>
> *Although practicing in a variety of public and private organizations, all public health nurses focus on one or more populations. A population may be defined as those living in a specific geographic area (e.g., neighborhood, community, city, or county) or those in a particular group (e.g., racial, ethnic, age, disease) who experience a disproportionate burden of poor health outcomes.* (ANA, 2007, p. 5)

The new Public Health Nursing standards, released in 2013, converge economic, political, and social factors including Healthy People 2020 and the Patient Protection and Affordable Care Act (ACA) to provide a directive for improving the health of populations. *(ANA, 2013)*

FACTORS INFLUENCING COMMUNITY HEALTH NURSING IN THE 21ST CENTURY

All health professions are being influenced by the changes occurring in our health care system. Some relevant factors shaping 21st-century community health are summarized in Box 2.3 and are elaborated below.

Health Care

That health care is in flux is obvious every day. Read a newspaper or watch the news: health care reform and the passage of the Affordable Care Act (ACA) have captured the imagination and attention of all thinking health care professionals and the public as well. What triggered the need for this sweeping reform? The APHA provides the answers in a comprehensive, easy to maneuver web page from www.apha.org. Several salient points will be summarized here.

The critical need for health care reform stemmed primarily from five factors: (1) the high rate of uninsured Americans under the age of 65 (approximately 50 million); (2) unsustainable health care spending that represented almost 18% of our gross domestic product; (3) a lack of emphasis on prevention (7 of 10 deaths in the United States are related to preventable diseases, and 75% of our health care dollars are spent on treating such diseases); (4) poor health outcomes (reflected in our high spending on medical care with a ranking of 24th among countries in terms of life expectancy); and (5) health disparities (well-documented disparities

---

Box 2.3   Factors Shaping 21st-Century Health

Health care "reform"
Demographics
Globalization
Poverty and growing disparities
Violence, injuries, and social disintegration

in the high death rates of African American women in heart disease, breast and lung cancer, stroke). As the APHA points out,

> *The ACA won't solve all of these problems overnight, but it's an important step forward. By making health coverage more affordable and accessible and thus increasing the number of Americans with coverage, by funding community-based public health and prevention programs, and by supporting research and tracking on key health measures, the ACA will begin to reduce disparities, improve access to preventive care, and improve health outcomes and reduce the nation's health spending.* (American Public Health Association, n.d.)

One innovative program aimed at our fragmented system serves as an example of how health professionals can partner to affect the health of our citizens. This program, Turning Point, was begun in 1997 with funding from the Robert Wood Johnson Foundation and additional funding from the W. K. Kellogg Foundation. Threats to our nation (bioterrorism and emerging infectious diseases, along with obesity, violence, and tobacco-related illnesses) require a strong public health system, and currently, 23 states practice the philosophy of Turning Point. It behooves community health nurses to be aware of such innovations and to support those that prove effective in improving health. Tools for improving practice and collaboration are readily available through the W. K. Kellogg Foundation website (www.wkkf.org), and positive outcomes, such as the establishment of local health departments to cover all of Nebraska, for example, are being reported regularly (Berkowitz, Nicola, Lafronza, & Bekemeier, 2005).

Demographics

Many countries with very large populations have shown great progress in lowering their birth rates. However, the very size of their current populations means that, in absolute terms, their populations will continue to increase for many years. As large numbers of young people become sexually active, they, in turn, will place greater pressures on local health services, schools, and employers. In the United States, certain ethnic and cultural groups with young populations are presenting similar challenges to local education and social service systems.

Family structures and living arrangements are also changing rapidly in much of the world. Fewer people live in traditional family groups or have extended family support networks. The stress that often results from these changes, along with the growing disruption of traditional cultural patterns, is another factor adding to the erosion of social support systems and people's burden of disease.

Two significant demographic factors shaping the future of community health nursing and all health care are age and increasing ethnic diversity. Studies predict that by 2040, one out of five Americans will be 65 years or older. The graying of America will continue to shift the focus of medical care from acute to chronic illness and challenge the development of new and effective health-promotion strategies for this population. Quality of life, not merely a long life, will become the priority. There is no debate about the growing ethnic diversity of this country. Changes in immigration laws and differential fertility rates and age patterns among minority groups have dramatically altered the ethnic makeup of the United States. Nationwide, Asians and Pacific Islanders will constitute the fastest growing ethnic group, but Hispanics will comprise the largest ethnic "minority" group. These changes have many social and health implications for community health nursing.

Globalization

The major factor affecting communities today and in the foreseeable future is the phenomenon of globalization. Globalization represents a global market that brings together capital, technology, and information across borders to create what some call a global village.

When global financial markets go up or down, when trade agreements are negotiated, when recessions threaten the countries that purchase the products made in our towns and communities, we and our communities can be at risk. When recession or political instability occurs in other countries, foreign companies often lower their prices to make their products more competitive. They are able to do this and still make a profit because the levels of local unemployment create conditions in which those competing for jobs are willing to work for less and less. When this happens over a period of time and is widespread, companies and factories, once considered sources of stable employment in our communities, close their U.S. operations and move to countries where salaries are lower and labor laws are weak or nonexistent. Anyone doubting this trend needs only to look at the labels on the clothes, electrical appliances, toys, food, flowers, and other merchandise in our local stores.

With the growing strength of organizations such as the World Trade Organization (WTO) and trade pacts such as the North American Free Trade Agreement (NAFTA) with their emphasis on free trade, free financial markets, and economic profits, governments—especially those of resource-poor nations—find themselves losing the ability to define and control their own futures. Political scientists and sociologists warn of the declining strength of the "nation state" and the questionable future of international organizations such as the United Nations (UN) and its related units such as the World Health Organization (WHO). If many countries are weakening in relation to powerful international forces, what does this mean for the development of our local communities? How are they affected by the emphasis on profit—usually for a few privileged individuals and companies?

Globalization, however, can have many positive consequences in our lives. New technologies bring almost instant communication with other parts of the world. Today, mobile phones bring nearly instant access to previously remote areas. Cyberspace, with its internet electronic mailing lists and chat rooms, allows us to learn of other people's realities—their dreams, needs, and challenges. In education, for example, there was a proposal to launch the iNet Global Village program. This program included a series of activities and events aimed at preparing schoolchildren to become competent and productive citizens in a world that is increasingly global and virtual (Zhao, 2006).

How can these same advances in technology and information be used by communities in their struggles for health, social justice, and equity for all? Review Chapter 1 for a comprehensive overview of globalization.

Poverty and Growing Disparities

The developing world has already attained the first Millennium Development Goal target to cut the 1990 poverty rate in half by 2015; however, "even if the current rate of progress is to be maintained, some 1 billion people will still live in extreme poverty in 2015" (World Bank, 2013). People's health and well-being suffer the most when they are unable to secure appropriate employment and can no longer access adequate "social safety nets" and supportive services. Gaps between rich and poor continue to widen so that access to good schools, health care, electricity, safe drinking water, and other critical services becomes elusive for many.

Take Note

"Recognizing that health disparities are a moral wrong that needs to be addressed is . . . [a] step in the moral evolution toward fairness and equality of opportunity in our society." (Jones, 2010, p. S51).

Wherever people live, poverty has been identified as a major cause of malnutrition and illness, thus further undermining the efforts of health workers and health services. Whether at home or at work, the poor are often more exposed to pollution and other health risks than others. They frequently eat poorly, whether in quantity or in quality, and are more likely to smoke tobacco and be exposed to other harmful substances. Differences such as these are found throughout the world, including in the United States.

But poverty is not the only disparity. Additional disparities identified are geographic and racial or ethnic. Lack of health insurance is a major disparity. Although the percentage without health insurance decreased, the number of uninsured people in the United States is 48.6 million. The uninsured rate for children in poverty is 13.8%, and for the Hispanic population, the percentage in 2011 was 30.1 or 15.8 million (U.S. Bureau of the Census, n.d.).

Devoting entire issues of nursing journals to the topic reflects the importance of health disparities in the United States. *Nursing Outlook*, the Official Journal of the American Academy of Nursing, published a special issue on health disparities (American Academy of Nursing, 2005). The same year *Advances in Nursing Science (ANS)* and *Nursing Research* collaborated on a call for manuscripts addressing the problem. Editor Chinn of ANS reminds us that there is a long history of nurses reaching out to the underserved and advocating policies to improve health (Chinn, 2005). Recall earlier in the chapter when we spoke of Lillian Wald and others. May our legacy also represent our future.

Violence

Sexual violence, stalking, and intimate partner violence are major public health problems in the United States. Many survivors of these forms of violence can experience physical injury, mental health consequences such as depression, anxiety, low self-esteem, and suicide attempts, and other health consequences such as gastrointestinal disorders, substance abuse, sexually transmitted diseases, and gynecological or pregnancy complications. These consequences can lead to hospitalization, disability, or death.
(Black et al., 2011, p. 1)

The National Intimate Partner and Sexual Violence Survey (NISVS) quoted above clearly documents that violence is very much a part of our society, and underscores the heavy toll that sexual violence, stalking and intimate partner violence place on women, men, and children in the United States.

Violence takes many forms and ranges from highly visible armed conflict and teen street gangs to the 2.4 million people across the globe who are victims of human trafficking at any one time. Eighty percent of them are being exploited as sexual slaves. Actress Mira Sorvino, the UN goodwill ambassador against human trafficking, said at a General Assembly meeting, "modern day slavery is bested only by the illegal drug trade for profitability," but, it was reported, very little money and political will is spent to combat trafficking (Lederer, 2012).

Although it is very difficult to establish a cause-and-effect relationship between the number of guns available, the violence of the entertainment media, and the number of gun-related crimes committed by younger and younger people, communities have become increasingly concerned about violence. They are also concerned about the weakening of human relationships—in families, between generations, and in communities—that often result in social disintegration.

Internationally, the UN Convention on the Elimination of all Forms of Discrimination against Women (CEDAW) was created in 1979 as an important tool for all those who seek to end abuse of women and girls. The ANA is one of some 168 professional, religious, civic, and community organizations that support ratification of this International Bill of Rights for Women (UN Women, n.d.). Being aware of such documents and promoting their adoption is a way you can serve as an advocate for a violence-free community.

Take Note

"An estimated one in every three women worldwide experiences violence, with rates reaching as high as 70 percent in some countries. Gender-based violence ranges from rape to domestic abuse and acid burnings to dowry deaths and so-called 'honor killings.' Violence against women and girls—in peacetime and in conflict—knows no national or cultural boundaries." (Women Thrive Worldwide, n.d.)

CHALLENGES FOR THE FUTURE

Community health nurses in the future need to stretch their thinking and go far beyond traditional nursing practice in conventional medical and health services. They will continue to be teachers, advocates, monitors, catalysts, and enablers. They will be scientifically and technically skilled. They will be knowledgeable about economics, politics, and global issues. But, most of all, they will be partners with communities at local, regional, national, and international levels. Amelia Maglacas, Chief Nurse Scientist of the WHO at the time, pointed out that enabling people to increase control over and to improve their health will continue to be an integral part of all nurses' roles. This new partnership, involving nurses, communities, and their environments, involves a common search, based on personal choice and social responsibility, for a healthier future (Maglacas, 1988). Almost 30 years later, her words continue to ring true for community health nurses.

Summary

This chapter provides you with an overview of the role of the community health nurse and introduces you to factors influencing that role. Essential theories will be elaborated in subsequent chapters. Awareness of the global factors that affect health and of the essentials of community health nursing will arm you with tools and knowledge to work toward improving health in communities everywhere.

Critical Thinking Questions

1. Review the 10 essential public health services. How does the ACA affect these services? Is the community health nurse's role affected as well?

2. What health concerns in your community have resulted in death, disease, or injury recently? What could population-based community health nursing do to help prevent these problems?

3. Identify three factors that impinge on the health of the community in which you live. Prioritize these factors in terms of their impact and give the rationale for your choices.

REFERENCES

American Academy of Nursing. (2005). Health disparities [Special issue]. *Nursing Outlook, 53*(3), 107–166.
American Nurses Association. (2007). *Public health nursing: Scope & standards of practice.* Washington, DC: American Nurses Publishing.
American Nurses Association. (2013). *Public health nursing: Scope & standards of practice* (2nd ed.). Washington, DC: American Nurses Publishing.

American Public Health Association. (n.d.). *Health reform resources.* Retrieved July 6, 2013, from www.apha.org

American Public Health Association, Public Health Nursing Section. (1996). *Definition and role of public health nursing.* Washington, DC: Author.

Association of Community Health Nursing Educators. (2003). *Essentials of baccalaureate nursing education for entry level community/public health nursing practice.* Wheat Ridge, CO: Author.

Backer, B. A. (1993). Lillian Wald: Connecting caring with action. *Nursing and Health Care, 14*(3), 122–129.

Bekemeier, B., & Butterfield, P. (2005). Unreconciled inconsistencies: A critical review of the concept of social justice in 3 national nursing documents. *Advances in Nursing Science, 28*(2), 152–162.

Berkowitz, B., Nicola, R., Lafronza, V., & Bekemeier, B. (2005). Turning point's legacy. *Journal of Public Health Management and Practice, 11*(2), 97–100.

Black, M. C., Basile, K. C., Breiding, M. J., Smith, S. G., Walters, M. L., Merrick, M. T., … Stevens, M. R. (2011). *The national intimate partner and sexual violence survey (NISVS): 2010 summary report.* Atlanta, GA: National Center for Injury Prevention and Control, Centers for Disease Control and Prevention.

Centers for Disease Control and Prevention. (1999). Ten great public health achievements—United States, 1900–1999. *Morbidity and Mortality Weekly Report, 48*(12), 241–243. Retrieved July 6, 2013, from http://www.cdc.gov/nphpsp/essentialServices.html

Chinn, P. L. (2005). From the Editor: Nursing activism and scholarship to address health disparities [From the Editor]. *Advances in Nursing Science, 28*(3), 193.

Coss, C. (1989). *Lillian Wald: A progressive activist.* New York, NY: Feminist Press.

Feld, M. N. (2008). *Lillian Wald: A biography.* Chapel Hill, NC: University of North Carolina Press.

Jones, C. M. (2010, April). The moral problem of health disparities. *American Journal of Public Health,* 100 (Suppl. 1), S47–S51.

Lederer, E. M. (2012, April 3). Human trafficking victims: 2.4 million people across the globe are trafficked for labor, sex. *Huffington Post.*

Maglacas, A. M. (1988). Health for all: Nursing's role. *Nursing Outlook, 36*(2), 66–71.

UN Women. (n.d.). Convention on the Elimination of all Forms of Discrimination against Women. Retrieved July 6, 2013, at http://www.un.org/womenwatch/daw/cedaw/

U.S. Bureau of the Census. (n.d.). *Highlights 2011, health insurance.* Retrieved July 6, 2013, from www.census.gov

Women Thrive Worldwide. (n.d.). Retrieved July 6, 2013, from www.womenthrive.org

World Bank. (2013). *Poverty overview.* Retrieved July 6, 2013, from www.worldbank.org

World Health Organization. (1978, September). *Report of the international conference on primary health care.* Geneva, Switzerland: Author.

Zhao, Y. (2006, March 19). *iNet global village* [Concept paper]. East Lansing, MI: Michigan State University. Retrieved July 6, 2013, from www.docstoc.com

CHAPTER 3

Epidemiology, Demography, and Community Health

Judith McFarlane and Heidi Gilroy

LEARNING OBJECTIVES

After studying this chapter, you should be able to:

1. Interpret and use basic epidemiologic, demographic, and statistical measures of community health.

2. Apply principles of epidemiology and demography to the practice of community health.

Introduction

Epidemiology and demography are sciences for studying population health. To promote, restore, and maintain the health of populations, the community health professional integrates and applies concepts from these fields. Use of the epidemiologic process can significantly enhance community health practice, providing both a body of knowledge and a methodology for investigating health problems and evaluating health services. This chapter introduces epidemiologic and demographic concepts that are essential for the practice of community health nursing.

EPIDEMIOLOGY

The term *epidemiology* originates from the Greek terms *logos* (study), *demos* (people), and *epi* (upon)—literally, "the study of what is upon the people." Epidemiology is concerned with the distribution and determinants of health and diseases, morbidity, injuries, disability, and mortality in populations. Population in this context refers to people with a common characteristic such as gender, age, and place of residence. Although epidemiologic investigations examine conditions in population groups, it is important to remember that a population consists of individuals, each of whom is a person with a particular condition.

Epidemiology is the study of the distribution and determinants of health-related states or events in specified populations and the application of this study to improve health. Epidemiology is a quantitative discipline based on principles of statistics and research methodologies. Epidemiologic studies have made a significant contribution to the identification of risk factors, such as smoking and lung cancer. In addition, epidemiologic studies identify modifiable risk factors for heart disease resulting in lifestyle changes for individuals along with changes in public health policy. Thus, epidemiologic research methods are a powerful tool for investigating health-related events.

Early epidemiologic studies were concerned chiefly with the control of epidemics (an outbreak of an illness beyond the levels expected in a population). John Snow's study of a cholera epidemic in London in 1853 is a classic in epidemiologic history. At that time, the mode of transmission of cholera was unknown. Snow suspected it was spread by contaminated water. Applying epidemiologic principles, Snow determined that death rates from cholera were highest in areas served by two specific water-pumping systems. He learned that the water from these systems came from portions of the Thames River into which London sewage was discharged. Thus, this early epidemiologist was able to identify a waterborne mode of transmission of cholera and determine measures to control its spread (Snow, 1936).

Many epidemiologic studies have a disease morbidity/mortality focus; however, the dimensions of health and well-being extend beyond these components. Epidemiology as practiced today has expanded its scope to include investigation of lifestyles, health-promotion strategies, injury, environmental conditions, and other factors that influence health. Public health practitioners use the knowledge gained from the epidemiologic process to guide decision making and aid in developing and evaluating interventions for health promotion and disease prevention. The epidemiologic process is analogous to the nursing process in that critical analysis is required to gain further insight into public and community health issues.

Descriptive Epidemiology

Descriptive epidemiology focuses on the distribution of frequencies and patterns of health events with groups in a population. Descriptive studies examine disease patterns and other health-related phenomena according to "person" (who is affected?), "place" (where were they affected?), and "time" (when were they affected?). Descriptive statistics provide data, information, and insight into the characteristics present in a group or population with a disease or the absence of disease in unaffected groups or populations. The question addressed is "Are there characteristics present in the affected population that are not present in the unaffected population?" For example, why are breast cancer rates lower in women who have had children and breast-fed them than in women who have not had children? Descriptive statistics provide epidemiologic studies with data to develop rates, ratios, and proportions of morbidity and mortality statistics for use in public health and vital statistics. Data from descriptive studies suggest hypotheses for further testing and usually involve some form of quantification and statistical analysis. Descriptive studies generally precede analytic studies.

Analytic Epidemiology

In contrast to descriptive epidemiology, analytic epidemiology seeks to identify associations between a particular disease or health problem and its etiology. Analytic studies are directed toward finding answers to the "how" and "why" of health and disease to determine causality. Analytic studies are concerned with the determinants of disease and seek to identify the causes of the problem. They test hypotheses or seek to answer specific questions and can be retrospective or prospective in design.

DEMOGRAPHY

Demography (literally, "writing about the people," from the Greek *demos* [people] and *graphos* [writing]) is the statistical study of human populations with reference to size and density, distribution, and vital statistics. Demographic statistics provide information about significant characteristics of a population that influence community needs and the delivery of health care services. Demographic studies (i.e., demographic research) provide descriptions and comparisons of populations according to the characteristics of age, race, sex, socioeconomic status, geographic distribution, birth, death, marriage, and divorce patterns. Demographic studies often have health implications that may or may not be addressed by the investigators. The census of the US population is an example of a comprehensive descriptive demographic study conducted every 10 years.

LEVELS OF PREVENTION IN COMMUNITY HEALTH PRACTICE

The concept of prevention is a key component of modern community health practice. In popular terminology, prevention means inhibiting the development of disease before it occurs. For the community health practitioner, three levels of prevention—primary, secondary, and tertiary—guide practice.

Primary prevention applied to a generally healthy population precedes disease or dysfunction. Primary prevention is divided into two component areas: (1) general health promotion such as nutrition, hygiene, exercise, and environmental protection and (2) specific health promotion, which includes immunizations and the wearing of protective devices to prevent injuries. If a disease is environmentally induced, primary prevention can prevent a person's exposure to the environmental factor involved and thereby prevent development of the disease. Prevention is difficult to measure and demonstrate empirically; however, it is less costly both in terms of human suffering and in terms of economic expenditures than crisis intervention and treating disease and disabilities after they have occurred.

Secondary prevention is the early detection and treatment of adverse health conditions. The goal of secondary prevention is to detect and treat a problem at the earliest possible stage when disease or impairment already exists. Secondary prevention may result in the cure of illnesses that would be incurable at later stages, the prevention of complications and disability, and confinement of the spread of communicable diseases. Examples of secondary prevention include blood pressure screening for hypertension, audiometric testing for hearing impairment, skin test for tuberculosis, and phenylalanine test for phenylketonuria in infancy. On a community basis, early treatment of people with infectious disease, such as a sexually transmitted disease (STD), may protect others from acquiring infection and thus provides secondary prevention for infected people and primary prevention for their potential contacts.

Tertiary prevention is employed after diseases or events have already resulted in morbidity. The purpose of tertiary prevention is to limit disability and to rehabilitate or restore the affected people to their maximum possible capacities. Examples of tertiary prevention include physical therapy for stroke victims, social support programs for recovering alcoholics, exercise programs for heart attack victims, and mental health counseling for rape victims.

The goal of intervention at each of the three levels of prevention is to prevent the progression process. To plan appropriate methods of primary, secondary, and tertiary prevention, the community health nurse must initially assess the current health status of the community.

DESCRIPTIVE MEASURES OF HEALTH

Demographic Measures

Certain human characteristics, or demographics, may be associated with wellness or illness. Age, race, gender, ethnicity, income, and educational level are important demographics that may affect health outcomes. For example, men are more likely than women to develop certain heart diseases, and African American women are more likely than Caucasian women to deliver low-birth-weight infants (usually defined as infants weighing less than 2,500 g at birth). To plan for the health of a community, the nurse must be familiar with the demographic characteristics of the community and with the health problems associated with those characteristics.

Morbidity and Mortality

Although epidemiology describes the distribution and determinants of both wellness and illness states, wellness is difficult to measure. Therefore, many measures of "health" are expressed in terms of morbidity (illness) and mortality (death). An excellent source of morbidity and mortality data, by state and for select cities, is the Centers for Disease Control and Prevention (CDC), *Morbidity and Mortality Weekly Report* (http://www.cdc.gov/mmwr).

Incidence

The incidence of any health or disease condition refers to the number of people in a population who develop the condition during a specified period of time. Incidence rates measure the rate at which people without a disease develop the disease during a specific period of time (i.e., the number of new cases of a disease in a population over a period of time). Mathematically, incidence rate over a period of time is expressed as:

$$\frac{\text{Number of new cases of disease}}{\text{Total population at risk}} \times 100,000$$

The incidence rate uses the frequency of new cases in the numerator. The denominator for incidence rates is the population at risk. For example, to calculate the incidence rate of postmenopausal breast cancer, women who are still premenopausal would not be a part of the population at risk. Incidence is particularly important for analytic epidemiologic research because it allows the estimation of risk necessary to assess causal association (relative risk [RR]). The calculation of incidence generally requires that a defined population initially free of the disease in question must be followed over a period of time in what is called a prospective (forward-looking) study.

Prevalence

The prevalence of a disease or condition refers to the total number of people in the population who have the condition at a particular time. Thus, prevalence may be calculated in a "one-shot" cross-sectional (slice of time) or retrospective (backward looking) study. Mathematically, prevalence is expressed as:

$$\frac{\text{Number of existing cases of disease}}{\text{Number in total population}} \times 100,000$$

Prevalence, therefore, examines the extent of morbidity in a community and is influenced by the rate of new cases, the number of existing cases, effective new treatment modalities, and deaths. It can be classified as period prevalence (existence during a period of time, such as 32% of children at Camp North had diarrhea between June 10 and June 25) or point prevalence (a specific point in time, such as 10% of children at Camp North had diarrhea on June 15).

Understanding Incidence and Prevalence

Measures of incidence and prevalence provide different information. To understand the relationship between incidence and prevalence, consider the number of passengers on a train. The number of passengers represents prevalence (existing disease, old and new cases); the number of boarding passengers represents incidence (new cases of disease); passengers who get off the train represent individuals who either recover or die. Both the number of new cases entering and the number of individuals with disease who leave either through death or through recovery from the illness influence prevalence. The number of passengers on board will increase if the number of boarding passengers (new cases) is high, if the number of passengers exiting is low (fewer deaths or increased survival rate due to new treatment), or both occur. Conversely, prevalence will decrease when the number of new cases is low or when individuals die or persons are cured of disease or both.

Consider another example. You read about an increase in the prevalence of a certain type of cancer; this increase may mean that there are a higher number of people with this type of cancer in the population. This higher number may be due to more new cases (in other words, increased incidence) or because people with this type of cancer are living longer. In either case, the community may need to allocate additional resources toward cancer identification and treatment.

Ratios, Proportions, and Rates

In epidemiologic studies, data and statistics make comparison possible among populations. Therefore, it is necessary to convert raw data into ratios, proportions, and rates to provide a more valid description of health problems. A *ratio* is simply one number divided by another, in which there is no specified relationship between the numerator and the denominator. For example, of 1,000 motorcycle fatalities, 950 victims are male and 50 are female. The sex ratio is the number of males compared with the number of females (950/50 or 19 males to 1 female).

In contrast, a *proportion* is one number divided by another, in which the numerator is a subset of the denominator (i.e., it is included in the denominator) and is expressed as a percentage. Using the same data, you can calculate the proportion of males to females. Of 1,000 motorcycle fatalities, 950 are male and 50 are female. What percentage of fatalities is male? A proportion is expressed by the formula $X / (X + Y)$; thus, the percentage of males to females would be 950/1,000 multiplied by 100, which equals 95%. Neither ratio nor proportion has a population base or specific unit of time.

Because epidemiology is the study of population health, statistical measures must relate the occurrence of a health condition to the population at risk. To assess the probability that one group is at higher risk than another, rates are calculated. *Rates* measure the amount of disease, injury, disability, or death within a unit of the population and within a unit of time. Rates express a mathematical relationship in which the *numerator* relates to the number of persons experiencing the condition, and the *denominator* expresses the population at risk or the total number of persons who have the possibility of experiencing the condition. Rates improve the ability to make comparisons because they reduce the standard of comparison to a common denominator, the unit size of the population. For example, the crude death rates for heart disease in Florida and Texas were 222.6 and 153.6 per 100,000 persons, respectively. It appears that the death rate is higher in Florida compared with Texas. This difference may be due to population characteristics (e.g., age differences between the states) that can affect mortality experiences. Later in this chapter, specific rates are discussed that can be calculated for a subgroup of persons, such as death rate for heart disease in Florida and Texas for persons over the age of 65.

Do not confuse rates with other proportions that do not use the population at risk as the denominator. For example, the death rate from cancer is not the same as the proportion of deaths from cancer. In each, the numerator is the number of deaths from cancer. However, the denominator differs. In the death rate, the denominator represents all people at risk of dying from cancer. Therefore, the cancer death rate is an expression of the risk of dying from cancer.

In the proportion of deaths, also called proportionate mortality rate (PMR), the denominator is the total number of deaths from all causes. Mathematically, the PMR is expressed as:

$$\frac{Number\ of\ deaths\ due\ to\ a\ specific\ cause}{Total\ number\ of\ deaths\ from\ all\ causes} \times 100$$

Therefore, the proportionate cancer mortality simply describes the proportion of deaths attributable to cancer. For example, if the PMR of heart disease is 25%, this indicates that 25% of all deaths, regardless of age, sex, or race, are related to diseases of the heart. However, this statistic provides no indication of the rate for heart disease.

Calculation of Epidemiologic Rates

Rates are calculated by the formula:

$$Rate = \frac{Number\ of\ people\ experiencing\ condition}{Population\ at\ risk\ experiencing\ condition} \times K$$

K is a constant (usually 1,000 or 100,000) that allows the ratio, which may be a very small number, to be expressed in a meaningful way. The concept of rates can be understood more easily by applying this formula to the calculation of the infant mortality rate (IMR), which estimates an infant's risk of dying during the first year of life.

Example of a Rate: The Infant Mortality Rate

The IMR is usually calculated on a calendar year basis. The number of infant deaths (deaths before the age of 1 year) during the year is divided by the number of live births (infants born alive) during that year. The numerator represents the number of infants experiencing the "condition" of dying in the first year of life, and the denominator represents the population of infants at risk for dying in the year.

If within a given year 34,400 infant deaths and 4,084,000 live births were reported for the United States, these data would provide the numerator and denominator to calculate the IMR. Applying the formula for a rate, one would divide the numerator 34,400 by 4,084,000 and obtain a value of 0.0084, which would indicate that 0.0084 of the infants died during the first year of life. To obtain a meaningful rate, it is necessary to multiply by a constant, in this case 1,000, and find that 8.4 infants per 1,000 live births died during the first year of life (i.e., the IMR was 8.4 infant deaths per 1,000 live births). This IMR would be calculated as follows:

$$\frac{34,400}{4,084,000} \times 1,000 = 8.4\ infant\ deaths\ per\ live\ births$$

Interpretation of Rates

Rates enable researchers to compare different populations in terms of health problems or conditions. To assess whether one community is at greater or lesser risk for the problems or conditions, compare the rates for the community with rates from similar communities, from the state, or from the United States as a whole.

Caution is required in interpreting rates. Like most statistical measures, rates are less reliable when based on small numbers. This is important when assessing relatively infrequent events or conditions or communities with small populations.

The majority of rates are based on data from a calendar year, which may also present some difficulties. Populations may increase or decrease during a calendar year. To adjust for population changes over the year, the midyear population estimate is generally used because the population at risk cannot be determined accurately.

Commonly Used Rates

Box 3.1 summarizes a number of important rates. Note that the measures of natality and mortality are, in essence, measures of incidence of the conditions of "being born" and "dying." Study the various ways in which the denominator, or population at risk, is determined in different rates.

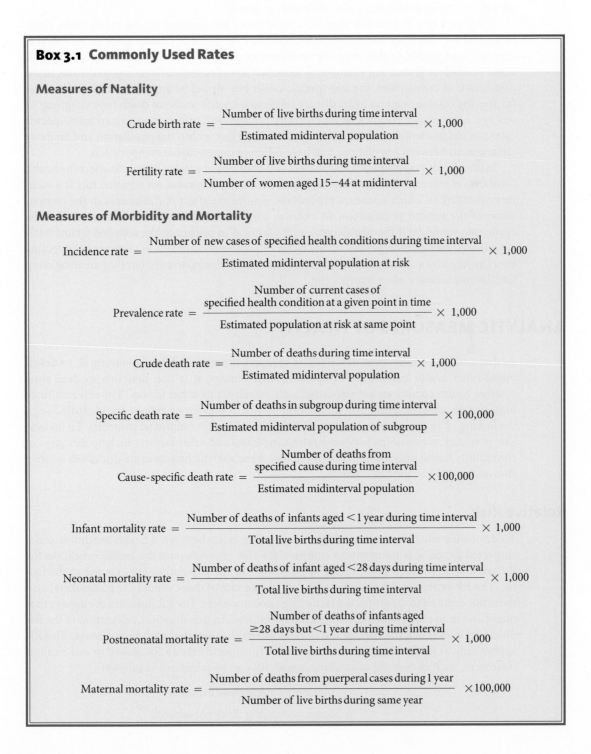

Box 3.1 Commonly Used Rates

Measures of Natality

$$\text{Crude birth rate} = \frac{\text{Number of live births during time interval}}{\text{Estimated midinterval population}} \times 1{,}000$$

$$\text{Fertility rate} = \frac{\text{Number of live births during time interval}}{\text{Number of women aged } 15{-}44 \text{ at midinterval}} \times 1{,}000$$

Measures of Morbidity and Mortality

$$\text{Incidence rate} = \frac{\text{Number of new cases of specified health conditions during time interval}}{\text{Estimated midinterval population at risk}} \times 1{,}000$$

$$\text{Prevalence rate} = \frac{\text{Number of current cases of specified health condition at a given point in time}}{\text{Estimated population at risk at same point}} \times 1{,}000$$

$$\text{Crude death rate} = \frac{\text{Number of deaths during time interval}}{\text{Estimated midinterval population}} \times 1{,}000$$

$$\text{Specific death rate} = \frac{\text{Number of deaths in subgroup during time interval}}{\text{Estimated midinterval population of subgroup}} \times 100{,}000$$

$$\text{Cause-specific death rate} = \frac{\text{Number of deaths from specified cause during time interval}}{\text{Estimated midinterval population}} \times 100{,}000$$

$$\text{Infant mortality rate} = \frac{\text{Number of deaths of infants aged} <1 \text{ year during time interval}}{\text{Total live births during time interval}} \times 1{,}000$$

$$\text{Neonatal mortality rate} = \frac{\text{Number of deaths of infant aged} <28 \text{ days during time interval}}{\text{Total live births during time interval}} \times 1{,}000$$

$$\text{Postneonatal mortality rate} = \frac{\text{Number of deaths of infants aged} \geq 28 \text{ days but} <1 \text{ year during time interval}}{\text{Total live births during time interval}} \times 1{,}000$$

$$\text{Maternal mortality rate} = \frac{\text{Number of deaths from puerperal cases during 1 year}}{\text{Number of live births during same year}} \times 100{,}000$$

Crude, Specific, and Adjusted Rates

Rates can be broken down into three categories: crude, specific, and adjusted. Rates computed for a population as a whole are *crude rates*. When calculating deaths in the total population, irrespective of age, the rate obtained is the *crude mortality rate* or crude death rate. With the crude mortality rate, there is no allowance for the age distribution of the population or comparisons between populations with different age groups.

Subgroups of a population may have differences not revealed by the crude rates. Rates calculated for subgroups are *specific rates*. Specific rates relate to demographic factors such as age, race, and gender, or they may refer to the entire population but be specific for some single cause of death or illness. For example, to eliminate the effects of different age structures in the population of comparison, the age-specific death rate would be appropriate. Mortality rates for specific diseases such as heart disease relate to a specific cause of death (any subgroup or any age, race, gender, religion, or for an entire population). Information gained from specific rates can aid in identification of groups at increased risk within the population and facilitate comparisons between populations that have different demographic compositions.

In comparing populations with different distributions of a factor known to affect the health condition of interest, the use of *adjusted rates* may be appropriate. An adjusted rate is a summary measure in which statistical procedures remove the effect of differences in the composition of the various populations. In essence, adjustment produces an estimate of what the crude rate would be if the populations were identical in respect to the adjusted factor. Rates are adjusted for age, race, gender, or any factor or combination of factors suspected of affecting the rate. Adjusted rates are helpful in making community comparisons, but they are imaginary. Caution is necessary when interpreting.

ANALYTIC MEASURES OF HEALTH

As discussed previously, rates describe and compare the risks of dying, becoming ill, or developing other health conditions. In epidemiologic studies, it is also desirable to determine whether health conditions are associated with, or related to, other factors. The research findings may provide the theoretical foundation by which preventive actions are identified (e.g., the linking of air pollution to health problems has led to environmental controls). To investigate potential relationships between health conditions and other factors, analytic measures of community health are required. In this section, three analytic measures are discussed: *relative risk, odds ratio*, and *attributable risk*.

Relative Risk

To determine whether a relationship or association exists between a health condition and a suspected factor, it is necessary to compare the risk of developing the health condition for the population exposed to the factor with the risk for the population not exposed to the factor. The RR expresses the risk ratio of the incidence rate of those exposed (e.g., smokers) and those not exposed to the suspected factor (e.g., nonsmokers). The RR indicates the benefit that might accrue to the person if the risk factor is removed. In this situation, calculation of the RR illustrates how much the risk for the smoker increases compared with nonsmokers. The RR applies only to studies that determine incidence (prospective data). RR is used to make causal inferences, such as *smoking causes lung cancer*. RR can be calculated as follows:

$$RR = \frac{\text{Incidence among those exposed}}{\text{Incidence rate among those not exposed}}$$

The RR indicates whether the rate in the exposed population is higher than the rate in the nonexposed population and, if so, how many times higher. A high RR in the exposed population suggests that the factor is a risk factor in the development of the health condition. RR does not indicate that someone with the factor will develop the disease. It is important to note that risk estimates are probability statements; therefore, (1) all those exposed to the factor do not develop the disease, but merely have an increased probability of doing so and (2) some people who have not been exposed to the factor will develop the disease. A RR of 1.0 means the risk of disease among the exposed is no different from the risk of disease among the nonexposed. A RR of 2.0 implies that risk is twice as high, whereas a RR of 0.5 indicates that the exposure factor is associated with half the risk of disease. For example, if the RR of postmenopausal breast cancer among women who breast-fed is 0.8, then breast-feeding can be considered a protective factor for postmenopausal breast cancer.

Internal and External Risk Factors

The concept of RR applies when one group of people clearly is exposed and another is not exposed to an external factor such as cigarette smoke, exercise, or foods high in saturated fat. However, it may be confusing to see RRs applied to internal factors such as age, race, or gender. Nevertheless, as can be seen in the following example, people are also "exposed" to intrinsic factors that may carry as much risk as extrinsic ones.

Relative Risk: Premature Death

Ma, Xu, Anderson, and Jemal (2012) studied death in men and women between the ages of 25 and 64. In 2007, working-aged men with less than 12 years of schooling died at a rate of 657.1 per 100,000. Men with more than 16 years of schooling died at a rate of 184.4 per 100,000. With this information, one can calculate the RR. The RR of death for working-aged men with less than 12 years of schooling compared with those with greater than 16 years of schooling may be calculated as follows:

$$RR = \frac{657.1 \, per \, 100,000}{184.4 \, per \, 100,000} = 3.6$$

In other words, the risk of dying prematurely increases more than three and a half times for men with less than a high school education. Clearly, lower educational attainment is a risk factor. Health care professionals may not be able to change past educational attainment of patients; however, the information can be used to plan interventions for populations at risk.

Odds Ratio

Calculation of the RR is straightforward when incidence rates are available. Unfortunately, not all studies are prospective as is required for the computation of incidence rates. In a retrospective study, the RR is approximated by the *odds ratio*.

As shown in Table 3.1, the odds ratio is a simple mathematical ratio of the odds in favor of having a specific health condition when the suspected factor is present and the odds in favor of having the condition when the factor is absent. The odds of having the condition when the suspected factor is present are represented by *a/b* in the table. The odds of having the condition when not exposed to the factor are *c/d*. The odds ratio is thus:

$$\frac{a/b}{c/d} = \frac{ad}{bc}$$

TABLE 3.1 Crosstabulation for Calculation of Odds Ratio

	Health Condition		
	Present	Absent	Total
Exposed to factor	a	b	a + b
Not exposed to factor	c	d	c + d
Total	a + c	b + d	a + b + c + d

In recent decades, changing social norms and increasingly effective infertility treatments have made assisted conception more common among live births. Types of assisted conception include in vitro fertilization (IVF), intracytoplasmic sperm injection (ICSI), or medications. Davies et al. (2012) used an odds ratio to measure the incidence of birth defects in women who did or did not use assisted conception to get pregnant. In this case, it may not have been practical to recruit women on a prospective basis because the researchers were interested only in live births and a large sample was needed. Therefore, birth defects were compared among existing cases of assisted conception and nonassisted conception. The authors found that babies born after assisted conception were more likely to have birth defects than babies born after nonassisted conception. Data in Table 3.2 can be used to calculate the odds ratio.

$$\text{Odds ratio} = \frac{ad}{bc} = \frac{513(285265)}{5690(17546)} = 1.47$$

An odds ratio of 1.0 implies that the odds of exposure are equal and suggest that a particular exposure is not a risk factor for the disease of study. Babies born after assisted conception were nearly one and a half times more likely to have birth defects compared with babies born after nonassisted conception.

Relative Risk and Odds Ratio: Caution in Interpretation

A high odds ratio or RR must be regarded with appropriate concern; however, the finding should not obscure the potential involvement of other factors. As illustrated in Table 3.2, 17,546 of the babies in the sample had birth defects although assisted conception was not used. In other words, assisted conception was not the sole cause of birth defects. The risk may also be offset by the potential benefit for mothers who need assistance to conceive. Women should be informed of increased risk when deciding on options for pregnancy.

Attributable Risk and Attributable Risk Percentage

Another measure of risk is *attributable risk* (AR), which measures the difference between the incidence rates for those exposed and those not exposed to the risk factor. The measure estimates the excess risk attributable to exposure to the risk factor. It shows the potential

TABLE 3.2 Birth Defects in the Presence or Absence of Assisted Conception

Assisted Conception	Birth Defects		
	Present	Absent	Total
Used	513	5,690	6,163
Not used	17,546	285,265	302,811

Data from Davies, M. J., Moore, V. M., Willson, K. J., Van Essen, P., Priest, K., Scott, H., . . . Chan, A. (2012). Reproductive technologies and the risk of birth defects. *New England Journal of Medicine, 366* (19), 1803–1813.

reduction in the overall incidence rate if the factor is eliminated. The AR is calculated by subtracting the incidence among those unexposed to a risk factor from those who were exposed:

AR = incidence rate in exposed group *minus* incidence rate in nonexposed group

AR usually is further quantified into attributable risk percentage:

$$\frac{AR}{\text{Incidence rate in exposed group}} = 100$$

This provides an estimate of the percentage of occurrences of the health condition that is potentially preventable if the risk factor is eliminated. For example, a study of the relationship between childhood adversities and physical dating violence before the age of 21 found that the AR associated with exposure to interparental violence was 10.7% (Miller et al., 2011). Thus, preventing children's exposure to interparental violence in the home has the potential to reduce physical dating violence among adolescents.

Point Estimate and Confidence Intervals

RRs and odds ratios provide a point estimate (a number) that identifies whether those in the exposed group will develop the disease or condition when compared with those not exposed. To apply the point estimate to decisions of community health, it is important to understand the relationship of the point estimate to the number one (1.0) and the range of numbers within the confidence interval (CI).

A point estimate is the mathematical calculation derived from the data, such as a RRs or odds ratio. Relationship of the point estimate, such as a RR of 3.0, to the number one (1.0) allows you to determine whether an association exists between the exposure and the condition. As you learned earlier, a risk of 1.0 means the person has no added risk. A risk of less than 1.0 suggests some protection from the exposure and a RR above 1.0 suggests increased risk of the disease or condition from the exposure.

After establishing the point estimate and the position of the RR in relation to 1.0, you must also assess the CI or range of point estimates around the RR. Most studies report a 95% CI. The relationship is statistically significant *only* if the entire CI is *above* or *below* 1.0 (Brucker, 2005). For example, a RR may be 5.0, but the 95% CI is reported as 0.45 to 10.8. The CI crosses, or encompasses, the number 1.0; therefore, the association is not significant. However, the RR of 0.21 with a 95% CI of 0.10 to 0.45 would be statistically significant, as the CI does not cross or encompass 1.0. In a study by McFarlane, Campbell, Sharps, and Watson (2002), the odds ratio for murder or attempted murder of women abused during pregnancy was 3.08 with 95% CI of 1.86 to 5.10. The CI did not include 1.0; therefore, the women abused during pregnancy were three times as likely to be murdered or have an attempt made on their lives compared with women not abused during pregnancy.

Cause and Association

Ultimately, community health professionals hope to determine causes of adverse health conditions so steps can be taken to improve health. In view of the complexity of the human body and human behavior, establishing causality is very difficult. Therefore, investigations of population health generally examine relationships or associations between variables. The *variables* are the characteristics or phenomena (such as age, occupation, or physical exercise), and the health conditions (such as heart disease) being studied.

Variables and Constants

An important requirement in any study is that the factors studied must have the potential to vary from person to person. If a factor cannot vary, it is not a variable but a *constant*. It is impossible to establish an association between a constant and a variable because the constant, by definition, cannot change when the variable changes. Thus, a study that looks only at men cannot establish an association between gender and, for example, heart disease; the study has made gender a constant. A study that looks only at people with heart disease cannot establish an association between heart disease and any other variable; heart disease has become a constant in the study.

Control or Comparison Groups

To ensure that associations between variables can be examined, control groups or comparison groups are essential. A study of heart disease might compare people with the disease with a control group of people without the disease. An investigation of a new treatment would study people who receive the treatment and a control group of people who do not receive the treatment.

Independent and Dependent Variables

The *dependent variable* is the outcome or result that the investigator is studying. The dependent variable can change (e.g., health status, knowledge, and behavior). The *independent variable* is the presumed "cause" of or contributor to variation in the dependent variable. For example, in the physical dating violence study cited earlier (Miller et al., 2011), the authors found that exposure to interparental violence, the independent variable, contributed to adolescent physical partner violence, the dependent variable. An independent variable may be a naturally occurring event or phenomenon such as level of usual physical activity, exposure to ultraviolet radiation, and type of employment, or it might be a planned intervention such as an exercise program, a medication, and a support group. An independent variable might also be an intrinsic quality such as age, race, gender, or genes. (Note that these intrinsic qualities, although they cannot vary within an individual, can vary from person to person; thus, they are studied as independent variables.)

Confounding Variables

When an association exists between variables, it is tempting—but incorrect—to assume that one variable causes the other. If, for example, a study found that communities with low salaries for public health workers had high crime rates, one could not conclude that low public health salaries lead to high crime rates. Common sense suggests that economic conditions might influence both salaries and crime (i.e., economic conditions intervene in the study and confound the results). Here is another example: Driving without seatbelts increases the risk of a fatal automobile accident. However, nonusers of seatbelts are likely to speed, and speeding is another cause of automobile fatalities. Therefore, some of the apparent benefits of seatbelts relate to differing driving speeds of users and nonusers of seatbelts. In this example, speeding is a confounding variable. Any factor that may influence a study's results is an extraneous, intervening, or confounding variable.

Criteria for Determining Causation

Association does not imply causation. If an association is found between variables, it means the variables tend to occur or change together (parallel increase or decrease); it does not prove that one variable causes the other. The first question to ask is whether a statistical relationship exists between the two factors. Before an association is assessed for possibility that it is causal, other explanations such as chance, bias, and confounding variables are considered. Statistical methods alone, however, cannot establish proof of a causal relationship in an association. Because of the possibility of confounded results, very strict criteria for determining causation exist. An association must be evaluated against all of the criteria; the more criteria that are met, the more likely it is that the association is causal. However, an association may meet all the criteria for causation and later be shown to be spurious (false or factitious association) because of factors that were not known at the time the study was done. For this reason, investigators must interpret results with great caution; they rarely consider a cause "proven." Six widely used criteria for evaluating causation are the following:

1. *The association is strong.* The strength of the relationship is usually measured statistically with RR or, alternatively, the odds ratio. The higher the RR or odds ratio, the greater the likelihood that the association is causal.
2. *The association is consistent.* The same association exists repeatedly in other studies, in other settings, and with other populations. The more the association appears under diverse circumstances, the more likely it is to be causal in nature.
3. *The association is temporally correct.* The hypothesized cause of the health condition must occur before the onset of the condition (i.e., exposure to the risk factor must precede the onset of disease). This criterion is definitely essential. It is the first and most important variable—if exposure did not precede the onset, the remaining facts are irrelevant because exposure could not have caused the disease.
4. *The association is specific.* The hypothesized cause should be associated with relatively few health conditions. Specificity measures the degree to which one particular exposure produces one specific disease—the uniqueness of the relationship. If the biologic response is variable, it is less likely to be causal.
5. *The association is not the result of a confounding variable.* Although not all potential intervening variables are identified, the alternate explanations for the association are examined carefully before considering an association causal.
6. *The association is plausible and consistent with current knowledge.* Any disease or injury causation association must be congruent and compatible with current biomedical and scientific knowledge and information. This depends on the state of scientific information at a given time. An association that contradicts current scientific views must be evaluated very carefully. However, associations may be inconsistent with current knowledge simply because current knowledge is not as advanced as a new discovery.

SOURCES OF COMMUNITY HEALTH DATA

To be an effective community health practitioner, it is essential to interpret and use data from various sources. This section reviews important sources of data.

Census

The census is probably the most comprehensive source of health-related data for the United States. Every 10 years, the Bureau of the Census enumerates the US population and surveys it for basic demographics. Census data provide a wealth of information about a community's characteristics, such as age, race, and sex, along with other factors such as employment, income, migration, and education. Traditionally, epidemiologists have used the census of the population as a reliable source for denominators in the calculation of rates.

Census information is analyzed and reported for the nation as a whole and in progressively smaller regions down to municipalities, census tracts, and blocks. Results are also reported in regions known as standard metropolitan statistical areas (SMSA). Census data are available online at http://www.census.gov. Only a limited number of questions are asked of the entire population. More detailed surveys are taken of selected samples of the population.

Although census data are comprehensive, bias does occur. For example, people may answer personal questions dishonestly. Perhaps more significantly, the census underrepresents low-income residents, minorities, and transients. These people are more difficult to locate, enumerate, and tend to be less likely to respond to census surveys.

Vital Statistics

Data that describe legally registered events such as births, deaths, marriages, and divorces are called vital statistics. Government agencies collect vital statistics on an ongoing basis. The CDC's National Center for Health Statistics collects and publishes vital statistics from individual states. Health professionals can use the data in examining trends over time and in establishing health improvement plans. The data are available on the internet at http://www.cdc.gov/nchs. The U.S. Public Health Service also gathers data from the states and publishes annual volumes, along with periodic reports on specific topics.

Beginning researchers tend to consider vital statistics "hallowed" because they are, after all, legal data. However, legality does not guarantee validity. For example, a person's race sometimes differs on birth and death certificates, and the manner in which cause of death is recorded on death certificates is inconsistent. The numbers of unmarried but cohabitating couples also demonstrate that marriage and divorce records are also not completely valid measures of reality. Despite their limitations, vital statistics are often the best available data.

Notifiable Disease Reports

The CDC/U.S. Public Health Service reports data collected by state and local health departments on legally reportable diseases, and periodically requests voluntary reporting of non-notifiable health conditions of special interest. Notifiable diseases are frequently referred to as reportable diseases. Criteria to determine whether a disease is notifiable are (1) the ability of the disease to cause death and (2) the communicability of the disease. Notification to public health officials of diseases posing a threat to large populations provides an initial starting point for local epidemiologic investigations. The concept of surveillance is essential to identification and control of notifiable diseases. Surveillance is the systematic collection of data pertaining to the occurrence of specific diseases, the analysis and interpretation of these data, and the dissemination of information about the data. The CDC weekly publication, *Morbidity and Mortality Weekly Report*, is a valuable resource for community health practice.

The major deficiency of this category of data for epidemiologic research purposes is the possible incompleteness of population coverage. Even legally mandated disease reports may not be representative of all cases of the disease. Thus, valid descriptions of the disease as it exists in the community may not be accessible. In practice, health care providers may also fail to complete the required reporting form.

Vital Record Linkage

Vital record linkage connects data and information contained in two or more medical, morbidity, or mortality records, and other vital event records. Record linkage systems provide excellent sources of information on the courses of diseases, demographic data, health care services utilization, fertility, maternal health issues, child health concerns, chronic disease tracking, and the natural history of specific disease or morbidity-related events. Record linkage is facilitated by the advent of modern computers. This system offers a potentially rich source of information and may facilitate research on measures of public health.

Medical and Hospital Records

Medical and hospital records provide valuable information for community health research. The increasing use of electronic health records (EHRs) among health care providers and hospitals has facilitated data mining or the use of large amounts of information from patient records. It is important to note that, though these records contain comprehensive information about patients seeking services, they do not provide a completely representative or valid picture of community health. Not all clients with health problems receive medical attention, so medical records are biased by including only those that do. Also, medical documentation is not always complete. Hospitalized patients are also more likely to have coexistent illnesses. This phenomenon, called Berkson's bias, creates the likelihood of finding a false association between the two or more illnesses.

Autopsy Records

Autopsy records have a very severe inherent bias: The patient may have been so ill that death occurred. Autopsies are not performed for all deaths. Autopsy records include a disproportionate number of cases of violent death and people for whom the cause of death was unknown until after autopsy (e.g., the manifestation of the illness was unusual). People who do not sanction autopsy are underrepresented. These factors influence the validity and representativeness of the findings of any study using autopsy records.

National Electronic Disease Surveillance System

The National Electronic Disease Surveillance System (NEDSS) provides an integrated surveillance system that transmits public health laboratory and clinical data via the internet. This process improves the nation's ability to identify and track emerging infectious diseases and potential bioterrorism attacks. Therefore, NEDSS is of particular importance to state health departments in investigating outbreaks and monitoring disease trends in that it is used for surveillance and analysis of notifiable diseases. For further information, visit http://www.cdc.gov/nedss.

SCREENING FOR HEALTH CONDITIONS

Screening can be defined as the presumptive identification of unrecognized disease or defects by the administration of tests, examinations, or other procedures that can be applied rapidly. Screening tests do not provide a conclusive diagnosis of a disease, but rather identify asymptomatic people who may unknowingly have a health problem. Anyone who shows evidence of symptoms of a disease through a screening program should have further medical diagnostic testing. The purpose of screening is to rapidly and economically identify people who have a high probability of having (or developing) a particular illness so they can be referred for definitive diagnosis and treatment.

Considerations in Deciding to Screen

Screening goes further than identifying groups at risk for illness; it identifies individuals who may actually have an illness. Screening carries an ethical commitment to continue working with these people and to provide them access to diagnostic and treatment services. In general, screening should be conducted only if

- Early diagnosis and treatment can favorably alter the course of the illness.
- Definitive diagnosis and treatment facilities are available, either through the screening agency or through referral.

- The group being screened is at risk for the illness (in other words, the group is likely to have a high prevalence of the illness).
- The screening procedures are reliable and valid.

Screening Test Reliability and Validity

Reliability (precision) refers to the consistency or repeatability of test results; *validity* refers to the ability of the test to measure what it is supposed to measure. A few considerations specific to screening tests are discussed below.

Test Reliability

A reliable screening test yields the same result even when administered by different screeners. Training for all screening personnel involved in the test is essential. Lack of reliability may suggest that the screeners are administering the test in an inconsistent manner.

Test Validity: Sensitivity and Specificity

To be valid, a screening test must distinguish correctly between those people who have the condition and those who do not. This ability to distinguish is measured by the test's sensitivity and specificity, as shown in Table 3.3.

Sensitivity is the ability of a test to correctly identify people who have the disease (i.e., to call a true positive "positive"). A test with high sensitivity will have few false negatives.

Specificity is the ability of a test to identify correctly people who do not have the disease, or to call a true negative "negative." If a test is not specific, people who do not actually have the disease will be referred for additional diagnostic testing. A test with high specificity has few false positives.

Ideally, a screening test's sensitivity and specificity should be 100%; in practice, however, screening tests vary in this regard. As shown in Table 3.3, sensitivity, or the true-positive rate, is the complement of the false-negative rate, and specificity, or the true-negative rate, is the complement of the false-positive rate. Thus, as sensitivity increases, specificity decreases. Therefore, decisions regarding screening test validity may require uncomfortable compromises, as discussed in the following section.

TABLE 3.3 Sensitivity and Specificity of a Screening Test

	Reality	
Screening Test Results	**Diseased**	**Not Diseased**
Positive	True positive	False positive
Negative	False negative	True negative
Total	Total diseased	Total not diseased

$$\text{Sensitivity (true-positive rate)} = \frac{\text{True positives}}{\text{Total diseased}}$$

$$\text{Specificity (true-negative rate)} = \frac{\text{True negatives}}{\text{Total not diseased}}$$

$$\text{False-negative rate} = \frac{\text{False negatives}}{\text{Total diseased}} \text{ or } 1 - \text{Sensitivity}$$

$$\text{False-positive rate} = \frac{\text{False positives}}{\text{Total not diseased}} \text{ or } 1 - \text{Specificity}$$

Decision Making in Screening: Practical and Ethical Considerations

In a community health setting, a screening program is necessary for a deadly disease that is curable only if detected early. The two tests available are one with a high sensitivity and low specificity and one with high specificity and low sensitivity. One must make a decision as to which test should be selected. To save the most lives, high sensitivity is essential (i.e., a low rate of false negatives [people who have the disease, but are not detected by the screening test]). However, if one selects the test with high sensitivity, its low specificity means that one will have a high rate of false positives (people who do not have the disease but whom the test falsely identifies as having it). With increased numbers of false positives, many people could be alarmed needlessly, resulting in unnecessary expenses by overreferral of people who are disease-free. Which test would you choose? Why?

How does the situation differ when one is screening for a deadly disease, but the diagnostic and treatment facilities in the community are already overloaded and further budget cuts are projected? To minimize unnecessary referrals of false positives, the test with high specificity would be preferable. However, owing to the low sensitivity of this test, it will be necessary to weigh the benefits of a low false-positive rate against the ethics of a high false-negative rate. Is it justifiable to lull the undetected diseased people into a false—and potentially fatal—sense of security? Which test would you select in this situation? Why?

Decisions regarding screening involve seeking the most favorable balance of sensitivity and specificity. Sometimes, sensitivity and specificity can be improved by adjusting the screening process (e.g., adding another test or changing the level at which the test is considered positive). At other times, evaluating sensitivity and specificity may result in a decision not to conduct a screening program because the economic costs of overreferral or the ethical considerations of underreferral outweigh the usefulness of screening. An understanding of the principles discussed in this section will help you make informed decisions regarding community screening.

EPIDEMIOLOGIC APPROACHES TO COMMUNITY HEALTH RESEARCH

Epidemiologic models guide investigators in examining the determinants of population health. This section describes four models and explains how each might guide the approach to the same problem.

Application of each model is illustrated using the problem of an increase in the IMR in a hypothetical community. The IMR is a particularly important health index that health professionals should understand even if their main concern is not maternal or child health. Because infant mortality is influenced by a variety of biologic and environmental factors affecting the infant and mother, the IMR is both a direct measure of infant health and an indirect measure of community health as a whole.

The Epidemiologic Triangle

The epidemiologic triangle or agent–host–environment model is a traditional view of health and disease developed when epidemiology was concerned chiefly with communicable disease. The model, however, is applicable to other health conditions. In the model, the *agent* is an organism capable of causing disease. The *host* is the population at risk for developing the disease. The *environment* is a combination of physical, biological, and social factors that surround and influence both the agent and the host. The epidemiologic triangle is used to analyze the role and interrelatedness of each of the factors (i.e., the influence, reactivity, and effect

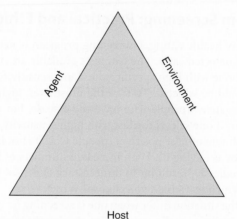

Host

FIGURE 3.1   The epidemiologic triangle is the traditional view, showing health and disease as a composite state of three variables.

each factor has on the other two). According to this model, the agent, host, and environment can coexist. Disease and injury occur only when there is an interaction or altered equilibrium between them.

Figure 3.1 shows the triangle in its normal state of equilibrium. Equilibrium does not signify optimum health, but simply the usual pattern of illness and health in a population. Any change in one of the factors (agent, host, or environment) will result in disequilibrium—in other words, a change in the usual pattern.

How could this model guide the investigation of increased infant mortality? To understand this, one must consider the three facets of the model.

Agent

If one thinks of the epidemiologic triangle model from an infectious disease perspective, it might appear that the investigation should focus on types of infections as agents that cause infant deaths. However, major causes of infant mortality in the United States include prematurity and low birth weight, birth injuries, congenital malformations, sudden infant death syndrome (SIDS), accidents, and homicides. Therefore, an investigator may try to determine whether there has been a change in any of the other agents.

Host

The characteristics of the host (the infant population) will be the second area of assessment. This assessment involves examining infant birth and death patterns in terms of age, ethnicity, sex, and birth weight. These characteristics have been shown to be important risk factors for infant mortality. By studying these factors, it may be possible to identify groups of infants who are at particularly increased risk of dying.

Environment

Lastly, the environment is assessed. The mother is a significant part of the infant's prenatal and postnatal environment. Therefore, the investigators will analyze birth and infant mortality patterns according to factors such as maternal age, ethnicity, parity (number of previous live births), prenatal care, and education or socioeconomic status. Analysis of these factors, which are also related to infant mortality, will help provide further identification of at-risk groups. Other conditions in the environment also need to be considered. For instance, has migration into the community from other areas increased? Has adult morbidity or mortality, particularly among pregnant women, increased? Have there been changes in health services, policies, personnel, funding, or other factors that could affect infant health?

Practical Application

The analysis of these three areas—the agent, host, and environment—should provide information regarding groups at risk for increased infant mortality and a means of reducing a risk factor. Thus, the epidemiologic triangle, although it was designed with a communicable disease orientation, can provide a useful guide for studying the multifaceted problem of infant mortality, along with other health problems.

The Person–Place–Time Model

In an epidemiologic study, variables can be considered in terms of person (who is affected), place (where affected), and time (when affected) relationships. The person–place–time model examines the characteristics of the people affected (the host in the triangle model), the place (environment) or location, and the time period involved (which could relate to the agent, host, or environment). In studying infant mortality according to this model, infant and maternal factors are considered traits of "person." Aspects of "place" are such factors as whether the community is rural or urban and affluent or poor. Aspects of "time" include seasonal or age-specific patterns or trends in mortality.

The Web of Causation

The web of causation (MacMahon & Pugh, 1970) views a health condition as the result not of individual factors but of complex interrelationships of numerous factors interacting to increase or decrease the risk of disease. The essence of this concept is the multifactorial nature in that a number of interrelated variables are almost always involved in the cause of a particular outcome. The web of causation attempts to identify all the possible influences on the health and illness processes. Creating the web identifies the most direct causes of conditions, factors contributing to those causes, factors influencing each of these factors, and so on.

Synergism and Factors in the Web

Central to the web of causation model is the concept of *synergism*, wherein the whole is more than the sum of its separate parts. For example, the effects of a *Shigella* infection of the infant, combined with the effects of poverty, youth, and low educational level of the mother, are more deleterious to infant health than the sum of the effects of the individual risk factors.

Use of the web of causation may result in a more expansive study of infant mortality than one guided by other models. Ideally, investigators using this model first identify all factors related to infant mortality. Next, they identify factors that are related to each of these factors. These two comprehensive steps provide the outline for the web of causation for infant mortality. Finally, the investigators examine the relationships among all the identified components of the web and attempt to determine the most feasible point of intervention to improve infant mortality in the community. Figure 3.2 depicts a web of causation for infant mortality.

Practical Application

This multifaceted approach taken in the web of causation model addresses the concept of causation in a manner consistent with current knowledge of human health. However, it may be overwhelming to carry out in everyday practice. In fact, it is more common to examine only a portion of the web, acknowledging that other relationships exist. Thorough examination of one portion of the web may provide sufficient information for initiation of useful actions to improve community health.

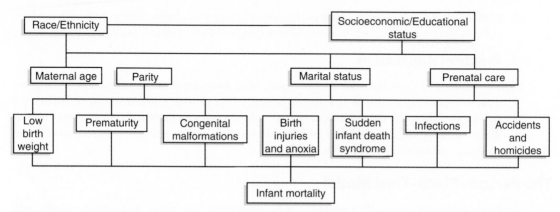

FIGURE 3.2   A web of causation for infant mortality, based on information available from birth and death certificates.

The Social Ecological Model

The social ecological model views health and wellness and disease as the result of interactions of factors at different levels within society. The word *social* describes an issue related to society. *Ecology* refers to the study of organisms and their interactions with other organisms and their environment. Most social ecological models place the individual at the center, with progressive layers radiating outward that include immediate relationships, communities, and society. While social ecological models may differ in number of layers or the words used to describe the layers, they have in common the idea that the layers interact to influence the individual at the center of the model. Figure 3.3 is an example of a social ecological model.

In order to understand how to use the social ecological model to understand the issue of infant mortality, it is important to understand each level of the model.

Individual

The individual is the center of the social ecological model. At this level, it is important to consider the traits, behavior, and past history of the individual. In the case of infant mortality, we may think about genetic predisposition or exposure to drugs in utero. As the most internal layer of the model, the individual level is influenced by the outer layers.

Microsystem

Individuals are most often influenced by the people and environments with which they have the most frequent and direct contact. For most people, this includes the household, school, workplace, or other setting such as a church or club. Their risk for death may increase or decrease due to interactions at the microsystem level. For example, exposure to breast milk in the mother–baby microsystem serves as a protective factor. On the other hand, violence in the home can serve as a risk factor for infant mortality.

Exosystem

The next layer of the social ecological model includes those factors that influence the microsystem in which the individual is functioning. The individual does not have immediate contact with the exosystem, so the influence is indirect. The workplace of the infant's parents may be an example of the exosystem. If the parent is exposed to toxins at work, it may affect the child when the parent comes home with the toxins on their clothing. A parent's access to

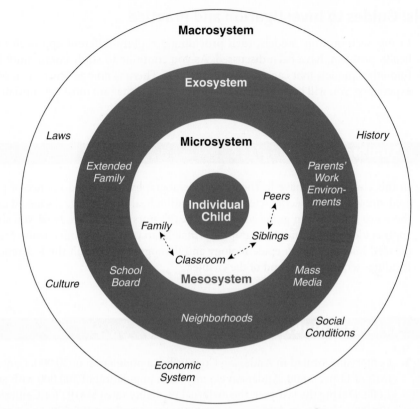

FIGURE 3.3   The ecological model for child development (Bronfenbrenner). (Copyright © 2008 Eisenmann et al.; licensee BioMed Central Ltd. Eisenmann, J. C., Gentile, D. A., Welk, G. J., Callahan, R., Strickland, S., Walsh, M., & Walsh, D. A. [2008]. SWITCH: Rationale, design, and implementation of a community, school, and family-based intervention to modify behaviors related to childhood obesity. *BMC Public Health, 8*[1], 223.)

health care or a breast-feeding mother's access to nutritious food is another example of how the exosystem can affect the infant's risk for death.

Macrosystem

The final layer is the most broad, ecompassing cultural values and beliefs that influence the exosystem, microsystem, and individual in the social ecological model. Bronfenbrenner (1993, p. 40) calls the macrosystem the "societal blueprint for a certain culture or subculture." Public policy, economic conditions, and history all play a role in forming the macrosystem. One might look at IMR data from different countries around the world to see the influence of the macrosystem on infant mortality. One might also look at disparities in IMR among cultural groups such as immigrants, individuals of low socioeconomic status, or racial and ethnic minorities. These differences in groups highlight the importance of society in health outcomes for individuals.

Practice Application

The social ecological model is used in a variety of forms to describe many different health issues, including intimate partner violence, nutrition, and child development. It can be useful in daily practice because all individuals interact with their society in this way, with direct, indirect, and overarching societal influences. Acknowledging these levels can make community health nurses more effective in practice.

Models: Guides to Investigation and Practice

In this section, four models, each providing a slightly different approach to a community health problem, have been discussed. As you continue to study community health, you will find other models that can guide your practice. There is no one "correct" model; as you gain experience, you will be able to choose or adapt those that are most appropriate for your work.

Summary

In this chapter, you have learned about demography (the broad science of population) and epidemiology (the specific science of population health). We have discussed examples of how these two sciences can guide community health nursing practice. Now, you should be able to apply epidemiologic and demographic principles to your community health practice. For more detailed information on epidemiology and demography, consult the References and Further Readings sections at the end of the chapter.

Critical Thinking Questions

1. Centerville, located in Anderson County, has a population of 30,000. Centerville has an IMR of 11 per 1,000. Anderson County has a population of 300,000 with an IMR of 6 per 1,000. During the last year, the maternal mortality rate (MMR) for Centerville was 9 per 100,000, whereas in Anderson County the rate was 7 per 100,000. How would the community health nurse interpret these data?
   a. Does the IMR in Centerville reflect a problem? If so, why?
   b. Does the MMR indicate a problem? If so, why?
   c. What do the IMR and MMR indicate about the health status of Centerville and Anderson County?

2. Select a health issue such as asthma, domestic violence, or cardiovascular disease, which affects a large number of people. Draw a web of causation that connects the different factors that may result in this health condition. Identify where the community health nurse can intervene.

3. An epidemiologic study investigates smoking as a contributing factor to lung cancer. The findings of the study are as follows: a RR ratio of 3.5 in the exposed group (smokers), an odds ratio of 4.0, and an AR of 10 cases per 100 people in 10 years. Which of the three measures of association would have significant implications for designing a prevention plan? Explain the rationale for your selection.

4. Incidence and prevalence rates provide different information about the same health condition.
   a. Which rate provides the most useful information about the risk of illness? Explain your answer.
   b. If you were a health agency administrator, in what situations would incidence rates be helpful to you?
   c. Under what situations would prevalence rates be helpful to the community health team?

5. You are an administrator in a community health center. A screening program is necessary for a deadly disease, which is *curable* only if detected early. The tests available are one

with a *high sensitivity* and *low specificity* and one with *high specificity* and *low sensitivity*. You must make a decision as to which test would be more appropriate.

   a. What are your concerns with the test with high specificity and low sensitivity?

   b. What are the considerations in the selection of the test with high sensitivity and low specificity?

6. Does fast food cause weight gain? A recent research study reported that eating at a fast-food restaurant two or more times a week was associated with a 10-pound weight gain over a 2-year period based on a RR of 2.5 (95% CI of 1.5 to 4.8).

   a. Is the research finding statistically significant?

   b. Does eating fast food cause obesity?

   c. Is the risk of weight gain increased or decreased for someone who eats two or more times a week at fast-food restaurants?

   d. What is the magnitude of increased risk compared with the average person: 2.5 times, 2.5%, or 25%?

REFERENCES

Bronfenbrenner, U. (1993). Ecological models of human development. In Gauvain, M. & Cole, M., (Eds.), *Readings on the development of children* (pp. 37–43). New York: Freeman.

Brucker, M. C. (2005). Providing evidence-based care: You can understand research and use it in practice. *AWHONN Lifelines, 9*(1), 47–55.

Davies, M. J., Moore, V. M., Willson, K. J., Van Essen, P., Priest, K., Scott, H., . . . Chan, A. (2012). Reproductive technologies and the risk of birth defects. *New England Journal of Medicine, 366*(19), 1803–1813.

Ma, J., Xu, J., Anderson, R. N., & Jemal, A. (2012). Widening educational disparities in premature death rates in twenty six states in the United States, 1993–2007. *PLoS One, 7*(7), e41560.

MacMahon, B., & Pugh, T. F. (1970). *Epidemiology: Principles and methods.* Boston, MA: Little, Brown.

McFarlane, J., Campbell, J., Sharps, P., & Watson, K. (2002). Abuse during pregnancy and femicide: Urgent implications for women's health. *Obstetrics and Gynecology International, 99*(7), 27–36.

Miller, E., Breslau, J., Chung, W. J., Green, J. G., McLaughlin, K. A., & Kessler, R. C. (2011). Adverse childhood experiences and risk of physical violence in adolescent dating relationships. *Journal of Epidemiology and Community Health, 65*(11), 1006–1013.

Snow, J. (1936). *Snow on cholera, being a reprint of two papers by John Snow, M.D., together with a biographical memoir by B. W. Richardson, M.D., and an introduction by Wade Hampton Frost, M.D.* New York, NY: The Commonwealth Fund.

FURTHER READINGS

Aschengrau, A., & Seage, G. R. (2008). *Essentials of epidemiology in public health* (2nd ed.). Boston, MA: Jones & Bartlett.

Chernick, K. M., & Friis, R. (2003). *Introductory biostatistics for the health sciences.* Hoboken, NJ: Wiley.

Cravens, G., & Mair, J. L. (1977). *The black death.* New York, NY: Dutton.

Crichton, M. (1969). *The Andromeda strain.* New York, NY: Alfred A. Knopf.

Dunne, T. L. (1978). *The scourge.* New York, NY: Coward, McCann, & Geohegan.

Everitt, B. (2003). *Modern medical statistics: A practical guide.* London: Oxford University Press.

Fowler, J., Jarvis, P., & Chevannes, M. (2002). *Practical statistics for nursing and health care.* New York, NY: Wiley.

Friis, R., & Sellers, T. (2013). *Epidemiology for public health practice* (5th ed.). Burlington, MA: Jones & Bartlett.

Merril, R. (2012). *An introduction to epidemiology* (6th ed.). Burlington, MA: Jones & Bartlett.

Savitz, D. (2003). *Interpreting epidemiologic evidence: Strategies for study design and analysis.* New York, NY: Oxford University Press.

Selvin, S. (2004). *Statistical analysis of epidemiologic data* (3rd ed.). New York, NY: Oxford University Press.

CHAPTER 4

Environment and the Health of Communities

Robert W. McFarlane

LEARNING OBJECTIVES

The community health nurse needs to have an understanding of the environmental factors that affect the health of communities.

After studying this chapter, you should be able to:

1. Understand the ecologic mechanisms that affect human health.

2. Identify physical, biologic, chemical, and gaseous hazards to human health.

3. Describe health effects of environmental conditions on human populations.

4. Apply principles of ecology to promote the health of communities.

Introduction

Environmental health refers to freedom from illness or injury related to exposure to toxic agents and other environmental conditions that are potentially detrimental to human health. (Pope, 1995, p. 3)

Florence Nightingale emphasized the importance of clean and safe environments for proper recovery to health (Nightingale, 1969). Her emphasis was on pure air, pure water, efficient drainage, cleanliness, and light.

Good health lies in recognizing that each of us is part of a wider web of life. No one person or community is an independent entity. Each is intimately linked to the environment, frequently in ways we have never imagined. Thus, the environment influences health, directly and indirectly, through subtle, indirect pathways. Conversely, human activities affect the health of the environmental system. One aspect of human ecology is the study of these linkages. Let's explore the ways in which interconnections, transport mechanisms, and constant change combine to affect health.

POLLUTION

Pollutants are the residues of things humans make, use, and throw away. Nondegradable pollutants either do not degrade or degrade very slowly in the natural environment. Biodegradable pollutants can be rapidly decomposed by natural processes unless input exceeds decomposition or dispersal capacity. Degradable pollutants that provide energy or nutrients may increase the productivity of an ecosystem by providing a subsidy when the rate of input is moderate. However, high rates of input can cause productivity to oscillate, whereas additional input may poison the system completely.

When any pollutant is introduced into the environment, we must be concerned about both the fate of the pollutant (where it goes and how it gets there) and its effect on humans or any of the ecosystems on which we depend. We must always keep in mind that any effects that pollutants have on other species are early-warning signals that something is amiss in the ecosystem and that humans may well be the next to be affected.

Major Pollutant Mechanisms

Living organisms have a hierarchical organization. Atoms link to form molecules, then macromolecules and cells are created. Cells link to form tissues, then organs and organ systems, and finally an independent organism. Numbers of self-replicating organisms create populations. Interacting populations of different kinds create an ecologic community, combining with the flow of nutrients and energy to form an ecosystem. Unicellular and multicellular organisms capable of photosynthesis combine carbon dioxide and water with sunlight to create complex carbon molecules, store energy, and release oxygen to the atmosphere. The photosynthesizing green plants and algae are eaten by myriad creatures, large and small, which are also eaten, in turn, by others. This pattern of consumption creates a food web, with links in numerous directions. Each exchange constitutes a trophic level within the food web. At each level, the consumer builds nutrients into its own body, burns most of the consumed energy for its own existence, and stores a small portion of the energy. In this manner, the self-organizing ecosystem creates an efficient mechanism for gathering and moving nutrients and energy from one organism to another. Pollutants are incorporated into this distribution system as readily as nutrients. Five pollutant mechanisms are of particular concern: transport, transformation, bioaccumulation, biomagnification, and synergism.

Transport

Transport of the pollutant, once it is introduced into the environment, is generally accomplished by way of wind patterns or aquatic systems. Pollutants can be dispersed aerially as particulates or in a gaseous state; they can travel long distances before falling to earth as dust or being carried in rain water. Ironically, the construction of increasingly tall smokestacks to relieve local pollution generally results in greater dispersal, thus enlarging the area affected without diminishing the amount of pollutant released. Once air pollutants have settled to earth, they frequently continue their movement by traveling along waterways. After a single heavy rainfall, storm water runoff can mobilize more suspended particulates than may be transported during the rest of the year. Dissolved pollutants may be transported long distances before settling onto the bottom sediments through some precipitative mechanism.

Pollutants generally exert greater influence on aquatic ecosystems than on terrestrial environments. Air pollutants may enter a person's lungs or settle on vegetation and then be eaten with the plants. Water, though, is nature's best solvent, and many pollutants go into solution in aquatic ecosystems, with the result that aquatic animals and plants live in a weakly polluted "soup." Many chemicals enter the biota directly through the skin or across gill surfaces, because there is no escape from a dissolved pollutant. The effects of a given one-time polluting event, such as an accidental spill, are, therefore, exerted for a longer time in aquatic than in terrestrial ecosystems. Not only is a greater portion of the pollution incorporated into and cycled within the biotic nutrient pool, but material that settles into the sediment can also be resuspended and redistributed with every major storm event. The dispersion of pollutants is also more restricted in aquatic than in terrestrial systems because movement is always downstream, until the pollutants reach the ocean. The efficacy of ocean transport has been demonstrated by the ubiquitous spread of several insecticides throughout the world; their area of distribution even includes the Antarctic continent.

Transformation

Transformation of a pollutant within an ecosystem takes place in many ways. Harmful substances can be rendered innocuous or even helpful during the biodegradation process. But occasionally, a relatively harmless substance is transformed into a noxious form. A classic example is the transformation of metallic or inorganic mercury, which is relatively immobile, into methylmercury by microorganisms living in aquatic sediments.

Methylmercury is readily incorporated into detrital food chains, which may terminate with human consumption of contaminated fish and shellfish, producing the neurologic disorder known as Minamata disease. Nonbiogenic chemical transformations are more common in the environment (e.g., the conversion of sulfur dioxide and nitrous oxides in the atmosphere to form sulfuric and nitric acids and create acid rain).

Bioaccumulation

Bioaccumulation refers to the introduction of substances into ecologic food webs. Chemicals that behave in a manner similar to essential elements are most susceptible to rapid uptake and retention. Chiefly because of humans and their activities, the ecologist must now be concerned with the cycling of nonessential elements. For example, the radionuclides of strontium and cesium, whose chemical behavior is analogous to calcium and potassium, respectively, are introduced into the environment by nuclear reactors and represent a potential health hazard.

Biomagnification

Biomagnification results when the accumulation of a pollutant greatly exceeds the rate at which an organism eliminates it. The pollutant is concentrated in organisms at a low trophic level, where it is further concentrated and passed to the third level, and so on. For example, polychlorinated biphenyls (PCBs) are a large class of 209 separate chemical compounds that held many industrial applications before 1976, when they were banned in the United States. Each of these compounds has a different type and degree of toxicity, bioaccumulates at different rates, and behaves differently when free in the environment. In the 1970s, these PCB compounds were associated with adverse health effects in people eating fish from the Great Lakes. The PCBs were acquired by phytoplankton that innocuously acted as tiny scavengers of the pollutant, reaching levels of only 2.5 parts of PCB per billion parts of phytoplankton. These were then eaten by zooplankton, which, in turn, were eaten by larger zooplankton, in which PCB concentrations increased nearly 50-fold, reaching 123 parts per billion. The zooplankton were eaten by small fish, rainbow smelt, with PCBs increasing ninefold to 1 part per million (ppm). Next, the smelt were eaten by lake trout, which reached 5 ppm PCB, and finally consumed by humans (or other end-chain carnivores). At each step, the PCBs were sequestered in the fatty tissue of the carrier and stored. The final concentration of PCBs in herring gull eggs, which are rich in stored fat and sometimes consumed by humans, was 124 ppm, or 50,000 times greater than the original concentration in the phytoplankton.

Synergism

Synergism is the simultaneous action of separate substances or agencies that together produce a greater total effect than the sum of their individual effects. It is common to discover that a given substance behaves in one fashion in a controlled laboratory environment and in quite another when introduced into a natural ecosystem, where it interacts with a number of physical and chemical properties of the environment.

Toxic Substances

In recent years, toxic substances have received a great deal of attention in governmental regulations and the news media. Any chemical can be toxic, including table salt, sugar, and the chlorine in drinking water. Toxic substances are generally considered to be any chemicals or mixtures of chemicals, either synthetic or natural, poisonous to humans, plants, or animals under expected conditions of use and exposure. There are four major categories of toxic substances: pesticides, industrial chemicals, metals, and substances with radiation-emitting isotopes. Pesticides are lethal chemicals specifically designed to kill weeds, fungi, insects, mites, rodents, and other pests. Four pesticides have been banned from further use in the United States: DDT, aldrin, dieldrin, and chlordane. Industrial chemicals are particularly numerous, and a few have proven especially dangerous (e.g., asbestos, benzene, vinyl chloride, and PCBs). A number of metals, such as arsenic, lead, cadmium, and mercury, have also proven to be very toxic in the environment. The fourth category includes those substances with isotopes that emit various types of radiation, such as strontium, cesium, and iodine.

Chemical toxicity occurs when a chemical agent produces detrimental effects in living organisms. The effects of a toxic substance can be immediate or long term and can harm selected tissues or the entire organism. Both the toxicity of the substance and the expected exposure to the organism must be considered to define the anticipated risk. Neurotoxins are likely the most significant toxic substances in both prevalence and severity that pose a risk to human health. Epidemiologically, a relatively small fraction of major neurologic disorders are inherited; most neurologic diseases appear to be associated with environmental factors. Many commercial chemicals used in very large amounts and known to persist in the environment have neurotoxic properties. In fact, insecticides, designed to have neurotoxic properties, are manufactured for deliberate release into the environment.

Ecologic Principles

Knowing how pollutants move in the environment and how they can be transported or transformed, how they accumulate or magnify to affect health, we need to review some basic ecologic principles.

Law of gravity. In recent history, the interdependency of the human species and the natural world has been too frequently overlooked or ignored. As we seek ways to alleviate problems associated with health, it is imperative to be cognizant of nature's operating principles. The "laws of nature" have not been repealed, and knowledge of these laws is vital to understanding the origin of health problems and in successfully designing strategies to reduce them. The law of gravity is particularly important to the ecologic system. Everything that goes up, including pollutants, must come down, and everything dumped on the surface of the earth must ultimately flow downhill. Water and even land masses, such as mountains, move slowly to the sea. It is imperative that we learn to design with nature, exploiting these principles to our advantage, rather than expending resources in a useless struggle, because nature always wins. It is important to remember three commonsense observations that are frequently overlooked because of their inherent simplicity.

Everything is connected to everything else, but some things are connected more tightly than others. This observation is the least obvious. As we go from a climate-controlled workplace to a correspondingly pleasant home, insulated from the vagaries of the weather even while en route, it is easy to forget that working in a climate-controlled environment is a very recent phenomenon, restricted to a minority of the world population. As we select foodstuffs from the bounty of 24-hour supermarkets, we seldom stop to wonder where a particular item came from; what chemical abuses it may have suffered during its growth, harvest, or transportation; or what unsuspected surprises may lurk beneath the protective cellophane.

Everything has to go somewhere. Although this observation is readily acknowledged, "somewhere" is generally considered synonymous with "away" and is not considered to be a problem until the "away" becomes your living space. This may produce the now-familiar "NIMBY" reaction (not in my backyard!). As human populations and industrial development grow, pollutants are produced in greater quantities and dispersed over longer distances. At the same time, unpopulated areas are diminishing. Some pollutants are conspicuous and readily detected. Others, perhaps more insidious, are detected only when sought; the search frequently requires elaborate instrumentation and methodology.

Everything is constantly changing. Although constant change is universally recognized, the nature and rate of change are generally unappreciated. The natural environment undergoes continual change. Some changes seem irreversible, permanent, or barely detectable from our perspective in time (e.g., geologic transformations and continental drift). Other changes are cyclic (such as the seasonal climate) or transient (floods or droughts). However, changes produced by the actions of human beings have become more prominent. Significant human-induced changes began with the domestication of animals and the development of agriculture. These led to the growth of large human settlements, soon followed by deforestation and the depletion of local resources. The rate of change increased greatly as muscle power was replaced by mechanical power and renewable energy resources (wood, wind, and water) were replaced by energy derived from fossil fuels. Today, human populations dominate the earth's ecosystems. Nearly one half of the earth's land surface has been modified by human activity. More than half of the accessible fresh water is used by humans for various purposes. Humans have become a global change agent.

Pollutants and Human Population Size

All of the environmental processes described so far can influence human health. Any pollutant or toxic substance introduced into the environment is subjected to these processes, many of which lead directly to human beings. Pollution of the environment occurs when these pollutants overwhelm the capacity of the environment to assimilate them without being thrown out of balance. Thus, pollution is a rate function involving a quantity of pollutant introduced over a period of time. This rate is directly correlated with population size.

It can be said that all pollution is the result of population growth. A single family, living on a subsistence level in the wild, burning wood as their fuel, and discarding rubbish and human wastes on the landscape, would seldom be a polluting factor in their environment. The population of a small village would denude the landscape of wood fuel, pollute the air with smoke from numerous wood fires, and litter the ground with rubbish and human wastes randomly dispersed. Cities, with more numerous inhabitants, totally overwhelm the environment with rubbish and human waste, necessitating the development of sewage and garbage disposal systems. Industrial development increases the number of pollutants and environmental insults. Our past practice of handling pollutants has been to just dump them, taking further action only when the natural systems have been overwhelmed. We need to reverse this practice and remove the bulk of pollutants before inflicting them on nature. Then the natural ecosystem can work for us by removing the final bit of pollution that always proves so difficult and expensive to neutralize.

Demographic changes can rapidly alter the stress inflicted on the environment. As population grows, the stress increases. If the population moves, both the nature and the intensity of an environmental problem can shift. For example, the recent decline of industrial productivity in the northeastern United States has resulted in a shift in the population caused by the exodus of workers (particularly young families) and an improvement in the surface water quality. The growth of population in the South, especially the arid Southwest, is increasing water pollution and straining the overall water supply.

The solution to one environmental problem may be the creation of another. Pollutants do not disappear. Sulfur that is scrubbed out of powerplant smokestack gases ends up as a sludge stored on the ground, where it may threaten water quality. Pollutants removed from wastewaters by precipitation end up in the bottom sludge, which also requires disposal. Unfortunately, if the sludge is burned, the pollutants may be released into the air to settle and become incorporated into the water or land once again. If the sludge is buried in a landfill, it may threaten surface water or groundwater supplies. Sewage treatment plants that aerate water as part of the process may discharge substantial amounts of volatile toxic substances to the air. Disposable plastic containers and bedpans used in the hospitals are often incinerated and go into the air. *Everything has to go somewhere.* What goes up, comes down, and eventually enters the air, the water, and the ground.

In summary, virtually any pollutant that is introduced into the environment will subsequently be transported away from its point of entry. It may be transformed into another chemical form, either less or more hazardous. It will probably be accumulated by biologic organisms, possibly becoming magnified in its concentration. It is likely to react with other chemicals or physical processes and to produce unanticipated effects. Distinct and efficient chemical cycles and pathways that have evolved over millions of years ensure that toxicants will enter biologic systems and eventually reach humans or other organisms on which they depend. *Everything is connected to everything else, and everything has to go somewhere.* There is nowhere to hide. The only solution is to stop the pollution.

ENVIRONMENTAL ISSUES AFFECTING HEALTH

We are losing habitat that is the home to many plants and animals. The clearing of forests to create crop lands results in *deforestation*. This is most often done by cutting down and burning trees. Increasingly warm climates result in the disappearance of entire forest types and more frequent and intense forest fires. Deforestation contributes to soil erosion, a change in climatic conditions, and air pollution. Climate change results in increased *desertification*. Fertile land becomes desert because of hotter but not wetter conditions. Climatic change is achieved by altering the rain cycle by reducing forest area. Desertification also results from poor land management (i.e., an overgrowth of crops depletes essential nutrients from the soil). A loss of biodiversity results in the extinction of certain species of plants and animals and thus deforestation, desertification, and reproductive changes.

There has been an overall increase in temperatures throughout the world. The "greenhouse effect" is a contributing factor to this *global warming*. The greenhouse effect occurs from an increase in atmospheric carbon dioxide. The increase in atmospheric carbon dioxide is caused by burning fossil fuels and oil, which releases carbon dioxide into the atmosphere. This carbon dioxide allows sunlight to pass through the atmosphere to the earth to heat it, but also traps the heat that is reemitted by the earth. The increased temperature has contributed to an increase of certain vectorborne diseases, such as malaria and dengue fever. There is also an increase in heat-related mortalities and in premature labors. The community health nurse should help promote cost-effective strategies, such as a decrease in the use of fossil fuels for energy and an increase in the use of clean fuels such as sunlight and wind. Use of more efficient lights and appliances will also help to decrease the use of fossil fuels.

The protective atmospheric layer of ozone is gradually becoming depleted. This results from chemical interactions between air pollutants and ozone. The major source of air pollutants is chlorofluorocarbons (CFs). CFs are widely used in refrigeration, air-conditioning, and aerosols. Ozone is a pollutant when found in ambient air, but it is not a pollutant in the stratosphere. Without an ozone layer in the atmosphere, it is estimated that skin cancer incidence rates would increase 60% and 20,000 more fatalities would occur in the United States every year because of the excess ultraviolet (UV) radiation penetration. UV light exposure contributes to cataracts and the depression of the immune system (there is a reduction of lymphocyte production and susceptibility to infectious diseases). It is estimated that two thirds of all cancers are caused by environmental factors (U.S. Department of Health and Human Services, 2003).

An accumulation of a variety of wastes and their environmental effects results in planetary toxification. Contributing factors include air pollution, water pollution, acid rain, and accumulation of solid and hazardous wastes. Each household in the United States produces approximately 87 gallons of solid waste weekly. Thirty percent to forty percent of this waste comes from packaging materials. Health problems such as heavy metal poisoning and infectious disease can result from exposure to toxic wastes from illegal dumping.

Environmental Hazards Affecting Health

Physical Hazards

Physical hazards to health include radiation, lead, other heavy metals, and noise.

Ionizing radiation is found naturally in soil and rock. It can also be found in building materials such as granite. X-rays are a form of ionizing radiation. Radiation risks also include nuclear power emissions and nuclear weapons. Health hazards to humans from ionizing radiation include birth defects; increased rates of cancer, stroke, diabetes, cardiovascular, and renal disease; and immune system damage. *Nonionizing radiation* does not result in ionization when atoms are passed through the body. Sources of nonionizing radiation include electromagnetic fields, UV radiation, visible light, infrared light, and microwaves. Radiation leaks from microwave ovens that have improperly fitted seals can cause fatigue and headache.

Lead and other heavy metals are present in soil, water, and air. Lead is considered by the U.S. Environmental Protection Agency (EPA) as the greatest chemical risk to health. Sources of lead include vehicle emissions, burning coal, and decomposition of solid waste. Young children are at an increased risk of lead poisoning because of their propensity to put things into their mouths, such as lead paint chips. Exposure to lead is associated with learning disabilities in children. Lead poisoning in humans has been known for 5,000 years. Progress has been made since the phasing out of leaded gasoline began in the 1970s. In the United States, atmospheric lead concentrations have fallen 89% and blood lead levels in children have fallen 91%. That represents real progress, but such blood lead levels are still 100 times higher than natural background levels. There is no lower lead level for toxicity, and lead continues to be released through the burning of coal, and spread around the world in the atmosphere.

Mercury, a powerful neurotoxin, can be found in paint and some traditional medicinal remedies. Symptoms of mercury poisoning include listlessness and irritability. It concentrates in the kidneys, liver, and brain. Currently, some hospitals are trying to eliminate use of products containing mercury. Arsenic, which is found in pesticides, herbicides, and some over-the-counter poisons, causes nausea and vomiting, diarrhea, and abdominal pain in humans. Another heavy metal, cadmium, found in water supplies owing to contamination from rechargeable batteries, causes nausea and vomiting, diarrhea, and prostration in humans. Exposure to small quantities causes kidney damage and bone demineralization.

Noise affects hearing, and prolonged exposure contributes to anxiety and emotional stress. It may cause insomnia, skin problems, swollen ankles, and heart disorders. Common sources of noise pollution are industries, vehicles, subways, and loud music. Hearing loss can occur from the excess noise produced by airplanes in neighborhoods that are near airports.

Biologic Hazards

Biologic hazards can be infectious agents, insects, animals, and plants. Common indoor biologic pollutants include animal dander, dust mites, cockroach parts, fungi/mold, bacteria, viruses, and pollen. Infectious agents are primarily transmitted by way of water or an infected person. Contamination of water supplies can occur from septic tanks and untreated sewage, rainwater flow, and medical waste. Air becomes polluted from improperly cleaned air-conditioning and heating systems. Biologic pollutants can be found in dirty air conditioners; humidifiers; bathrooms and kitchens without vents or windows; dirty refrigerator vent pans; laundry rooms with unvented dryers; unventilated attics; carpets; and water damage around windows, roofs, or in basements.

Humans are hosts to a number of disease-causing pathogens and parasites. Some act directly, transmitting from one human to another (e.g., smallpox, measles). Others require an intermediate vector, typically a biting insect or other arthropod (mosquitoes—malaria, yellow fever, dengue fever; biting flies—Leishmaniasis, trypanosomiasis, onchocerciasis; fleas—plague; ticks—Lyme disease, tick-borne encephalitis; or snails—schistosomiasis). Each additional link in the transmission cycle allows for greater environmental influence, typically related to temperature or moisture. For example, the prevalence of malaria increases with higher temperatures and high amounts of rainfall.

Chemical Hazards

Chemical and gaseous hazards include poisons and air and water pollution. Poisoning occurs through cumulative exposure to insecticides, herbicides, fungicides, and rodenticides. Exposure can occur at work on farms and in industry, in the home through accidental ingestion, and from eating animals that have been exposed. Poisons cause sarcomas, lymphomas, myelomas, and respiratory and prostate cancers.

Air pollution, which occurs inside and outside, kills approximately 3 million people every year (outdoor 1 million and indoor 2.5 million). Contributing factors include automobiles, large industries, and small businesses, such as dry cleaners, household products, geography, and urbanization. Health effects from air pollution are many and include respiratory disorders, eye irritation, fatigue, and headaches. Indoor air pollution is most severe in buildings that are airtight and designed for energy conservation. Formaldehydes, carbon monoxide, nitrogen oxides, asbestos found in furniture and the structural compounds of buildings, aerosol deodorants, certain types of cooking and heating, and cigarette smoke are trapped inside buildings and cause nose and throat irritations, heart disease, central nervous system (CNS) damage, and certain cancers. Air pollution is linked to reduced lung function in children. Lung function growth in children who live in areas with increased air pollution in the form of acid vapor (found in smog) is decreased when compared with that in children who live in cleaner communities. Decreased lung function growth can lead to chronic respiratory problems in adulthood.

Water pollution is caused by acid rain, manufacturing, mining, septic tanks, salt and deicing chemicals on highways, sewage sludge, and certain chemicals. Less than 1% of the water on this earth is available for human consumption. Numerous health complaints are associated with water pollution, including bladder and colorectal cancers, CNS effects, skin irritation, alopecia, peripheral neuropathies, seizures, hepatitis and cirrhosis, infertility, congenital anomalies, developmental disabilities, anemia, renal failure, heart disease, and gastritis.

Global Climate Change and Human Health

Although change is a constant, the rate of climate change has quickened beyond doubt. Warming of the earth's climate system is indisputable (Intergovernmental Panel on Climate Change, 2007). Global average air and ocean temperatures have increased. Glaciers and polar ice caps are melting, and the sea level is rising. Temperature increases have been greater at higher northern latitudes, and land regions have warmed faster than the oceans. Precipitation has increased in some parts of the globe but declined in others, characteristic of shifting weather patterns. Climate change has resulted from increases in the release of greenhouse gases (carbon dioxide, methane, nitrous oxide, and certain aerosols), changes in land cover because of human activity, and changes in solar radiance that have altered the energy balance of the climate system.

Climate change has concatenating consequences. For example, climate and soils determine the prevailing vegetation for any area. In turn, the vegetation ameliorates the microclimate of the ecoregion. Ecosystems influence climate by changing the energy, water, and greenhouse gas balance of the atmosphere (Chapin, Randerson, McGuire, Foley, & Field, 2008). Ecosystems both create and consume oxygen and carbon dioxide. They augment the water cycle through evapotranspiration, moving large quantities of water from below ground to the atmosphere. Ecosystems also affect the albedo, or reflectance, of the earth's surface, absorbing or reflecting various wavelengths of solar energy.

Climate change directly and indirectly impacts human health (Haines, Kovats, Campbell-Lendrum, & Corvalan, 2006). For example, climate change affects regional and local weather patterns. It can increase extreme weather events such as heat waves and cold spells, storms, floods, and droughts. Storms and flooding may cause direct mortality and injury, displace large numbers of people, disrupt transportation and rescue efforts, and despoil productive cropland, leading to crop failure and malnutrition. Standing water may increase water-related diseases such as cholera and malaria. Higher air temperature may lead to an increase in heat-related illnesses and deaths during summer but a decrease in cold-related illnesses and deaths in winter. In urban areas, high temperatures can create air-inversion and stagnant air, decreasing the dispersal of air pollutants and increasing air pollution-related health effects.

Climate change affects both native vegetation and cultivated crops. Warming may lengthen the growing season, increasing crop yield but also augment pollen production of allergenic plants, increasing the incidence of allergic diseases. Precipitation may increase (causing flooding) or decrease (leading to desertification, crop losses, malnutrition, and population migration).

In the human population globally, 335 infectious diseases emerged or increased in incidence between 1940 and 2004 (Jones et al., 2008). These diseases include newly evolved strains of established pathogens (e.g., multi-drug-resistant tuberculosis, chloroquine-resistant malaria), pathogens that have affected humans for the first time (e.g., HIV-1, severe acute respiratory syndrome [SARS] coronavirus), and human pathogens that have increased in incidence (e.g., Lyme disease, now estimated at 300,000 new cases each year in the United States). In 2009 a new disease, the Heartland virus, was first recognized, and ticks were identified as the vector. Sixty percent of these emerging infectious diseases have involved a nonhuman, animal source (e.g., SARS, Nipah virus). Further, 23% of these emerging infectious diseases involved an animal vector. It is hypothesized that climate change is driving the emergence of diseases with vectors sensitive to changes in rainfall and temperature. Another new disease, coccidiomycosis, or valley fever, is an airborne fungal disease that has become epidemic, with 22,000 cases reported annually in the southwestern United States, especially in California and Arizona.

All animals occupy specific geographic ranges that expand or contract over time, occasionally in response to changes in climate. Expansion may bring infected vectors into contact with host populations that lack prior exposure and have not developed immunity or resistance to the disease. Human population density has been a good predictor of these emergent disease events. Wildlife biologists have identified a dozen pathogens that may spread into new regions as a result of climate change: avian influenza, babesia, cholera, Ebola hemorrhagic fever virus, intestinal and external parasites, plague, Lyme disease, red tides, Rift Valley fever, sleeping sickness, bovine tuberculosis, and yellow fever. Wildlife diseases may enter domestic animal populations, where minor diseases may become major infectious agents due to high-density crowded conditions. Prominent diseases of domestic animals may affect wildlife populations, and both may cross over to humans when domestic and game animals are handled and consumed (Jones et al., 2008).

Nursing Interventions to Decrease Environmental Influences on Health

Primary Prevention

A nurse can use primary prevention to decrease pollution in a number of ways:

- Reduce/eliminate environmental hazards, such as with enforcement of legal codes and standards
- Educate community residents, business owners, and government officials on how to avoid environmental hazards, such as the routine application of sunscreen and use of ear plugs and safety glasses
- Become involved with political actions that provide strategies to minimize environmental exposure in populations
- Promote routine immunizations to minimize diseases caused by biologic agents

For example, an environmental community action group, in collaboration with citizens of its community, is conducting a public education project on pesticide use in their community. Their goals are to increase public awareness of pesticide use and their environmental and health impacts, provide the public's right to know about pesticide use, and take steps to reduce pesticide use and health risks, particularly to children. Strategies they use in their project are similar to conducting a community assessment. First, they collect information regarding pesticide use in the area; then, they seek changes in pest management practices to reduce chemical pesticide use, and they build support in the community for implementation of new policies. They utilize parent–teacher organizations to build support in the community and to support their pesticide reduction campaign's legislative agenda.

Secondary Prevention

The nurse can use many techniques involving secondary prevention:

- Monitor for signs of hazardous environmental conditions such as blood lead levels
- Assess for signs of illness related to environmental hazards in the community such as increased incidence of asthma and mental retardation
- Decrease environmental pollution (refer to the section earlier in this chapter)
- Treat and monitor disorders caused by environmental conditions such as asthma and blood lead levels in children

With funding from the U.S. EPA, state departments of health are working with local public health units to conduct lead screenings of children. Because most funding in the past has targeted children on Medicaid, the new program targets non-Medicaid children 1 to 6 years of age who have never been screened and who live in homes built before 1950. Lead poisoning in children affects growth and development and can cause nervous system and kidney damage, learning disabilities, attention deficit disorder, decreased intelligence, speech and language problems, poor muscle coordination, decreased muscle and bone growth, hearing damage, convulsions, coma, and even death. Screening is a first step to detecting problems associated with lead poisoning.

Tertiary Prevention

The following are some ways to use tertiary prevention to keep the environment clean:

- Eliminate environmental hazards to prevent reexposure, such as removing asbestos, lead, and mold from buildings

- Help communities to manage the long-term effects of conditions that are caused by environmental hazards, such as the extra-care costs associated with mental retardation and asthma
- Participate in political activity that reduces environmental hazards, including strict adherence to emission regulations and air and water quality standards

Here is what one community did at the tertiary prevention level. In 1999, it was learned that two public schools had been built on land contaminated with a variety of toxic industrial chemicals. Although some cleanup of the site had occurred, a variety of carcinogenic and other hazardous chemicals remained, and according to the state pollution control board, there was a potential health risk to people using the site. Although the control board's approval was not required for the site cleanup, parents learned that the site had never received a clean bill of health, despite the fact that it was used by over 800 schoolchildren. As a result, Citizens for a Better Environment, working with individuals, the state EPA, and the state pollution control board, proposed changes to the state Site Remediation Program that would ensure that site cleanups receive certification before schools are built and occupied by children, and that they remain safe after schools are occupied (Citizens for a Better Environment, 2002).

NURSING ACTION FOR HEALTHIER COMMUNITIES

Change begins at the community level by making residents aware of the environmental issues and hazards present in their community. The community health nurse focuses on the concerns of the community residents and targets the problems that the people choose to address. The responsibility of the community health nurse is to make the community aware of the environmental health risks and the actions necessary to reduce exposure and potential health problems. The community health nurse works with the community to develop strategies for change and reduce resistance to change. Development of coalitions is important. The community health nurse assists the community to contact and partner with environmental organizations for help in improving the community's health. The community health nurse encourages communities to become involved in political action required to eliminate, avoid, and reduce exposure to environmental hazards. Assisting a community group in drafting an editorial for the local newspaper or writing a letter to an agency or congressional representative is the first step toward political action. If asked to describe the specific health effects associated with environmental exposures, where can you find information regarding environmental exposures in your community?

In one community with heavy toxic air emissions from chemical plants, a librarian decided to make a difference. She offered classes for citizens on how to use the internet to learn more about toxic air emissions. She taught residents how to study their potential health risks from exposures in their community. The citizens were exposed to various inhalant toxins such as benzene, 1,3-butadiene, and chloroform. The citizens learned that benzene can cause drowsiness, rapid heart rate, headaches, tremors, confusion, and unconsciousness. Long-term exposure (365 days or more) can cause leukemia and cancer of the blood-forming organs. 1,3-Butadiene is made from the processing of petroleum and is used to make synthetic rubber. Breathing small amounts for a short time can cause damage to the CNS, blurred vision, nausea, fatigue, headache, decreased blood pressure and pulse rate, and unconsciousness. Lower levels cause adverse effects such as eye, throat, and nose irritation. Chloroform is used to make other chemicals and can be formed when chlorine is added to water. Long-term inhalation exposure in high levels can damage the liver and kidneys. Both 1,3-butadiene and chloroform are considered possible carcinogens. In this community of 50,000 citizens, 61% of the population reported eye, nose, and throat irritation, but only 50% perceived a negative impact on their health from air pollution. The informed citizens wanted to share the information about the harmful effects of toxic air pollutants with all the citizens in their community. What strategies would you recommend to the citizens for informing the community? To which community groups would you suggest the informed citizens ask to make a presentation? What role does the community health nurse have in promoting the efforts of these concerned citizens? In addition to the health effects of environmental toxins, what other important information can the community health nurse assist the citizens in retrieving?

Community Health Nursing Actions for Healthy Air

Air pollutants can make asthma symptoms worse and trigger attacks, especially in children. Air pollution makes it hard to breathe and causes symptoms such as coughing, wheezing, chest discomfort, and a burning feeling in the lungs. There are two pollutants in the air that affect asthma: ozone and particle pollution. Ozone, found in smog, is often worse on hot summer days in the afternoon and early evening. Particle pollution, found in haze, smoke, and dust, increases when the weather is calm, and pollutants are able to build up in the air. Particle levels are highest near busy roads, during rush-hour traffic, near factories, and when there is smoke from wood fires in stoves or fireplaces and burning vegetation.

As a community health nurse, what interventions can you advise to citizens at risk for the adverse effects of air pollution? Where can citizens go to find up-to-date information about local air quality? People with asthma should exercise because regular exercise is important for health. Exercising in the early morning and away from busy roads or industrial areas should be recommended, and so should exercising indoors when pollutants are especially high outdoors. Trying a less intense outdoor activity, such as walking instead of jogging, on high ozone level days will reduce the amount of pollution inhaled. The community health nurse can stress the importance of access to quick relief medication when active outdoors, especially for those beginning an activity program that is more intense than usual. Sources of information about air quality and asthma can be found on the websites listed in Box 4.1. Free EPA brochures on ozone, particle pollution, and air quality can be obtained by calling 1-800-490-9198.

Community Health Nursing Actions for Healthy Water

Water is essential for life. According to the World Health Organization (WHO, 2006), 1.8 million people die from diarrheal disease each year, and 88% of these deaths are linked to contaminated water. Annually in the United States there are 900,000 illnesses and 900 deaths linked to poor water quality (Chalupka, 2005).

Natural disasters such as the tsunami in Asia in 2004 and hurricanes Katrina and Rita in the United States in 2005 destroyed water and sanitation systems. Subsequently, diseases including cholera, typhoid, dysentery, and diarrhea may result. Provision of uninterrupted safe drinking water is one of the most important preventive measures toward which community health nurses can contribute following a natural disaster.

Even in nondisaster situations, local water supplies are threatened by organic and synthetic contaminants. Private wells are affected by runoff from herbicides sprayed on vegetation.

Box 4.1 Web Resources for Information on Air Quality and Asthma

http://www.epa.gov/airnow
http://www.cdc.gov/asthma
http://www.epa.gov/asthma

Half of all Americans obtain their drinking water from surface water sources (lakes, rivers, streams), the other half from groundwater. Natural and synthetic hormones and pharmaceuticals often pollute surface waters. There are two sources of water pollution: point and nonpoint. Point sources are easily discernible sources that discharge chemicals into the environment (factories). Nonpoint sources are less discernible, carrying agricultural runoff or industrial runoff (melting snow, paved roads).

Community health nurses play key roles in assessing causes of illness from water contamination in any situation: disaster, local water supply, or private well system. Specific responsibilities for the community health nurse include education and advocacy to decrease the risk of waterborne illness in vulnerable populations and to improve the local drinking water supply. The nurse must become knowledgeable about the situation, counsel family members on how to protect their household water supply, consider the possibility of waterborne illness when encountering acute gastroenteritis of unknown etiology, and take steps to safeguard the community water supply. The following resources will assist you in assessing and working with communities toward healthy water.

- Local drinking water information: http://www.epa.gov/safewater/dwinfo/index.html
- Ground water and drinking water information: http://www.epa.gov/safewater/index.html
- Information on recognizing waterborne disease and the health effects of water pollution: http://www.waterhealthconnection.org

Excellent target objectives for promoting community health include the national health objectives related to environmental health in Healthy People 2020 available at http://www.healthypeople.gov/HP2020.

THE COMPLEX HUMAN ENVIRONMENT

The preceding sections described humans interacting with the physical world and other species in a simplistic fashion. The complete human environment is difficult to comprehend because of the multiplicity of interrelated elements. The delivery of health care sometimes goes awry because the influence of certain elements is underestimated or unappreciated. A conceptual model of the human environment from an ecologic viewpoint can often illuminate the problem and guide efficient intervention.

An ecologic model (Fig. 4.1), like most models, proposes a framework from which to study and understand a phenomenon. The environment surrounds people wherever they go, whatever they do. An ecologic approach to the study of human health relates the biologic, physical, sociocultural, and politicoeconomic components of an individual's environment to any deviation from a state of health. The model can be applied to study the health of any defined subpopulation (e.g., infants, children, adolescents, and the elderly).

Environmental systems not only act on the individual person but also interact with one another, and a change occurring in one system will frequently affect others. Each system consists of components that act with and on other systems to bring about equilibrium or disequilibrium within the system.

Conceptually, both the subsystems and environmental systems are in a constant state of interaction (everything is connected to everything else and is constantly changing). Enumerating the variables within the systems and measuring the interaction among them are the keys to operating the model. In Figure 4.2, environmental systems and subsystems are displayed in a tabular arrangement, with variables boxed according to the systems most acutely affected by their interaction. Certain variables, such as migration and consumption of basic needs, equally interact with all systems as they affect the family and individual's functioning. Other variables, such as birth statistics (mother's age at birth, sex, birth order, and condition), are primarily

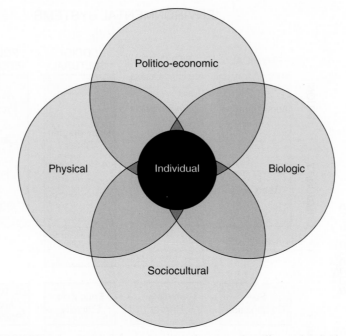

FIGURE 4.1 Model of the environmental systems that affect each individual.

within one system, affecting one developmental stage (the child) of one subsystem (the individual). Lines encasing variables are not set boundaries; rather, they serve as a guide to identify the system and subsystem most affected by variable manipulation.

The purpose of the conceptual model is to offer a framework from which to select significant variables related to the health status of a chosen individual. The variables that appear in Figure 4.2 are a synthesis of the epidemiologic, demographic, and social health indicators consistently proposed, tested, and recommended as valid and reliable indices of child health. Application of this model is described in the regional case history that follows.

Application: A Regional Case Study

The Problem

The following study concerns children with infection and their shared environmental variables. Much is known about the effects of infection; the morbidity and mortality statistics are salient testimony to the impact of infection on child growth, development, and survival. Surprisingly little is known, however, about the ecologic milieu that shrouds infected children or the causal paths by which the environmental variables interact to determine child health.

Epidemiologic studies of infection are plentiful, but their focus is usually on the incidence and seriousness of the problem, with little attention to the associated social or cultural forces. Similarly, sociologic analyses of infection focus on behaviors and attitudes, usually skirting the biologic as well as the economic and political factors. The objective of explaining this study is to demonstrate the usefulness of an ecologic model to identify and quantify the physical, biologic, sociocultural, and politicoeconomic variables related to infection among children.

Health statistics for children in rural communities, especially children of indigenous heritage, reveal that they have more problems than urban children. For example, in Chile, infant mortality rates in rural communities are more than twice those of urban communities. When risk is matched for ethnicity, indigenous children have a far higher risk, which is reduced

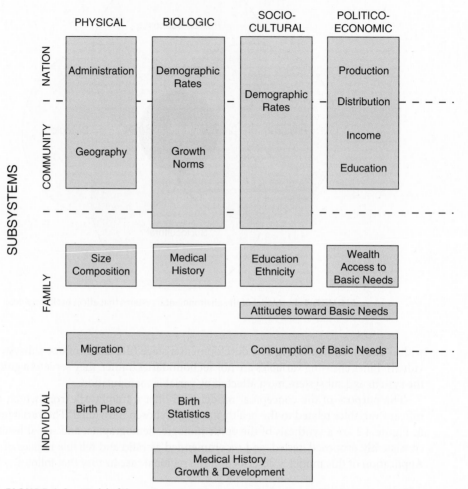

FIGURE 4.2   Model of the environmental systems and subsystems affecting human health.

somewhat if they live in urban areas but still remains substantially higher than that of non-indigenous children living in rural areas. The chance for indigenous children to attain the same mortality rate as nonindigenous children is directly correlated with years of maternal education.

In developing countries, income determines food consumption. With inadequate income, nutrient intake suffers. Malnutrition, defined as a deficiency of the essential nutrients required to support normal physiologic functions, has startling effects on health. The Pan American Health Organization found that a preexisting nutritional deficiency or immaturity (defined as a severe growth deficit) was the underlying or associated cause of death in 57% of deceased preschool children in the Americas. Infection was the leading (58%) cause of death, and 61% of those children who died of infection also had a nutritional deficiency (McFarlane, 1985). Malnutrition and infection demonstrate a synergistic and compounding relationship. Infection, a state in which microorganisms reproduce and cause damage to the host, is a radically different and more lethal process in a child than in an adult. Malnutrition and infection affect the vast majority of children in developing countries.

When a community seeks to maximize its resources of health personnel and capital goods to service the greatest number of children, it requires a tool that will (1) appraise the impingement of biopsychosocial variables that surround the child and (2) establish the relationships that link these variables to health status indicators such as the presence or absence of infection. Because infection is usually a short-term problem, whereas malnutrition is a chronic state of ill health, age-specific prevalence rates of infection are considered crucial indicators of health status and are used to measure health condition in this study.

Population and Methods

The Multinational Andean Genetic and Health Survey assessed the health status of the indigenous population living in Chile's northern province of Tarapacá. Northern Chile is geographically divided into three ecologic zones—the lowland coast, mountainous sierra, and highland altiplano—which differ radically in topography and climate. Associated with the differences are biotic changes that determine the type of agroeconomics, and thus lifestyle, that can be practiced. The health status of 988 children and 1,108 adults in 12 communities was determined; these people represented 70% to 90% of the people in any given village.

The International Classification of Diseases codes were used. Children with one or more diagnoses of infection were considered "infected," children with one or more noninfectious disorders were categorized as "noninfected," and children without coded diseases were considered "well" and "free of disease." In addition, family health variables were abstracted from census data collected concurrently. Family wealth was scored according to the number of animals and amount of acreage owned. Four anthropometric measurements—weight, height, arm circumference, and subscapular skinfold—were used to study the relationship between growth and present health status. From known surnames, ethnicity was determined: non-Aymara (Spanish), Mestizo (mixed Spanish and indigenous), or Aymara (indigenous).

The people studied were primarily agriculturists who derived their livelihood from the land. Inhabitants of the highlands had little arable land, but large expanses of grazing pasture were available. They used their livestock (goats, llamas, and alpacas) to convert the inedible (to humans) natural vegetation into animal products (meat, milk, cheese, and fibers) suitable for human use. Conversely, residents of the sierra had more arable land, more irrigated fields, more diverse livestock (adding sheep and cattle) and agricultural crops, and thus more available foodstuffs. Coastal residents had the least arable land (desert stream floodplains) but benefited from a favorable climate and subsidized irrigation. Plant production was high and diverse on the coast, but animal products were restricted.

Population Characteristics

The physical examinations of children of all three ecologic zones revealed that 40% of them had one or more infections, 18% exhibited one or more noninfectious disorders, and 42% were well and free of disease. Infection did not decrease appreciably with age. Non-Aymara children living on the coast were most likely to be well and free of disease, whereas highland children had the highest rates of infection. The prevalence of noninfectious disorders showed little ethnic variability and no appreciable difference between coast and altiplano regions.

A complex clustering of interacting variables prevailed at the family level. Some, such as the number of people in the household, influenced child health directly (the larger the family, the more potential reservoirs for the incubation and transmission of infection). Other variables exerted their influence indirectly, acting through a web of interrelationships. A primary problem in understanding the ecologic determinants of child health is deciding how to assess the extent to which a given variable acts within the family's environment, directly or indirectly, to affect health status. Analysis of socioeconomic variables (maternal age, education, and health; paternal occupation and health; and family wealth) revealed that well children were likely to have a mother with secondary education and that infected children were likely to have a mother with no education.

Additionally, children with one or more infections were more likely to be cared for by a mother who was also infected, who was younger than 35 years, and who had minimal or no education. A large number of infected children in the altiplano resided in homes below the median wealth index, but neither wealth nor the father's occupation differentiated the health status of coastal or sierra children. Only among sierra children did the father's health correlate significantly with the child's health. Most early child and maternal health factors varied as a function of region but not of ethnicity.

When compared with well children, infected children consumed fewer foods and, regionally, altiplano children consumed the fewest foods. Region of residence with associated access to food, shelter, education, and health care proved more connected to child health than culture and associated lifestyle behaviors. Child health was determined by environmental factors operant at the individual, family, and community levels.

Model Application

Most children in developing nations (and some children in developed nations) reside in abject poverty, resulting in inadequate dietary intake and significant prevalence of infectious disease. The dilemma facing health workers and planners in all countries is how to use existing resources to the greatest benefit of the largest number of children. To promote child health, causal determinants of infection and malnutrition as well as cost-effective interventions must be identified. The problem is how to define and measure the crucial variables of child morbidity.

Most assessment models are linear, unidirectional, and not designed to look beyond the child or immediate family for health indicators. The ecologic determinants responsible for the prevalence, severity, and duration of the infection–malnutrition cycle are practically unknown. In developing countries, almost all pediatric morbidity data are obtained from hospital records; consequently, they offer uncertain direction for regional or community health planning, especially in rural areas where people have limited or no routine access to medical care.

The Chilean study used an ecologic model to sort physical, biologic, sociocultural, and politicoeconomic variables that impinged on child health. Descriptive and multivariate analyses were used to delineate the variables that exerted an appreciable effect on child health. Using ecologic concepts and the variables found to be important links to child health, a model of the ecologic chain of events has been constructed (Fig. 4.3). This "ecologic map" begins with the geographic region of residence—the community.

The region, or community, surrounds the child with a given set of physical forces, including climate, water supply, and topography. These forces interact with demographic structure and political and economic organization to determine the nutrient productivity of the land. Food production in any region is conditioned by economic forces (resources allocated to food production and food distribution); social forces (land tenure); and political edicts (policy and legal implication of land ownership and use). These forces unite and determine the quantity and quality of land used for food production; the people and technology applied to the land to maximize production; and the diversity, nutritive value, and distribution of the produce. The physical, biologic, sociocultural, and politicoeconomic forces within each region determine the quantity and quality of nutrients available to the family for consumption.

The family consists of a clustering of interacting variables, many of which serve as gates, acting to impede or facilitate members' access to available nutrients. Simultaneously, infection

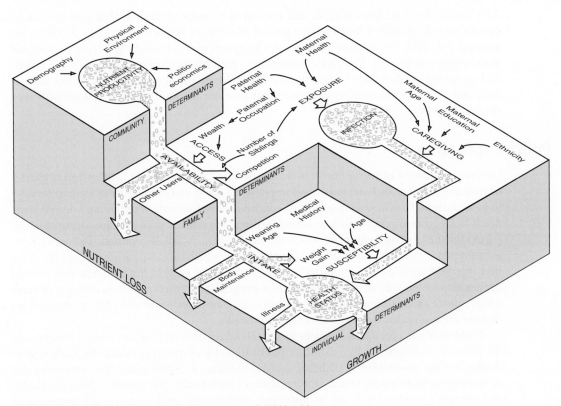

FIGURE 4.3   Model of the ecologic determinants of child health.

risk factors abide within the household, variables that mitigate or accentuate the child's risk of illness. Both nutrient intake and infection risk concurrently determine health status, which is reflected in growth patterns.

The web of interconnection continues even further. Paternal health influences paternal occupation, which determines family wealth and, in turn, defines purchasing power and access to available nutrients. The number and age of siblings influence both access to food (through competition) and infection risk (through exposure). In addition, poor maternal health not only exposes the child to illness but also acts as a deterrent to adequate caregiving. Caregiving is also affected by maternal ethnicity, age, and education. Each factor determines the mother's knowledge and experience regarding basic health-promoting acts, such as hygiene practices, appropriate solid foods, and needed nutrients and physical care during illness. When the caregiver lacks knowledge or is ill, the child's risk of infection increases.

The child is a composite of risk factors that interact with familial and regional variables to set his or her health status and subsequent growth. The quantity and quality of nutrients consumed by the child determine weight gain and nutritional status. Weight gain is a product of both nutrient intake and a risk variable for infection. The malnourished child has impaired immunocompetence and is prey to infection. Also influencing a child's weight gain are weaning age and first solid foods; both affect the child's nutritive status and susceptibility to infection. Finally, the child's age and past medical history decrease or accentuate susceptibility to infection. In this study, it was the young, preschool children, ill within the last 2 weeks, who experienced the bulk of morbidity.

For most children, the interaction of nutritive intake and infection determines growth. Infection is wasteful and has a negative effect on nutrient absorption, metabolism, and use.

As a result, the child loses weight, and growth is halted or retarded. Low nutrient intake equally retards growth. Children have greater nutritional needs relative to body mass: the younger the child, the more kilocalories per kilogram of body weight is needed for normal metabolism and growth. The risk of infection is high for all children, especially for infants and preschool-aged children, regardless of their nutritional status; however, when adverse infection–risk factors combine with marginal nutrient intake, the result is morbidity and delayed growth.

Policy Implication

Current assessment of world health indicates that lack of basic needs is the primary barrier to wellness. To provide basic needs and improve access to and availability of human services (e.g., education, health, sanitation), most countries have focused on providing selected basic needs to designated groups, such as school feeding programs or prenatal care. Unfortunately, regard for the environment, from which the needs arose, is usually omitted. To focus on selected needs without assessing the environment from which the needs arose ignores the complex interrelationships of the biopsychosocial system and negates the structure that created the health problems. Basic-needs intervention programs that do not address ecologic dynamics can create an illusion of success and allow continuation of social and political inequalities that are themselves major contributors to poor health.

Child health is ecologic and relates to the total environment that surrounds children and the physical ecosystem, as well as social, political, and economic organizations. Each system determines the production, availability, and distribution of resources and the eventual access of children to basic needs, which, in turn, dictates both health and growth. Children's health and nutrition problems will not be improved substantially until measures are instituted to eradicate poverty.

Using an ecologic model to identify and sort the determinants of infection among children in northern Chile, researchers found that the region of residence consistently emerged as a significant correlate of health. Region embraces politicoeconomic factors as well as a set climate and demographic state that determine nutrient productivity and access. Once the child acquires food, whether the nutrients are used to maintain and promote growth or are degraded by infection that retards growth and development depends on the family milieu, especially the mother's health, age, and education. Additional risk factors include family wealth, ethnicity, and paternal health. No one risk factor can be addressed independently of the others. Infection is promoted or hindered by a maze of intercorrelated variables, and to address only one or two does little more than vibrate the web of causation.

The root determinants of child health lie deep in the social, economic, and political fiber of the people. Child health cannot be improved independently of changes in the environment surrounding the child. To focus on selected prevention programs (such as improved nutrition or adequate housing) without simultaneously attending to the environment from which the deficits arise (such as existing political and economic policies) negates the determinant values of health and is an inappropriate use of time, money, and personnel.

Summary

Where does this knowledge of ecologic processes leave us? As practitioners of community health, how does this information aid us?

First, we must be aware that the health of any population can be affected by its surrounding environment. Next, be skeptical of any claims of perfect disposal schemes for pollutants;

they do not exist. Remember that pollutants can travel long distances and remain undetected. Water treatment systems usually precipitate pollutants to a bottom sludge. Eventually, the sludge must be cleaned out. If it is burned, will the pollutants go back up the smokestack, only to settle into another watershed? If it is buried in a landfill, will the pollutants remain in place or seep into a groundwater reservoir, only to surface at your kitchen faucet? Everything—including pollutants—has to go somewhere, and it may be difficult to keep them in any one place.

Finally, as a consumer or a public advocate, do not demand perfect disposal schemes. Demand honest and realistic estimates of the risk that invariably accompanies any plan, no matter how appealing. Beware of flowcharts that indicate perfect control of pollutants at all stages of the cycle. Remember that it is people who handle pollutants, and the people factor can overwhelm every other part of any plan. It is people who load, transport, and dispose pollutants. It is people who operate and maintain pollution control systems. It is people who give illegal orders for "midnight dumping and roadside disposal." In some instances, particularly involving the ultimate disposal of nuclear wastes, we may be planning caretaking operations that exceed the realm of past human experience. Our oldest civilizations generally have not persisted for more than 5,000 years, and individual nations typically survive for far shorter periods. Can we honestly listen to glib talk of storing radioactive materials that will require maintenance for 10,000 years or longer—and take such plans seriously?

Boxes 4.2 and 4.3 offer more examples of how the environment is connected to human health. Consider the role of the community health nurse in each example.

Box 4.2 Everything Is Connected

Japan is located on the "ring of fire," the rim of the Pacific Ocean basin where earthquakes and volcanic activity are commonplace. On March 11, 2011, the most powerful earthquake ever to strike Japan created tsunami waves that reached 133 feet in height and traveled up to 6 miles inland. This natural disaster resulted in 16,000 deaths, 6,000 injured, more than 2,000 people missing, and 1 million buildings totally or partially collapsed.

The Fukushima Daiichi nuclear power complex endured a direct hit. Three of the six nuclear reactors were operating at the time. These reactors automatically shut down when the earthquake occurred, and emergency generators came online to power the electronics and coolant systems. The tsunami that followed flooded the electrical connections, and the critical pumps that must circulate coolant water through the reactors failed.

The overheated reactors generated hydrogen gas, and several explosions occurred. Radioactive gases were released, and residents within a 12-mile radius of the power plant were evacuated. There were no deaths due to radiation exposure, but some experts predict a future increase in thyroid cancer among the exposed population. Within a few days, radioactive cesium, iodine, and xenon products were detectable in North America, Europe, and Australia. Two years after the accident the nuclear reactors are still too radioactive to approach, radioactive water is leaking into the adjacent coastal waters and contaminating fishes, and most fish and seafood from the coast have been barred from domestic markets and export. Radioactive iodine has been found in milk 18 miles away, and in spinach grown 50 and 65 miles distant.

An independent commission investigated the event and concluded that the nuclear disaster was "manmade" and the direct causes of the accident were all foreseeable. The operating company had been warned for years that the plant was vulnerable to a large tsunami, but corrective actions were only partially implemented or ignored completely. The "people factor" was operative before and following the concatenating events. Poor decisions, indecisive reactions, obfuscation, and nontransparency were apparent at every step.

Box 4.3 Unintended Consequences

Hydraulic fracturing, commonly known as "fracking," is a technique developed several decades ago to release oil and natural gas from deep layers of shale rock. Drillers inject highly pressurized water containing chemicals that reduce friction and sand to prevent cracks from closing. Some of the chemicals may be toxic and most are proprietary secrets. Fracking has created an economic boom by enhancing the recovery of natural gas. It has also unleashed a contentious dialog between drillers and local residents fearing that their water supplies may become contaminated with toxic chemicals. It has been difficult to establish a direct causative connection between fracking activity and the contamination of well water. Drinking water is typically obtained just a few hundred feet beneath the surface. Fracking activity occurs thousands of feet below the level of aquifers. Of course, the gas wells must pass through the aquifers to reach the gas-bearing shale rock below. Drillers maintain that their wells are appropriately sealed to protect the aquifers, and that the water carrying their chemicals will respond to gravity and flow downward, not upward. Their opponents suggest that injecting chemicals under high pressure will create cracks and leaks (after all, that is what it is designed to do). On the other hand, methane gas will rise to the surface and seems to frequently find an outlet at a handy water tap. The economic pressures to promote fracking are enormous, and politicians follow the money.

Anecdotal evidence that links fracking activity to well water contamination is plentiful (see McDermott-Levy, Kaktins, & Sattler, 2013). Consider this scenario: a family with healthy children moves to an area of active fracking for employment opportunities. Subsequently, the children, and perhaps the adults as well, exhibit fatigue, burning eyes, dermatologic irritations, headaches, and upper respiratory, gastrointestinal, or neurologic problems. Local health providers note that these symptoms have been on the rise since the burst of fracking activity and advise the family to leave the area. The family relocates and health returns. No direct causative connection has been established, but that family does not need one.

Fracking currently occurs in a dozen states and is being considered in a half-dozen more. Vermont has permanently banned the practice, while New York and North Carolina have temporary bans. There seems to be little questioning that fracking can be done safely, for the most part (Schrope, 2012). But all oil and gas wells are eventually abandoned. Will they be properly sealed? Will the seals persist? There are numerous examples of old wells gone bad. While the fraction of bad wells may be very small, as the number of holes punched deep into the ground rises into the thousands, so does the potential for leaky wells and opportunities for short-cuts. Once again, the "people factor" comes into play.

Critical Thinking Questions

1. Florence Nightingale recognized the connection of environmental conditions to human health. Based on what you have learned from this chapter, what are the major environmental conditions affecting the health of people in your community?

2. Exposure to lead and asbestos can happen at the worksite and then be transmitted on workers' clothing to the home, where it can affect family health. Think about the industries in your community, and identify potential sources of occupational exposure to substances that could be transmitted at home and affect family health.

3. Choose an environmental hazard, such as "ozone," and use the internet to learn about the health effects of exposure to this hazard. What populations are at highest risk of health problems? What are the health problems? What can be done in the community to reduce exposure?

4. What information about health risks can you determine are present for a residential community near a chemical plant? What approaches can you take to obtain this information?

5. What can community members concerned about environmental toxins do to protect their health? What resources can you suggest to concerned citizens to assist them with a healthy action plan?

6. What are potential environmental health risks to patients, staff, and the citizens living and working near a large urban medical center? What are some specific strategies to decrease environmental health risks to these population groups?

7. How might a community health nurse respond to questions posed regarding the safety of well water versus public drinking water versus bottled water?

8. Choose an existing environmental health problem in your community, such as lead levels in old homes; poor air quality related to ozone or smog; or an environmental threat posed by the construction of or an existing landfill, airport, or housing development. (This is a good time to read the local newspaper and note the environmental issues.) Once you have chosen an environmental health problem, research the health effects and strategies to minimize the effects. Outline a 15-minute presentation suitable for a group of parents of school-aged children, a group of seniors, or a group of pregnant women. (Of course, any interested group is just fine. The important point is to know your audience and tailor your presentation to the needs of the audience. Frequently faith communities and civic associations provide opportunities for interested citizens to gather.) Include references and sources for further information. Ask to make your presentation. Evaluate the responses of the audience. What questions were asked? What further information is needed? What action steps were discussed? What can be your continuing role in working with the group?

REFERENCES

Chalupka, S. (2005). Tainted water on tap. *American Journal of Nursing*, 105(11), 40–52.

Chapin, F. S., III, Randerson, J. T., McGuire, A. D., Foley, J. A., & Field, C. B. (2008). Changing feedbacks in the climate-biosphere system. *Frontiers in Ecology and Environment*, 6, 313–320.

Citizens for a Better Environment. (2002). Pesticide use reporting and reduction project. Retrieved September 6, 2006, from http://www.wsn.org/pesticides

Haines, A., Kovats, R. S., Campbell-Lendrum, D., & Corvalan, C. (2006). Climate change and human health: Impacts, vulnerability, and mitigation. *Lancet, 367,* 2301–2309.

Intergovernmental Panel on Climate Change. (2007). Climate change 2007: Synthesis report, summary for policymakers. Retrieved March 23, 2010, from http://www.ipcc.ch/pdf/assessment-report/ar4/syr/ar4_syr_spm.pdf

Jones, K. E., Patel, N. G., Levy, M. A., Storeygard, A., Balk, D., Gittleman, J. L., & Daszak, P. (2008). Global trends in emerging infectious diseases. *Nature, 451,* 990–994.

McDermott-Levy, R., Kaktins, N., & Sattler, B. (2013). Fracking, the environment, and health. *American Journal of Nursing, 113*(6), 45–51.

McFarlane, J. (1985). Use of an ecologic model to identify children at risk for infection and to quantify the expected impact of the risk factors. *Public Health Nursing, 2,* 12–22.

Nightingale, F. (1969). *Notes on nursing.* New York, NY: Dover.

Pope, A. M., Snyder, M. A., & Mood, L. H. (Eds.). (1995). *Nursing, health & the environment.* Washington, DC: National Academy Press.

Schrope, M. (2012). Fracking outpaces science on its impact. *Environment Yale.* Retrieved from http://environment.yale.edu/envy/stories/fracking-outpaces-science-on-its-impact

U.S. Department of Health and Human Services. (2003). Cancer and the environment: What you need to know, what you can do. Retrieved March 23, 2010, from http://www.cancer.gov/images/Documents/5d17e03e-b39f-4b40-a214-e9e9099c4220/Cancer%20and%20the%20Environment.pdf

World Health Organization. (2006). Water, sanitation and hygiene links to health. Facts and figures updated November 2004. Retrieved December 29, 2005, from http://www.who.int/water_sanitation_health/publications/facts2004/en/print.html

FURTHER READINGS

ANA RN No Harm Training and Pollution Prevention Kit for Nurses: http://www.nursingworld.org

Collaborative on Health and the Environment: http://www.cheforhealth.org

Health Care Without Harm and the Nurses Work Group: http://www.noharm.org

University of Maryland School of Nursing's Environmental Health Education Center: http://www.enviRN.umaryland.edu

U.S. General Services Administration. (continually updated). Code of Federal Regulations. Title 40—Protection of the environment, part 50. National primary and secondary ambient air quality standards, part 129. Toxic pollutant effluent standards, part 141. National primary drinking water regulations, part 143. National secondary drinking water regulations. Washington, DC: U.S. Government Printing Office.

CHAPTER 5

Ethical Quandaries in Community Health Nursing

Susan Scoville Walker

LEARNING OBJECTIVES

Effective partnership with communities requires sensitivity to the tension between the beliefs, perceptions, and priorities of the community and those of the health care professional.

After studying this chapter, you should be able to:

1. Identify essential elements of health care ethics.

2. Describe ethical implications of the community-as-partner model.

3. Analyze community health proposals in consideration of ethical principles.

4. Formulate ethically sound decisions in partnership with communities.

5. Evaluate ethical decisions within the context of human needs.

Introduction

This chapter reviews the general domain of ethics in health care to clarify the principles most often threatened or affirmed in health care decision making. Within the context of alternative approaches to ethical decision making and varying philosophical frameworks for defining the relationship between clients and health care providers, these principles are applied to the specific context of community health nursing. Finally, the concept of *community-as-partner* is reaffirmed as a guiding principle to unraveling the dilemmas encountered in the field of community health nursing.

WHAT IS ETHICS?

Ethics is a philosophical pursuit originating in an ancient discourse on the definition of "the good." To maintain a clear focus on ethics, it is helpful to contrast its domain to that of law, in order to avoid the tendency to confuse the two or to simplify the moral struggle to do the right thing by seeking a legal reason for action. The essential points of comparison are the following:

- Whereas ethics considers people as inherently good, law presumes them to be basically bad;
- Therefore, ethics proposes what a person *should* do, whereas law specifies what one *must* do;
- In fact, although one may be chastised if found in violation of ethical principles, there are no definite sanctions, whereas law imposes penalties in terms of fines and imprisonment.

Another point of confusion arises because the popular press often confuses the two terms or at least uses them interchangeably. Press coverage of the "ethics violations" of public officials actually deals with infractions of laws intended to bridge the gap between the two arenas and influence people to act in the "correct" way. The law is often seen as a way to enforce the current ethical values of a society because it responds more quickly to changing circumstances (O'Keefe, 2002).

Finally, ethics includes many levels of discourse, but the division of ethics most useful to health care decision making is that of applied ethics. The function of applied ethics is to provide a systematic, logical framework for analysis, discourse, and decision making that helps ensure that decisions are grounded in the philosophy of "good" actions.

APPROACHES TO ETHICAL DECISION MAKING

Although many philosophical approaches are discussed in the literature, two contrasting approaches are most helpful in applied ethics: deontology and teleology. Briefly, deontology is a rule-based approach, in which decisions are made by applying a set of rules of good conduct. Examples of such rules include personal moral codes and professional codes of ethics, such as the American Nurses Association (ANA, 2001) Code of Ethics for Nurses and the American Public Health Association (APHA, 2002) Public Health Code of Ethics. Deontology is grounded in the philosophy of Immanuel Kant and in the central precept of his teaching, that no person should be treated as the means to an end (Fry & Veatch, 2010; Petrini & Gainotti, 2008).

The contrasting approach is teleology, or outcome-based decision making, based on the philosophy of John Stuart Mill. Decisions are made on the basis of the greatest good for the greatest number (Fry & Veatch, 2010; Petrini & Gainotti, 2008). In actuality, the application of ethics to health care decision making usually involves a combination of these two approaches. Thus, the available options are evaluated, first, to determine what option would be of greatest benefit to most of the parties involved and, second, to ensure that the rights of all involved parties are respected.

The adequacy of either approach to health care ethics has come under scrutiny in recent years, however, as fundamental inequalities across geographical regions, strata of society, and age groups complicate the analysis (Daniels, 2006).

FRAMEWORKS FOR HEALTH CARE ROLES

Most people who enter the health care profession cite altruism as one of the reasons for their career choice. Given their desire to help others, the traditional framework of the relationship between health care professionals and the people they care for has been one of paternalism. In a traditional, literal rendition of this relationship, the physician holds the role of the father, the nurse is the mother, and the patient is the child. Indeed, this framework is inherently implied by those health care professionals whose chosen term for those in their care is "patient." Frequently, these health care professionals work in areas such as trauma, intensive care, and critical care, where they care for people who are often in acute distress and may not be able to be active participants in making decisions regarding their care.

In settings in which people can be active participants, a philosophy of contractualism applies. In these settings, the client and health care professional share in determining the options and selecting the best choice for that person.

Finally, in elective situations, such as plastic surgery, the balance of authority in decision making shifts away from the provider to the user of health care services, and the operative framework becomes one of consumerism, in which the consumer is clearly in control of choices among available options. Community health nursing is best understood within this framework, as exemplified in the model of community as partner. Effective, lasting community health nursing interventions depend on the ability of the community health nurse to relinquish decision-making control to the community and to trust its ability to make responsible decisions.

THE ROLE OF THE HEALTH CARE PROFESSIONAL

New roles of the health care professional within the framework of community as partner reflect an increasingly balanced participation between providers and recipients of health care. One role, developed and elaborated by nurse ethicist Sally Gadow, is that of advocacy. In her philosophical discourse, advocacy involves understanding the world view, life circumstances, and priorities of those requesting or receiving care and exploring the possible options with them in light of their preferences. In contrast to a strict contractualist or consumerist approach, however, the health care professional tries to imagine experiencing the situation of the person seeking care and offers an opinion of the best choice in full consideration of the other party's individuality (Gadow, 1990). The concept of advocacy has been refined by Racher (2007) to describe action within political, economic, and social systems on behalf of health interests of communities.

Another conception of the role of the health care professional, particularly applicable to community health nursing, is that of catalyst. In this model, the community is seen to contain all the necessary qualities and resources for change, and the role of the health care professional is to provide the spark that will initiate change, as desired by the community and on its terms.

Both of these models clearly establish the primacy of the community and the fact that lasting change depends on the investment of the community. However, it is important to underscore that the health care professional is an active, concerned, supportive, sometimes challenging participant in the process. As an advocate or catalyst, the community health nurse can make the difference between success and failure of a community's efforts to improve the quality of life of its members.

SEVEN PRINCIPLES ESSENTIAL IN HEALTH CARE ETHICS

The process of ethical decision making involves analysis of alternative actions in light of moral and ethical principles. In health care ethics, seven pervasive principles are useful in making conscientious decisions. These are the principles of autonomy, respect for people, beneficence, nonmaleficence, justice, veracity, and fidelity (Box 5.1). In this section, each principle is defined and then applied to situations typical of those encountered in community health nursing.

Box 5.1 Ethical Principles in Health Care

1. Autonomy
2. Respect for people
3. Beneficence
4. Nonmaleficence
5. Justice (distributive and retributive)
6. Veracity
7. Fidelity

Autonomy

The right of individuals to self-determination (autonomy) is the core value of western European and American law and ethics. In application to health care, it means that decisions should be made by those most affected, be they individuals, families, groups, or communities. Clearly, autonomy is the umbrella concept of the community-as-partner model. Many health care professionals will come and go, and any outside program, no matter how worthy, will endure only as long as those professionals remain active in the community, unless the community makes an autonomous investment to endorse and adopt the idea behind the program.

The altruistic nature of health care professionals presents a central challenge to the autonomy of those who receive their care. Often, the desire to care is so strong, and the appreciation of those who benefit from that caring so rewarding for the provider, that the result is a system of giving and taking that leads to increased dependency. It is striking to visit a remote community after a community assistance project of some kind has been operating there and be greeted with "Who are you and what are you going to give us?" For some community health care providers, it seems that the urge to help is so strong that it can get in the way of empowering people to help themselves. The classical field of community development, as exemplified by the Peace Corps and other relief organizations, assists people to develop the skills needed to improve their own circumstances. Thus, in contrast to programs focused on providing goods or services, these programs operate at the grassroots level. Outside helpers work as catalysts with people in communities to discover their potential and as advocates to help the community learn how to access resources needed to move toward their goals.

Respect for People

The second essential ethical principle, respect for people, recognizes that every person and community has intrinsic value. Applying this principle to community health directs health care professionals to evaluate the effect of proposed initiatives in light of their implications for all who might be affected.

One example of applying the principle of respect for people might be to encourage a community to reevaluate its proposal to resolve its solid waste or toxic waste problem by transporting this waste to another community. The benefit to people in one community creates potential harm for those in another. Another example would be to give careful consideration before introducing Western medical practices and ideals that might conflict with a community's cultural norms and folk-healing practices. Other examples will be discussed in more detail in the next sections in relation to justice issues and programs that are restricted to serve only a portion of the community in need.

Beneficence

The desire to act in the best interest of others, beneficence, is perhaps the strongest guiding ethical principle of health care professionals. Most people who enter the helping professions do so because of an altruistic desire to help others. Because of the desire to help people, to take care of them, and to alleviate their suffering, health care professionals often find themselves faced with conflicts between their desire to help (beneficence) and their respect for the other person's right to choose (autonomy). In fact, the principles of beneficence and autonomy are so often at odds that it is all but impossible to imagine an uncomplicated example of beneficence as applied to community health nursing. Even a community health initiative as apparently benign as an immunization campaign to protect community members from a communicable disease may conflict with the autonomy of people whose religious beliefs do not support the practice. The complexity of communities makes it unlikely that any community-wide activity will be uniformly beneficial to all sectors.

Nonmaleficence

Nonmaleficence, the avoidance of harm, is the silent partner of beneficence. Often, health care decisions may offer no really good option that will provide positive results, but at least there may be a choice that does not cause any outright harm. When proposals are considered for community health initiatives, it is important to evaluate not only what positive good (beneficence) may come from the activity, but also what harm might result, particularly if, as in the example above of solid waste and respect for people, the same initiative may well be beneficial for some community members and harmful to others. If a community attracts more industry to the area, the results may include increased job opportunities and better economic conditions for its residents, but there may be counterbalancing health risk factors such as environmental harm and decreased water and air quality.

Justice

The principle of justice has two aspects, both of them applicable to health care decision making. Most often, discussions of health-related justice center on *distributive justice*, the fair distribution of rights and resources. These discussions often center on allocation of scarce resources in ways that are fair and of greatest benefit to the most people. In this context, community health care providers and advocates argue for increased governmental support for preventive health programs that lead to better quality of life (beneficence) for the greatest number of people in the community (respect for people).

Well-meaning community programs designed to improve access to health services raise issues of distributive justice. In one example, a community coalition of diverse clinical providers and health care organizations developed a series of community health fairs in different neighborhoods in and near a small city. Initiated as a means of improving child immunization rates, in the early years the fairs were small and community oriented, combining health services and some aspects of a street fair, including games, food, raffles, and children's activities. Events were held three times a year, and the late summer fair was always the largest, because many children needed immunizations or athletic physicals before the start of school. Over time, civic groups joined in to provide school supplies for the back-to-school fair and other incentives for the other fairs. Incentives brought an ever-increasing number of people to the health fairs, including many people who came because of their need for the supplies (paper, pens, food, and blankets) rather than a need for health services. Because the intent of the organizers was to provide health services, there was often a requirement that participants receive a certain number of services to be eligible for the incentives. Service records from the fairs indicate that a number of participants traveled to health fairs in several communities and participated in repeated health screenings to receive the incentives.

Grant-funded community health research projects also raise issues of distributive justice when random houses in a particular neighborhood are selected for a project. A neighbor may be visiting on the porch at the time the field investigator visits and offers members of the selected household a stipend in return for participation. Culturally sensitive, caring field researchers who are invested in the community are known to dip into their own pockets and provide equal treatment to the neighbor even though the data will never be included as part of the study.

There is a second branch of the principle of justice, that of *retributive justice*, the arena of reward and punishment. Because of their generally altruistic nature, health care professionals may be reluctant to address this principle. However, the application of this darker side of justice is often tied closely to distributive justice. Allocation of resources is very often determined politically, and resources are awarded to those who have provided support to those in control of the resources. Thus, in poor communities everywhere, political candidates may provide transportation to the polls, along with assurances of improved living conditions should they be elected. At the same time, grants and projects often come to communities that have demonstrated a strong voting record for those in power.

Many community health programs are funded by local, state, or federal government grants. Often, communities are selected to receive grant-funded services through the political and legislative process. Therefore, it is important for community health nurses to be active and to help community residents establish a voice within the local, state, and national political arena. Starting with knowing their own city, county, and state representatives, effective community health nurses can serve as a link between the community and its elected representatives and can facilitate interaction and support as a two-way process. If the community (including the nurse) can find ways to support politicians (photo opportunities, voting, attending rallies), it is more likely that politicians will reciprocate by funding needed programs.

Veracity

Veracity is the commitment to tell the truth. In community health nursing, veracity centers on honesty about who you are and what you bring to the community. In some communities, many programs and researchers have come and gone, and a cynical materialism has arisen in the community. Community health nurses may find themselves entering communities that have become accustomed to outsiders bringing in programs, goods, or services. It is difficult but necessary to be clear from the beginning that, in the spirit of community as partner, the only gift brought by the nurse is the gift of self, offering advocacy and energy to support the community.

Community health research raises issues of veracity. Many communities, particularly those with underrepresented population groups, are frequently visited by teams of researchers who screen residents for any number of health conditions or risk factors, including chronic illness and toxic exposure. Community health nurses, as community advocates, should help ensure that they and other researchers are honest with the community about exactly what is to be provided. All too often, residents do not understand that the only benefit from participation in a research study is the screening itself. Access to the results of health screening raises a separate issue of veracity, as well as issues of beneficence and nonmaleficence. It is of little benefit to know of a serious health condition if there is no access to treatment for it.

Fidelity

The last of the seven essential principles is fidelity, or faithfulness. To work with communities or individuals, the health care professional must be careful in making promises and steadfast in keeping them. This obligation may be embodied as simply as making and keeping appointments. It may also extend to keeping a pledge to report back to community leaders on the outcome of a project.

As discussed above in the section on veracity, community health research raises serious questions of fidelity as well as veracity in projects that involve health screening. To be effective on a long-term basis in a community, a community health nurse needs to network with health care providers in the community to obtain treatment for people made aware of serious health conditions by community health screenings. Much of the work of the community health nurse, then, involves building relationships to advocate effectively for treatment for community members diagnosed with serious health conditions. It is important to be aware of the reciprocal nature of this relationship and how it relates to issues of retributive justice and political involvement. Thus, if the community health nurse expects another health care professional to respond to a community and its needs, the time will come when the health care professional is entitled to ask for a favor in return. An effective approach is to consider what one's community, one's associates, or oneself might have to offer in advance of asking the favor. It is also good to know about tax incentives, public relations, referrals, and other nonaltruistic motives as well.

ETHICAL QUANDARIES IN COMMUNITY HEALTH

The diversity and complexity of communities inevitably lead to a plethora of conflicts between and among these principles. In this section, several examples will be discussed to illustrate some common quandaries that complicate community health partnerships.

Quandaries Regarding Autonomy and the Public Good

The potential conflict between autonomy and the public good (beneficence) is a prominent feature of many of the Healthy People 2010 and Healthy People 2020 National Health Goals. As delineated by the U.S. Department of Health and Human Services (2000, 2010), the health indicators used to measure progress toward reaching these goals include the following: physical activity, overweight and obesity, tobacco use, substance abuse, responsible sexual activity, and immunization. Clearly, with the exception of immunization and substance abuse, these indicators are health behaviors that carry no mandates. On the other hand, they represent expressions of personal freedom that are highly cherished and protected by a society that values individual freedom and respect for a person's right to choose. However, the purpose of the National Health Goals and the establishment of indicators that can be used to measure progress toward goal attainment is to reduce the human and economic cost of preventable, disabling health conditions prevalent in the United States today. The health effects of a fast-food diet and inactivity are well documented, yet it remains a matter of personal choice for individuals to change behaviors that harm only the individuals themselves and that can be modified only if the individual desires. Nevertheless, the community health nurse can act as an advocate and catalyst by helping a community look at overall resources and alternatives that can promote health and a healthy lifestyle. Whether or not all individuals have free choice regarding health behavior decisions is open to discussion, considering the long-standing correlation of healthy behavior choices with socioeconomic status (Blacksher, 2008).

Quandaries Regarding Respect for People, Autonomy, Justice, and Beneficence

Although health care professionals desire to help improve people's lives and health status, they are often challenged to respect the rights of individuals or communities to choose other alternatives. For example, in many communities, a faltering economy has led to severe cuts in human services programs, often on the basis of perceived worth of the individuals. Among the first population groups to lose funding are the mentally ill and those with substance abuse disorders.

An example that illustrates the conflict between beneficence and respect for people concerns the activities of a group of community health nursing students who worked in a small, rural community on the Texas–Mexico border. The community is located on the Rio Grande River and has a population of around 3,000, including many migrant farm worker families. The community has an independent civic government, but a very limited economic base and a weak infrastructure. On arrival in the community, the students conducted a detailed community assessment, in keeping with the community-as-partner model, using the community assessment wheel as a guide. As they discussed their findings, the students noted the young population of the community, with a preponderance of children and youth, the proximity to the river, and the safety issues inherent in children swimming and fishing in the polluted river. The students thought that a high priority for the community would be safety, and they were prepared to teach parents and children about the health risks of the river. However, as they got to know the community better and community members spoke up, it was clear that the community had much the same concern but a very different perspective on what to do about it. Although their primary concern also related to the children and youth, they focused on the need for recreation, in particular the need for an informal ballpark on the riverbank.

Another example of ethical issues of justice, beneficence, and respect for people focuses on the choice and condition of goods delivered to impoverished areas as part of public health relief efforts. Often, as winter approaches, appeals go out for blankets and warm clothing. Although the appeals specify that donated items should be new or in excellent condition, all too often, organizers receive bags of clothing unfit for any use other than cleaning rags. Another notable example relates to food supplies sent to cultures with no appreciation for how to use them. Peanut butter was airlifted to Afghanistan to relieve hunger; it was unacceptable to the people, who did not have a taste for it, but who did find that some of their domestic animals were willing to eat it. In another instance, bulgur wheat, a Middle Eastern staple, was shipped to South America, where it was unknown and went unused.

Quandaries Regarding Autonomy and Beneficence: The Case of Scarce Water

Probably the most frequent source of conflict faced by community health nurses is the desire to help people whose values are at odds with those of the person desiring to help them improve their health status. In an acute care setting, chronic tobacco smokers defy the best attempts to improve their health status unless they are invested in the process. In community health, a similar situation exists. Community health workers starting a new outreach program to identify people at risk for human immunodeficiency virus/acquired immunodeficiency syndrome (HIV/AIDS) found that they needed first to provide information and access to basic needs like housing and food. Community members were more concerned about immediate risks than the long-term possibility of AIDS.

Similarly, a group of community health nursing students was assigned to an isolated rural community near the Texas–Mexico border. The water supply of the community was known to contain a high level of naturally occurring arsenic. The students were eager to learn about the community's perception of their health risk and to help find ways to remediate the situation. Students were surprised by the results of their comprehensive community assessment. Community members acknowledged the natural presence of arsenic in their water and the potential for long-term undesirable health effects. However, they compared that unknown risk with the outright lack of an adequate water supply of any kind in a neighboring town. They weighed the risks and benefits and considered themselves fortunate to have water in an arid region.

The health issue of highest importance identified by the community was the lack of accessible health services and the accompanying risks of traveling 50 miles each way on a dangerous highway to access services.

Quandaries Regarding Autonomy, Beneficence, and Justice: Access to Care

As the cost of health care increases, so does the population of uninsured and underinsured. Combined with the cost of litigation and extravagant settlements, open access to care is coming into question. When data showed a decrease in the number of eligible low-income families choosing to enroll their children in The Children's Health Insurance Program (CHIP), the low-cost, government-supported health insurance program, research revealed the most common explanation given by those who failed to reenroll was that they did not want to pay the $50 enrollment fee either because their children were not currently sick or because they could go to the emergency room when a child was sick and receive free care. Emergency rooms, on the other hand, have started to look more critically at their role in the health care system and treat only those cases that qualify as emergencies; other cases are evaluated and offered a referral to a primary care clinic for a nominal fee.

Communities are also beginning to explore strategies to encourage or even to force families to participate in some form of health insurance or other payment plan. As resources become scarcer and demand increases, these discussions are becoming more common and more frightening in their implications for other aspects of children's overall health when they include suggestions such as restricting access to recreational facilities or even public education.

Examination of access to care issues uncovers the hidden health disparity between rural and urban patients and families (NRHA, 2013). Usually, the discussion of health care disparities centers on ethnicity or socioeconomic status. Little if any attention is given to the disparity between rural and urban health care services. As part of planning for health care reform, however, researchers have tracked and compared health outcomes for urban and rural elderly clients (NAC, 2011; Smith, 2010). Results show more rural elderly being sick, more receiving care in hospitals and nursing homes rather than at home, and fewer surviving similar health conditions (Hutchison, Hawes, & Williams, 2005).

Philosophical and political differences play a part in these disparities. In some communities, home care agencies are ready to support rural as well as urban clients with home nursing and other services, like physical therapy, delivered in their own homes. In other communities, the agencies refuse to bring services into the home, insisting that the patient and family come into town for therapy several times a week, or move out of their own home environment and live in town for an extended period of time, in order to receive "in-home" services.

Quandaries Regarding Autonomy, Beneficence, and Nonmaleficence: The Case of the Tarahumara

In northwestern Mexico, in the beautiful Sierra Madre mountain range, is the spectacular natural wonder called the Copper Canyon, home to one of the world's last remaining indigenous cultures, the Raramari, also known as the Tarahumara Indians. They live a simple life, based on a philosophy of harmony with nature. As civilization has taken over more and more of Mexico, the Tarahumara have moved into more and more rugged and inhospitable regions, and are now isolated deep in the canyons of the Sierra Madre. The Tarahumara prefer to sleep out under the stars, weather permitting, but they maintain small huts or cave dwellings both on the rim and at the base of the canyon. Owing to the great variation in temperature from the rim to the base, they stay on the rim in summer to catch the cool breeze and move to the warmth of the canyon floor in the winter. The canyon is crisscrossed with paths used by the Indians to maintain communication with others in the community. The Tarahumara live in isolated family units and come together occasionally for special events. They are world-renowned long-distance runners, owing to their dependence on foot travel on the steep mountain trails to maintain communication between families. They maintain a subsistence lifestyle, carving out steep fields on the mountainside in which they grow the corn that serves as the staple of their diet.

During the past 50 years, "progress" in the form of industrialization and modernization led to the development of one of the greatest engineering marvels of the world, the Chihuahua al Pacifico Railroad, running through the Copper Canyon on its way from Chihuahua, near the United States–Mexico border, to Los Mochis and Topolobampo, across the Gulf of California from Baja, California. With the railroad has come world accessibility to the natural wonder of the Copper Canyon and alternatives to the traditional subsistence farming lifestyle of the Tarahumara.

Scholars admire the beauty of this vanishing lifestyle and fear the effects of increasingly greater accessibility to the region and increased interest of outsiders in "improving" the lot of these people (Fontana, 1987; Gorney, 2008). Electricity has moved farther into the canyon, bringing with it washers, dryers, and television. Convenience foods have introduced hypertension, and increasing contact with outsiders has exposed the people to communicable diseases for which they have no immunity. One proposed development plan would bring commercial air travel into the area, while resort hotels would require as much water for one day as a Tarahumara family might use in a year.

Some say the world is entitled to be inspired by visiting one of the most beautiful unique regions on earth (autonomy), but also has an obligation to preserve a unique culture (respect for people). On the other hand, increased tourism has offered the Tarahumara an easier means to survive by surrounding the train and hawking their carvings and beautiful pine needle baskets to the tourists as they come through. The Tarahumara themselves express no qualms about enjoying some modern conveniences.

The effects of a persistent drought lasting several years prompted a thoughtful newspaper article in late 2012 in which the need for food relief (beneficence) was carefully analyzed with respect to its impact on autonomy and self-reliance of the Tarahumara people and their culture (MacCormack, 2012). Internationally published reports of high suicide rates turned out to be inaccurate, and general conditions appeared similar to those in other drought years. Persons with years of experience working with the Tarahumara expressed regret that the relief efforts focused on distribution of goods rather than plans for the future (MacCormack, 2012).

EVALUATION OF ETHICAL DECISIONS WITHIN A HUMAN NEEDS FRAMEWORK

Another interesting approach to examining ethical issues within the community-as-partner model is to use a human needs framework to evaluate the merit of a particular choice of action. In this context, the most basic (and perhaps, therefore, the highest priority) need would be physiological need, followed by safety, then belonging, self-esteem, and finally self-fulfillment (Maslow, 1970). It is arguable, however, whether this hierarchy also reflects a scale of priorities for any particular individual. The ethical dilemma may come down to valuing an individual's right to development of his or her fullest potential (autonomy) against the physiological or safety needs of the larger community. This dilemma is best illustrated in a discussion of access to and use of a scarce commodity: water.

Does an individual or group have the right to enjoy water for its beauty, while the community as a whole is in danger of running out of water for basic needs such as sanitation and drinking? The classic example is an upscale community in a desert region with a waterfall feature that loses substantial amounts of precious water through evaporation. Unrestricted home landscaping choices may also require excessive amounts of water; however, those plants may have particular significance and give a sense of well-being to people who have moved to a strange area. What responsibility does a developer have in terms of water infrastructure to ensure adequate water pressure to the adjoining community? How might water be fairly allocated if it is to be rationed—should each individual or each household be allowed a particular number of gallons? Should water conservation be required as a feature of all new construction?

Is access to water a right? Some unscrupulous developers have sold parcels of land with no infrastructure. Community activism has focused on bringing in water lines at no cost to the residents. But some residents do not want to pay for the hookups, nor for water usage at the going rate. Alternatives to sewer hookup include septic systems and solar composting toilets. However, well-meaning community development workers may run afoul of regulations, ordinances, and cultural preferences in trying to implement reasonable programs without sufficient research and background preparation.

Another example of conflict between individual self-fulfillment and community basic needs is the involvement of an increasing number of people in so-called extreme sports and other high-risk behaviors. For example, in addition to scuba diving, horseback riding, mountain climbing, ski jumping, and motorcycling, America's active, affluent adventurers are showing increased interest in personal light aircraft, mostly made at home and not inspected or requiring a pilot's license to operate. All these activities provide an outlet for self-actualization and stress relief. However, the costs to the emergency medical system are immense when the resources involved in a search-and-rescue mission are calculated, along with the costs of medical care. At what point does the individual assume the risk, and at what point do emergency medical services determine that the cost and risk are just too great to pursue a rescue? As the affluent population becomes larger and their leisure-time activities expand, this question will become evermore critical.

The second level of human need is security—one of the most common areas of concern identified by community residents on community assessment surveys. In the past, proposed interventions to improve public safety centered on close collaboration among law enforcement agencies in the community. However, as the level of violence has escalated, communities have started feeling less confident in the law enforcement's ability to manage the situation. One community reportedly passed an ordinance requiring all adult citizens to be armed. After publication of this ordinance, the crime rate markedly decreased.

Increased drug and migrant-related activities along the United States–Mexico border have left many residents disillusioned with the federal agencies charged with securing the border. Citizens complain about receiving no response when they call to report groups of individuals trespassing on private property. Concern for their personal and economic safety and security has led to the development of controversial groups of volunteer patrols that pledge to make the designated agencies respond by observing, notifying, and monitoring the response. The controversy centers on whether these groups actually are peaceful observers, as they claim, or vigilantes, and how they will be perceived by the federal agencies, the local landowners, and the persons they are seeking to apprehend. Some unfortunate incidents in the past have raised questions about how the groups will conduct themselves and how they will interface with the community and its law enforcement agencies.

Local residents also wonder about the motivation of people from other parts of the country who participate in this activity. Do they come as a patriotic gesture in the interest of homeland security or as participants in a thrill-seeking extreme sport substitute? Are they prepared for the climate, terrain, and culture of the area? What sort of training do they have? How will they handle the boredom of watching and waiting and the frustration of observing and not taking action? What will be the demands on local resources for both infrastructure and emergency response?

Summary

Working in partnership with communities requires careful consideration of all seven primary ethical principles and the interplay among them. Autonomy, respect for people, and nonmaleficence are the principles most often threatened by the community health nurse's commitment to beneficence. Conscious awareness of this risk and application of the principles of justice, both retributive and distributive; veracity; and fidelity will assist community health nurses to analyze the ethical principles at stake at any given decision-making point in their work with communities. Their actions, then, will reflect the best possible application of the principle of community as partner and will promote the optimal overall health of a community within its own culture.

Critical Thinking Questions

1. As a nurse, how do *you* define the relationship between yourself and those for whom you care? What word do you use to describe the other(s) in that relationship? Why? Which ethical values are supported and which are threatened by your concept of this relationship?

2. Analyze the ethical implications of a community health initiative to decrease the rate of teenage pregnancy by means of health education in the public schools. Consider the following ethical principles in your analysis: autonomy, beneficence, nonmaleficence, and justice.

3. Imagine that you live in a community with a large number of homeless people. The climate is mild, and people live openly in the streets and parks. A proposal is to come before the city council to strengthen the vagrancy ordinance in order to promote tourism. As a community health nurse working with the homeless, you have been asked to provide testimony. What will your position be and how will you defend it ethically? Prepare a 3-minute public testimony to address the issue.

4. What role might a community health nurse play in the community's deliberations regarding the presence of a volunteer security patrol group? How might you help the community prepare for likely sequelae?

5. As a nurse and business partner in a home health agency, how do you respond to a request for home health services for an 85-year-old client living 50 miles from any town? Will you be for or against providing such services in the client's home? Define the ethical, economic, and therapeutic reasons for your position.

REFERENCES

American Nurses Association. (2001). *Code of ethics with interpretive statements*. Washington, DC: Author.

American Public Health Association. (2002). *Public health code of ethics*. Washington, DC: Author.

Blacksher, E. (2008). Carrots and sticks to promote healthy behaviors: A policy update [Electronic version]. *Hastings Center Report, 38*(3), 13–16.

Daniels, N. (2006). Equity and population health: Toward a broader bioethics agenda [Electronic version]. *Hastings Center Report, 36*(4), 22–35.

Fontana, B. (1987). *Tarahumara: Where night is the day of the moon*. Tucson, AZ: University of Arizona Press.

Fry, S., & Veatch, R. (2010). *Case studies in nursing ethics* (4th ed.). Sudbury, MA: Jones & Bartlett.

Gadow, S. (1990). Existential advocacy: Philosophical foundations of nursing. In S. Spicker & S. Gadow (Eds.), *Nursing images and ideals* (pp. 79–101). New York, NY: Springer.

Gorney, C. (2008). A people apart: Modernity looms for the Sierra Madre's Tarahumara. *National Geographic, 214*(5), 78–101.

Hutchison, L., Hawes, C., & Williams, L. (2005). Access to quality health services in rural areas: Long term care. In L. Gamm & L. Hutchison (Eds.), *Rural healthy people 2010: A companion document to healthy people 2010* (Vol. 3). College Station, TX: The Texas A&M University System Health Science Center, School of Rural Public Health, Southwest Rural Health Research Center. Retrieved from www.srph.tamhsc.edu/centers/rhp2010

MacCormack, J. (2012, September 28). Mexico's Tarahumara are a people in need. *San Antonio Express News.*

Maslow, A. (1970). *Motivation and personality.* New York, NY: Harper & Row.

National Advisory Committee on Rural Health and Human Services. (2011). Reducing health disparities in rural America: Key provisions in the Affordable Care Act [Policy brief]. Retrieved from http://www.hrsa.gov/advisorycommittees/rural/publications/healthdisparities.pdf

National Rural Health Association. (2013). *What's different about rural health care?* Retrieved from www.ruralhealthweb.org/go/left/about-rural-health

O'Keefe, M. (2002). Ethics in nursing. In M. O'Keefe (Ed.), *Nursing practice and the law* (pp. 58–93). Philadelphia, PA: F. A. Davis.

Petrini, C., & Gainotti, S. (2008). A personalist approach to public-health ethics [Electronic version]. *Bulletin of the World Health Organization, 86*(8), 624–629.

Racher, F. (2007). The evolution of ethics for community practice [Electronic version]. *Journal of Community Health Nursing, 24*(1), 65–76.

Smith, M. A. (2010). *Access to health care among the elderly.* Retrieved from www.webnponline.com/articles/article_details/access-to-health-care-among-the-elderly/

U.S. Department of Health and Human Services. (2000). *Healthy People 2010: Understanding and improving health* (2nd ed.). Washington, DC: U.S. Government Printing Office. Retrieved from www.Healthypeople.gov/2010

U.S. Department of Health and Human Services. (2010). *Healthy People 2020: Improving the health of Americans.* Retrieved from www.healthypeople.gov/2020

CHAPTER 6

Community Empowerment

Bruce Leonard

LEARNING OBJECTIVES

Community empowerment provides a foundation for community health nurses to build partnerships with communities. This chapter provides an overview of how community health nurses may apply the theoretical components of empowerment in practice.

After studying this chapter, you will be able to:

1. Understand a framework for empowering communities through building partnerships with community members.

2. Develop an understanding of empowerment as an important concept in the development of community partnerships to resolve problems, create change, and increase community action to address health and social issues.

3. Apply a bottom-up, top-down approach through participatory research as a pathway to community empowerment for improved community health status.

Introduction

Partnerships between community members and health care professionals are critical for collaborative decisions that promote awareness and understanding of a community's health needs. Community health nursing has the potential to create relationships beyond the individual and develop program interventions that affect the community as a whole. Nurses have long been at the forefront of integrating health resources by forming partnerships with clients, families, and communities. Through the application and use of relationship building concepts such as empowerment, we can influence and reshape the environment to address health disparities among those who are most vulnerable in our society. The process by which nurses develop positive relationships in the community reflects interactions among the four major constructs of the nursing paradigm: health, environment, client, and nurse. Community health nurses serve a vital function in developing relationships that promote health and empower others to engage community members in collaborative efforts, partnerships, and coalitions.

This is essential to their professional practice to engage community members in collaborative efforts that affect their well-being.

Community health nursing focuses on health, caring, and relationship building among community members. Community involvement is one of the critical elements of successful problem solving with communities. A basic component of community empowerment is that the community defines its own agenda. The role of the community health nurse involves collaboration and forming partnerships to address problems related to health and social issues (Kulbok, Thatcher, Park, & Meszaros, 2012). Community participation is a crucial element to engage community members to develop agendas that serve as a cohesive force to mobilize community toward a process of change. For social change to be long term and relevant to the needs of a community, it must come from the community members themselves (Laverack, 2006). Community empowerment works like a catalyst in creating a sense of readiness to mobilize forces among community members or groups to engage in active community interventions to build relationships.

PERSPECTIVES ON COMMUNITY HEALTH PARTNERSHIPS

Community partnership programs have not always been equitably distributed nor thought of as essential to community members. Many community health programs of the 1960s emphasized processes of community participation led by academic experts who were in control of health programs and who set the agenda for the types of programs offered within communities (Hanks, 2006). These programs often failed because they lacked true community commitment and involvement. A major lesson learned from failures in the past has been that effective partnerships require active community participation, community ownership and control of programs, and continual relationship building.

More recently, community health professionals have placed a new emphasis on having communities solve their own problems with guidance from experts by forming partnership alliances. The ideas of community participation as a model for community health initiatives in the 1960s and 1970s now focus upon ideas of partnership, collaboration, community empowerment, and community capacity (Fraser, Dougill, Mabee, Reed, & McAlpine, 2006). Rather than allow self-interests of experts to guide a community, partnerships work by integrating the community's ideas, people, and resources in both the development and implementation processes. A community's level of commitment and involvement may be increased by capacity-building in allowing them to gain knowledge, learn skills, and gain confidence to improve their health through partnerships (Raeburn, Akerman, Chuengsatiansup, Mejia, & Oladepo, 2007). The act of creating partnerships is a complex process of bringing together academics, community leaders, and health care providers to accomplish change. Effective partnerships require a sharing of power and decision making along with feedback mechanisms to assure understanding among all parties for successful implementation of community health promotion programs (Hanks, 2006). We will examine how nurses might use these concepts to expand upon nursing interventions for initiating social change.

Partnerships not only are important in implementing community-based programs, but must also be culturally sensitive to ensure success. When implementing a program, we need to assist communities in ways that match their perception of health problems. Partnership programs often fail if there is conflict between the health care provider's and the community's belief systems. We define our own health and illness beliefs based on our cultural and ethnic backgrounds, and on our own perceptions of how to be healthy or recognize illness (Drew, 2011).

Historically, nurses have had a rich practice in the community, transforming both individual and public health for the poor and disenfranchised through political advocacy. Lillian Wald (1915), who coined the term *public health nurse* in 1893, provides probably our prime example of working with communities to improve health. During the latter half of the 20th century, however, nurses have primarily been employed in hospitals rather than in communities. Our historical focus of nursing in the community has been replaced by "site-managed care systems" such as hospitals, and primary care clinics that require the client to come to a facility rather than the nurse providing care within the community. Although many nurses today are employed by organizations that provide home health care, community health nursing is more than just providing health care to an individual, but focuses upon the aggregate population in providing *primary health care* as opposed to primary care. The concept of *primary health care*, as defined in Chapter 1, embraces the ideals of the World Health Organization's Alma-Ata declaration (World Health Organization, Health for All, 1978) of providing essential health care based on the needs of the community emphasizing health and well-being as a fundamental right for all.

Modern health care emphasizes individualized medical care as opposed to providing aggregate community-based health care. Our present "system" of health care has not served our profession well, and has resulted in fragmented programs and limited return on improving the overall health in communities. In many respects, modern day nurses who work for large hospital-based institutions whose focus of care has been on the individual have lost their unique voice, innovation, and drive to be proactive in community affairs. Nurses frequently remain silent to what is going on around them in the community; however, what goes on in the community is really the pulse that drives our health care needs. Our challenge as community health nurses is to transform our health care system into one that reflects the values and needs of our communities based on the concepts of *primary health care.*

Community nurses may transform our fragmented system of individualized health care by reformulating a vision for the future. We must look beyond our past and explore new avenues aimed at improvement of health for all. Rather than focusing on disease-specific problems, we should explore developing new programs with a community focus on providing primary health care. People in communities deserve comprehensive nursing care aimed at improvement of health and quality of life. Health in this country cannot be improved just by providing health services, but needs to be based on principles of equity, participation, and involvement of communities in making decisions about health care. Successful participation implies negotiation without manipulation and equity in relationships between community members and health care workers who embrace common goals in providing health care with accessible programs and service for all.

EMPOWERMENT THROUGH COMMUNITY PARTICIPATION

Community participation is a social process involving people from specific geographic localities who share common values in identifying their needs (Rifkin, 1986). Participation in formulating the framework for primary health care in a community may lead not only to better services but also to services based on existing socioeconomic conditions. Rifkin (1986) described three approaches to community participation in health programs commonly used by different countries (Fig. 6.1). One is the medical approach, which is focused on curing diseases and is controlled by the medical profession. The second is a health services approach, which mobilizes people to take an active role in the delivery of services based on modifying unhealthy behaviors. The third is a community development approach in which people are involved in the decision-making process to improve health. The first two approaches to health care are top-down approaches where experts prescribe their values of health care for the public. The third approach is a grassroots approach in which members within the community determine what health care services should be provided. It is more consistent with the principles of primary health care.

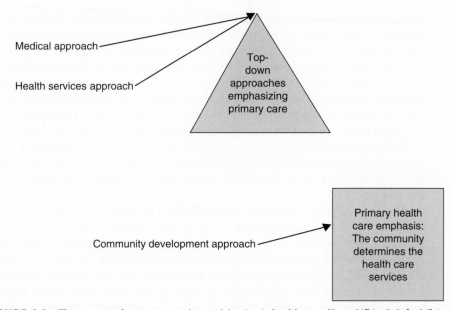

FIGURE 6.1   Three approaches to community participation in health care. (From Rifkin, S. B. [1986]. Lessons from community participation programs. *Health Policy and Planning, 1*, 240–249.)

Essential components for community participation include the following: (1) a framework to define the community; (2) shared awareness by members of the community; and (3) mechanisms to mobilize the community to recognize its needs and develop a culture of participation (Meleis, 1992). Through empowerment, community health nurses can enable people to make decisions and to act on issues they believe are essential to their health or well-being.

Empowerment through participation has three essential components to which nurses must be sensitive in order for community transformations to occur (Box 6.1). First, participation is an active process, not a process where one group or organization imposes its values on the community, but a process of mutuality where all have a voice. Second, participation involves choice, implying people have the right and the power to make decisions that affect their lives. Third, the decisions made through participation must have the possibility of being effective, and there are social systems to allow decisions to be implemented. Community participation, according to Rifkin, Muller, and Bichmann (1988, p. 933), "is a social process whereby specific groups with shared needs living in a defined geographical area actively pursue identification of their needs, make decisions and establish mechanisms to meet these needs."

The role of the nurse in community empowerment is to build effective partnerships through community participation. Only our imagination, vision, and moral or ethical values limit the climate of empowerment we create. Central to professional nursing is building human relationships that preserve human dignity of human-to-human caring (Watson, 2006).

Box 6.1 **Essential Elements of Community Empowerment**

- Active process (one that is nonjudgmental and characterized by mutuality)
- Choice (right to make decisions)
- Effective participation (decisions are implemented)

DEVELOPING RIGHT-RELATIONSHIPS

Nurses relate to clients, communities, and families on many psychosocial levels. In the development of a nurse–client relationship, nurses interact with clients and communities. For true relationships to develop, there must be a balance of unconditional acceptance between the nurse and the client as a whole person. The transformation of becoming whole is what Quinn (1997) identifies as the right-relationship among one or more levels of the human system. Right-relationship is defined "as any pattern of organization within the system that supports, encourages, allows, or generates actualization and self-transcendence—at any and all levels" (Quinn, 1997, pp. 2–3). Nurses play a critical role in the process of assisting communities, families, and individuals in the process of becoming whole as they facilitate right-relationships. The development of the right-relationship is not an ethical or moral judgment, but a pattern of organization that generates self-transcendence or self-actualization.

Communities are composed of many core groups and subsystems in the community-as-partner model. Community health nurses assist community members by transforming relationships. If relationships are limited or confined to the elements where "academic experts" maintain control of the health care resources through either medical or health care services approaches, as identified earlier by Rifkin (1986), that emphasize primary care, communities may not be able to maximize their human potentials to become proactive for positive outcomes to occur. Although the "primary care model" of health care strives for predictable outcomes in curing disease, people may be left out in the process. If nurses do not develop right-relationships with communities, community members may not be able to maximize their potential to become empowered.

In the traditional "primary care" approach to health care, community health care workers viewed community members as sources for data gathering or recipients of care. The conventional approach to health care has resulted in fragmented or unwanted programs, with community members as passive participants. Community health partnerships, by contrast, emphasize active participation by community members and health care workers not only from a variety of disciplines, but from every relevant segment of society. The goal for community health care workers, then, should be to empower community members to visualize their needs and actively participate in planning and implementing needed change—the tenets of primary health care.

TRANSFORMING COMMUNITIES THROUGH EMPOWERMENT

How can nurses assist communities to expand their resources? Empowerment means different things to different people and depends on the context. Community participation exists on many levels that may range from passive compliance by acceptance of the status quo to true shared decision making (Schwab & Syme, 1997). Empowerment is an avenue for communities to gain control of resources and transform inequities of power through social change. Only through the ability to organize and mobilize community forces can individuals, groups, and communities achieve social and political change necessary to rectify their powerlessness (Laverack & Wallerstein, 2001). Empowerment enables people to take control of their lives and community resources. Nurses work to empower communities not for domination or control of people, but rather to facilitate the development of others to promote change.

Dialogue is a critical element for community transformations to occur. All voices in a community are important. Paulo Freire (1997), a Brazilian educator, contributed philosophic and theoretical writings on empowering people through education to reverse the dehumanization and objectification of oppressed people. His concerns deal primarily with class oppression, but his philosophies have been applied to empowerment of professions such as nurses, feminist theory, and vulnerable populations among communities at risk for poor health.

Community partnerships develop through a process of empowerment. Four characteristics of an empowered community (conceptualized from Paulo Freire's *Pedagogy of the Oppressed*, 1997) follow:

- Faith in people
- Trust established through dialogue
- Hope in positive transformations benefiting the community as a whole
- Discussions grounded in critical thinking without fear of repercussions by those who are in power

Freire (1997) hypothesizes that dialogue or communication between people is the key to empowerment. Each of the empowerment characteristics is discussed below.

Faith in people implies that all people have the *potential* to provide a voice in community affairs. Faith in humanity encourages a commitment between community members to create and transform the bonds of human communities and interconnect those who live on the fringes or are the most vulnerable to the whole of society. Vulnerability includes individuals or communities who are camouflaged in our society, such as the homeless, chronically disabled, immigrants, or low-income single parents. Vulnerable populations are at great risk in society for harm to occur and are often those with the least social capital. The risk encountered by the vulnerable is generally not voluntary or under their control. The more risk encountered, the more vulnerable the person or population becomes. Vulnerability leads to symptoms of victimization, alienation, helplessness, or powerlessness, all opposite approaches to empowerment.

Freire (1997) believes that faith in people through dialogue is a primary component in transforming those who are most vulnerable to be empowered, but we cannot have dialogue without *trust*. Trust in people is founded on the principles of truth and integrity in our words. Many well-intentioned community projects have failed through false leadership of people saying one thing or designing projects for their own personal reality, ignoring those the project is intended to serve, or performing actions not congruent with their behaviors. Trust occurs when people meet in cooperation to transform ideas into a reality and are committed to making a difference or create change.

Hope is another vital component of empowerment (Freire, 1997). Hope engenders a sense of inner strength that propels people to act, mobilize forces, and envision a better tomorrow. Hope is all encompassing in providing people protection against despair, and gives them strength, as well as determination to live, when misfortunes in life occur. Empowerment through hope inspires an ability to move beyond the present difficulties and see a future with possibilities. Empowerment through hope is not an entity of imagination acquired while sitting still, but rather a transformational process fought for with conviction. Empowerment is not an instant transformation, but a slow process of weaving thin threads of society together through dialogue like a spider weaves a web.

Trust, faith, and hope are significant concepts that relate closely to developing relationships, but it is through the process of critical thinking and evaluation that people are ultimately empowered. For empowerment and communication to be successful, people must engage in critical thinking, continually evaluating and reevaluating the premises behind their thoughts (Freire, 1997). People need to be free to exchange ideas, weighing the positive and negative impacts of change on themselves or their communities. As new realities emerge, people must critically evaluate their world and not remain blind or naive to those who are most vulnerable in our communities. Naive thinking justifies maintaining the "status quo" or the continual oppression of those who are at the greatest risk for harm to occur. For social inequalities to change, we must develop new abilities through education to influence others and transform our communities.

Empowerment is gained through critical dialogue and reflection of critical thought, not necessarily from what is known. It is a process of going from the known to the unknown and reflecting on the possible, with hope for a better tomorrow. Without critical dialogue, true learning ceases to exist and only knowledge—not wisdom—is passed between the empowered and the oppressed. Critical thinking encourages the transformation of knowledge into wisdom for those who are most vulnerable. The wisdom gained through critical thought, faith, trust, and hope in humanity may transform social structures from ones of oppression to powerful communities with a voice (Fig. 6.2).

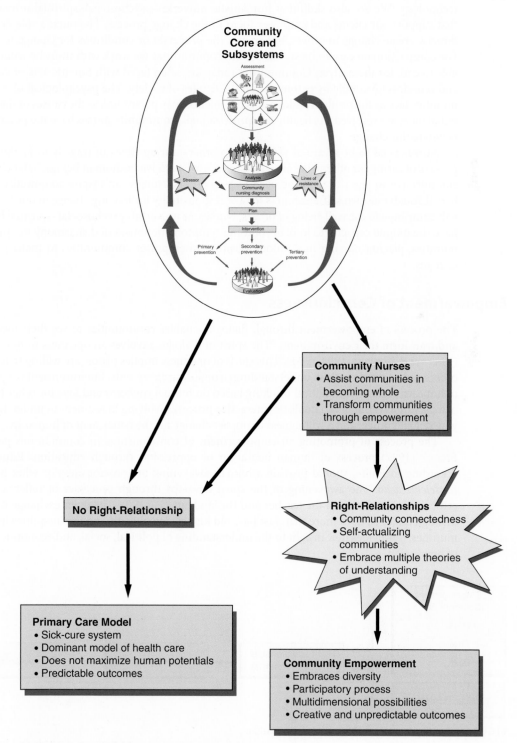

FIGURE 6.2   Model for community empowerment.

EMPOWERING COMMUNITIES

Community health nurses are responsible for caring for and supporting communities, families, and individuals as they respond to health, violence, or dissonance within society. Nurses are skilled in compassionate caring and the application of scientific knowledge and technology. We are also skillful at humanistic universal–psychosocial–spiritual interactions that support our clients and empower them in the change process. The nurse's role does not directly create change in others, but creates the processes or conditions for change to occur. For compassionate care to be sustained, the communities we work with must be willing and able to care for themselves. Communities today are often faced with horrific acts of violence and senseless loss of life by extremists on the fringes of society. The psychological scars communities face as the result of sudden acts of violence may persist unless the causes of the social imbalances are resolved. As health care professionals, community nurses have the potential to facilitate this change.

Nurses need to be aware of ways to help others during times of tragedy to facilitate the process of caring for others. We also need to care for ourselves as human beings, balancing our commitment to practice with the need to help others. Nurses can inspire community members through our own self-awareness to take responsibility for making change in our lives that will contribute to the well-being of others. Nurses, as universal–psychosocial–spiritual beings, have the unique capacity to look beyond the symptomatic causes of disharmony in our communities, placing nursing in a unique position to empower communities to make positive changes.

Empowerment of Consciousness

The process of empowerment through dialogue enables communities to see their inequities and transform their environment. "The spirit of dialogue involves an openness to new ideas" (Koerner & Bunkers, 1994, p. 51). This spirit of openness implies people are willing to listen to others and negotiate with an understanding of opposing viewpoints. Empowerment is a process of hope, trust, faith, and critical thinking based on mutual concerns and love for other human beings. Empowerment is a dualistic interactive process involving investment in understanding yourself and others and a willingness to impact change for the betterment of humanity.

The process of promoting an empowerment of consciousness in communities parallels Freire's (1997) process of human liberation of oppression through education. Education, according to Freire, should provide a human awakening of consciousness or what he calls *conscientizacao*. The awakening of the spirit develops through processes of reflection and critical thinking between the teacher and the students (Fig. 6.3). The open exchange of ideas through dialogue does more than just pass old knowledge in justifying the inequities in communities; it provides new insight to the understanding of political, social, and economic forces of oppression.

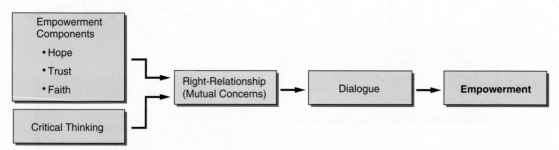

FIGURE 6.3   Key components for social transformation.

In the modern Western paradigm of the world, "a person is merely in the world, not with the world or with others; the individual is spectator, not re-creator" (Freire, 1997, p. 56). In the postmodern paradigm of community health nursing, only our imaginations and our own fears limit reality. Empowerment is essential to the nursing process. Nursing is a profession based on mutual understanding of clients, families, and communities. Empowerment provides the force of liberation for communities to reconcile forces of oppression and transform the human consciousness to awaken our capacities for humility, love, and cooperation. For empowerment to emerge as a new consciousness, community health nurses must engage in active, critical dialogue that promotes understanding, cooperation, and critical reflection of community aspirations. Nurses may institute global change through the application of the concept of empowerment and help our communities achieve their hopes and dreams.

Transformation of Global Community

The transformative process of empowering a community through the integration of humanistic relationships by community health nurses has the potential to change the global environment of health care and promote healthy environments for all. The community development approach to health care involves empowerment participation by all members of society regardless of culture, social status, gender, or ethnicity. As the world shrinks through instantaneous global communication, we are exposed daily, through the news media, to inequities in our global environment. We are able to witness firsthand the adversities of war, famine, drug abuse, unemployment, genocide, murder, and lack of health care worldwide. Community health nurses must not remain blind to these inequities, but advocate transforming our societies into communities based on principles of trust, hope, love, and faith in humanity.

Our unique vantage point as nurses is our ability to communicate, dialogue, and form partnerships with clients, families, and communities. Nurses are in a prime position to chart a new course for the delivery of health care and resolve many of the social injustices for the world's disenfranchised through empowerment.

EMPOWERING A COMMUNITY THROUGH PARTICIPATORY ACTION RESEARCH

One method community health nurses may employ in empowering a community to focus on health problems is participatory research. This is performed through collaboration between health professionals and community members. Participatory research is problem-focused or context-specific research centered on a particular problem involving all participants. Participatory research is similar to action research in which each person or group engaged in the process is committed to improvement through continuous interaction among dialogue, research, action, reflection, and evaluation (Hart & Anthrop, 1996). Individuals are active participants in change and are not passive objects. Through participatory research, community members can gain skills to critically think and analyze the health concerns of their community.

Participatory research is a form of emancipatory inquiry that addresses inequities and injustices in health and society. This is a research method community health nurses may employ in empowering a community to focus on health problems (Aston & Meagher-Stewart, 2009; Fraser et al., 2006). It incorporates conversations that produce both collaboration and self-awareness between nurses and their community. The methods of participatory research incorporate scientific research, education, and political action developed primarily out of the works of Freire (1997). Critical theory and feminist theory underlie the emancipatory process. Critical theory emphasizes a critical analytic approach to discussing social problems by active reflection and synthesis through continuous dialogue. In understanding the social and political patterns of oppression, community members may be able to facilitate change using processes of engagement, collaboration, cooperation, reflection, and evaluation (Corbett, Francis, & Chapman, 2007). Feminist theory shares many of the humanistic values of nursing based on concepts of caring, intuitiveness, and valuing others' worldviews and experiences (Meleis, 1997). A feminist perspective provides a powerful language to enhance our understanding or to provide insights for social change.

Wallerstein (1999) identifies six core principles of participatory and action research. These include: (1) the participants in the research project are the ones who determine the research agenda; (2) the research project should be one that benefits the community as a whole, and allows community members to make informed decisions and act collectively; (3) the relationship between health care experts and community members should be a collaborative effort based upon the principles of shared dialogue (Freire, 1997); (4) community members should have access to all information and knowledge from which they might normally be excluded; (5) the process should be democratic and empower the participation of a wide range of community members; and (6) community members and the researchers should strive to achieve mutual goals.

The goal of participatory research is social change, not just the advancement of new scientific knowledge. Emancipatory inquiry is designed to have a direct effect on the lives of all participants in the research process, not just the life of the researcher. Individuals involved in participatory nursing research are able to explore how inequities in society are linked to their own health and, therefore, are enabled to act on this knowledge through empowerment (Henderson, 1995).

The Nurse's Role in Participatory Research Programs

In instituting participatory research programs, nurses help communities identify, understand, find solutions, and determine common goals in resolving community problems. The problems examined through emancipatory inquiry are those that community members believe are important and not necessarily those identified by health professionals in the community. Nurses are challenged to awaken the spirit of social change among those who are most vulnerable in our communities. Emancipatory inquiry provides a framework to expand the political consciousness of the disenfranchised in a community. As Henderson (1995) reminds us, "The goal of emancipatory inquiry is neither prediction nor understanding, but emancipation, both within the research process and within society" (p. 64).

Community health nurses can be the eyes and ears of a community. We have considerable credibility in the community as health professionals. Our clinical and educational experiences guide us in assessing the pulse of our surroundings. We have numerous tools for implementing change in the community environment based on theory and experience. Nurses have strong interpersonal communication skills, understand the importance of client–nurse relationships, are willing to learn from others, and know how to maximize the health resources of a community. Through our professional encounters with clients, we learn to solve problems almost intuitively and attempt to fix them before harm occurs. Our solutions are not always the right answer if the end result is not congruent with the views or beliefs of those affected. A better solution is to empower the community to resolve its problems while at the same time expanding their resources. Participatory research is an excellent method for nurses to implement change, even on a small scale.

Developing a Participatory Research Program

An example of participatory research by the community health nurse might be your recognition of the importance of informing clients of influenza vaccines for seniors during the flu season while working at a senior center checking blood pressures in a low-income, African American neighborhood. In talking with clients, you may find that very few in this community have had flu shots, but many have friends who died last year or were seriously ill from influenza. The seniors seem very concerned in light of many news broadcasts predicting a major flu epidemic. You assess that this may be an important health issue to bring up at the monthly board of directors of the senior center meeting next week.

On the way back to the local public health department, you decide to stop by the epidemiology department to examine the community statistics related to influenza over the past few years. In analyzing the data, it is evident that low-income seniors in the county had a death rate 50% higher than those with higher income. The death rate for seniors living near the senior center where you were taking blood pressures was significantly higher than in the rest of the city. The data also indicate that there is an overall higher death rate for senior African Americans within the county. You feel compelled to act because this is a significant health problem where nursing might make a difference.

Over the next week, you do a literature search and put together a proposal to present to the senior center's executive board members to develop a participatory research influenza immunization program with the support of the public health department. You reflect on how to make your proposal successful, knowing there are several barriers. A potential barrier identified is to make the program culturally sensitive to the African American community. Many seniors around this senior center have limited access to health care, lack transportation, and have minimal understanding of the importance of influenza vaccinations. Your literature search, as well as the experience of your practice, reveals some key issues related to the African American communities. Religion is central in their lives; cultural beliefs and health practices are often underutilized, regardless of their impact on well-being; and family support networks and informal health care systems play important roles in maintaining health during periods of stress or crises (Russell & Jewell, 1992). The community health diagnosis for this proposal might be: decreased influenza immunization rate of senior African Americans living in this community related to (1) cultural barriers, (2) low socioeconomic status, (3) attitudes, and (4) lack of resources for health promotion and disease prevention, as manifested by statistical evidence of high mortality rates and low immunization rates.

Your proposal includes a conceptual framework for increasing the effectiveness of an immunization program for the senior center based on the components of the community-as-partner model. The plan incorporates African American cultural values relating to health and illness practices. The strategies include three main components. One involves increasing the active participation of community members from the senior center in the program design, implementation, and evaluation process. The second includes strategies to tap into the established formal and informal community networks, and the third is structuring the plan to be culturally sensitive with the assistance of the executive board of the senior center as well as religious leaders in the community.

A fundamental component of your proposal is how to empower senior African Americans to receive their flu immunizations through health promotion. Health promotion entails motivating the community, families, and individuals toward obtaining their optimum state of well-being, health, or happiness. The strategies should encourage the best quality of life, with goals toward continuous improvement in the overall health of the community. The health status of a community is directly related to the individual health-related behaviors and environmental conditions, and is indirectly affected by environmental factors, which influence health behaviors (Brown, 1991). Communities can directly influence their health status by targeting individual health-related behaviors and can change health-damaging environments to health-promoting environments. Brown states, "The ultimate objective of community action for health promotion must be to empower people to improve their individual and collective health" (p. 455).

Three essential elements of health promotion identified by Brown (1991) involve (1) encouraging individuals to change and sustain personal behaviors that prevent disease and promote healthy lifestyles, (2) encouraging health-promoting behaviors that discourage health-damaging behaviors of individuals, and (3) creating an environment that promotes health by eliminating health hazards from the physical environment. According to Brown, most health promotion programs focus on encouraging individuals to change their health behaviors, but seldom look at empowering people to change the lifestyle or environment that shapes their behavior and influences their lifestyle. The goal is to increase the number of seniors immunized against the flu, and the objectives are to assist seniors to overcome their fears of immunizations, increase seniors' knowledge about the flu, increase their political power, and improve their physical health. The community-as-partner model, the concepts outlined for developing a participatory action research plan, and Brown's theory of health promotion are several tools community health nurses can use to promote change.

With the approval of the executive board of the senior center, the nursing interventions to meet the objectives of the immunization project are focused on participatory research emphasizing education and focus group community interaction. The strategies addressed in the focus groups to make the program successful highlight clarification of information on flu immunizations, stressing healthy outcomes, keeping the message culturally sensitive, and decreasing fears of the vaccine.

The missing component in our discussion on developing a participatory research program for our immunization project is the ethic of connectedness or developing the right-relationship with the senior African American community members. We have mentioned the critical component of cultural sensitivity, but we need to focus our energies on building relationships in the process of participatory research. The relationships nurses develop in the processes of human interactions are critical to the success of all community programs. We cannot ignore the political, social, environmental, cultural, and economic relationships among all community members. How we interact with communities on all social levels has an impact on our ability to provide a voice to those who are most vulnerable in our society. Community health nurses are morally responsible to provide a voice that maintains a dialogue of caring and builds a dynamic of empowered connectedness within the community-as-partner model.

Summary

Community nurses can provide the critical conscience of health in a community. As a group, nurses can provide the bonding capital and bridging capital for community members to work together effectively to achieve common goals for improved community health and quality of life. Empowerment requires active community participation by community members and formal organizations to work together to achieve mutually agreed upon outcomes based upon trust. Empowerment is not just a program nurses create, but a process enabled by community health nurses to transform thinking through dialogue. Only through continued activism can nurses expose the social injustices that continue to contribute to powerless communities. Through community empowerment, nurses can provide a moral voice to inspire change to regain our historical roots as vanguards of the community.

Critical Thinking Questions

1. How might you apply empowerment in your community nursing practice?
2. What are the essential processes for empowerment to occur within a community?
3. As a nurse, how might you describe empowerment as a transformational process?

REFERENCES

Aston, M., & Meagher-Stewart, D. (2009). Public health nurses' primary health care practice: Strategies for fostering citizen participation. *Journal of Community Health Nursing, 26,* 24–34.

Brown, R. E. (1991). Community action for health promotion: A strategy to empower individuals and communities. *International Journal of Health Services, 21*(3), 441–456.

Corbett, A. M., Francis, K., & Chapman, Y. (2007). Feminist-informed participatory action research: A methodology of choice for examining critical nursing issues. *International Journal of Nursing Practice, 13,* 81–88.

Drew, J. C. (2011). Cultural competence: Common ground for partnerships in health care. In: E. T. Anderson & J. McFarlane (Eds.), *Community as partner theory and practice in nursing* (6th ed., pp. 103–118). Philadelphia, PA: Wolters Kluwer.

Fraser, E. D. G., Dougill, A. J., Mabee, W. E., Reed, M., & McAlpine, P. (2006). Bottom up and top down: Analysis of participatory process for sustainability indicator identification as a pathway to community empowerment and sustainable environmental management. *Journal of Environmental Management, 78,* 114–127.

Freire, P. (1997). *Pedagogy of the oppressed* (New rev. 20th-anniversary ed.). New York, NY: Continuum.

Hanks, C. A. (2006). Community empowerment: A partnership approach to public health program implementation. *Policy, Politics, and Nursing Practice, 7*(4), 297–306.

Hart, E., & Anthrop, C. (1996). Action research as a professionalizing strategy: Issues and dilemmas. *Journal of Advanced Nursing, 23*(3), 454–461.

Henderson, D. J. (1995). Consciousness raising in participatory research: Method and methodology for emancipatory nursing inquiry. *Advances in Nursing Science, 17*(3), 58–69.

Koerner, J. G., & Bunkers, S. S. (1994). The healing web an expansion of consciousness. *Journal of Holistic Nursing, 12*(1), 51–63.

Kulbok, P. A., Thatcher, E., Park, E., & Meszaros, P. S. (2012). Evolving public health nursing roles: Focus on community participatory health promotion and prevention. *Online Journal of Issues in Nursing, 17*(2), 1.

Laverack, G. (2006). Improving health outcomes through community empowerment: A review of the literature. *Journal of Health Population and Nutrition, 24*(1), 113–120.

Laverack, G., & Wallerstein, N. (2001). Measuring community empowerment: A fresh look at organizational domains. *Health Promotion International, 16*(2), 179–185.

Meleis, A. I. (1992). Community participation and involvement, theoretical and emperical issues. *Health Services Management Research, 5*(1), 5–6.

Meleis, A. I. (1997). *Theoretical nursing: Development & progress* (3rd ed.). Philadelphia, PA: Lippincott.

Quinn, J. F. (1997). Healing: A model for an integrative health care system. *Advanced Practice Nursing Quarterly, 3*(1), 1–6.

Raeburn, J., Akerman, M., Chuengsatiansup, K., Mejia, F., & Oladepo, O. (2007). Community capacity building and health promotion in a globalized world. *Health Promotion International, 21*(S1), 84–90.

Rifkin, S. B. (1986). Lessons from community participation programs. *Health Policy and Planning, 1,* 240–249.

Rifkin, S. B., Muller, F., & Bichmann, W. (1988). Primary health care: On measuring participation. *Social Science and Medicine an International Journal, 26*(9), 931–940.

Russell, K. J., & Jewell, N. (1992). Cultural impact of health-care access: Changes for improving the health of African Americans. *Journal of Community Health Nursing, 9*(3), 161–169.

Schwab, M., & Syme, L. (1997). On paradigms, commuinty participation, and the future of public health. *American Journal of Public Health, 87,* 2049–2052.

Wald, L. (1915). *The house on Henry Street.* New York, NY: Henry Holt.

Wallerstein, N. (1999). Power between evaluator and community: Research relationships within New Mexico's healthier communities. *Social Science & Medicine, 49*(1), 39–53.

Watson, J. (2006). Caring theory as an ethical guide to administrative clinical practices. *Nursing Administration Quarterly, 30*(1), 48–55.

World Health Organization, Health for All. (1978). *World Health Organization primary health care. Report of the international conference on primary health care.* Alma Alta, USSR: World Health Organization.

CHAPTER 7

Cultural Competence: Discussion and Tools for Action

Judith C. Drew

LEARNING OBJECTIVES

This chapter discusses the concept of cultural competence as a primary factor in providing quality health care to all people, regardless of their ethnic and cultural backgrounds. Theoretical perspectives on culture, ethnicity, diversity, and cultural health care systems are presented to provide health professionals with tools needed to build cultural competence in themselves, service agencies, and the larger community.

After studying this chapter, you should be able to:

1. Describe the influence culture and ethnicity have upon an individual's recognition of and responses to health and illness conditions.

2. Discuss the role cultural competence plays in meeting the overarching goals of Healthy People 2020 and specific objectives for health education and community-based programs.

3. Describe the characteristics of culturally competent individuals, health care systems, and communities at large.

4. Assess the role your own cultural identity has in the development of your cultural competence as a health professional.

5. Recommend specific changes that you, your employer, and the larger community can make to deliver culturally competent health care that achieves health equity, eliminates disparities, and improves the health of all groups.

Introduction

Cultural competence has gained attention over the past several decades as a vital strategy for improving health care quality for all people regardless of race, ethnicity, culture, and language proficiency. Affirming the need for cultural competence in all health care providers is the fact that cultural and ethnic diversity among health professionals has failed to keep pace with the ever-changing US population (Condon et al., 2013; Reyes, Hadley, & Davenport, 2013), thus laying the groundwork for health disparities, patient–provider misunderstandings, and poor health outcomes.

Cultural competency is evident when all people are treated in ways that respect their uniqueness and preserve their dignity. It goes beyond simple awareness of similarities and differences in ours and another's cultural beliefs and practices. Being culturally competent means that we understand how cultural and ethnic beliefs and practices influence our daily lives, and recognize that people with cultural backgrounds different from our own have unique values, life ways, health practices, and interpersonal styles (Betancourt, Green, Carrillo, & Park, 2005; Engebretson, Mahoney, & Carlson, 2008). The culturally competent health professional has the skills to use this knowledge effectively, to set aside "ethnocentric" views, and provide culturally sensitive care that improves the health of all people.

As health care providers, we must make the commitment to learn actively and use the knowledge and skills needed to work competently with culturally diverse clients, their families, and communities (Kleinman & Benson, 2006; Unger & Schwartz, 2012). Such imperatives are consistent with the goals and objectives of *Healthy People 2020* (*HP 2020*), our nation's health promotion and disease prevention agenda. During the past two decades, more and more emphasis has been placed upon the problem of health disparities, defined by the U.S. Department of Health and Human Services (USDHHS) as a type of health difference or disadvantage that adversely affects groups of people based on any characteristic historically linked to bias and discrimination (USDHHS, Office of Minority Health, 2010). An overarching goal in *Healthy People 2000* (*HP 2000*) was aimed at reducing disparities among Americans. In *Healthy People 2010* (*HP 2010*), the goal was expanded even further: to achieve health equity, eliminate disparities, and improve the health of all groups (USDHHS, Office of Disease Prevention and Health Promotion, 2013). Instrumental to the success of *HP 2020* is the continued growth of cultural competence education and implementation for professionals, agencies, and communities that can significantly improve access to quality care and reduce disparities by designing health promotion programs and illness intervention services that are available, acceptable, and appropriate to the cultures they seek to serve.

A growing body of evidence indicates that one of the major reasons that health services remain inaccessible and underutilized by some ethnic and cultural group members is that the services are not responsive to the needs of those they intend to serve (Alegria, Atkins, Farmer, Slaton, & Stelk, 2010; Renzaho, Romios, Crock, & Sunderland, 2013). The health services are not culturally competent. Reducing and eventually eliminating disparities depends on building common ground among clients, providers, agencies, and communities so that culturally competent health care services can grow in number and quality. Efforts to develop these competencies and partnerships must accelerate if we are to meet the health challenges of our ever-changing population demographics (American Association of Colleges of Nursing [AACN], 2013b; Loftin, Newman, Gilden, Bond, & Dumas, 2013; Siegel et al., 2011; Trickett, 2009).

The demographic composition of the US population will continue to change dramatically for the next several decades. Experts suggest that growth in racial and ethnic group diversity will continue at a rapid rate throughout the 21st century, causing descendants of European whites to become the *new minority* (U.S. Census Bureau National Population Projections [US-CBNPP], 2012). As a result of these trends, health care providers will interact more frequently with clients of diverse ethnic and cultural backgrounds whose health beliefs, languages, and life experiences differ greatly from their own. Therefore, to help us prepare to meet the health needs of our ever-changing population, this chapter offers descriptions of concepts and strategies that will assist you in building cultural competence, beginning with an enlightened awareness of diversity, ethnicity, and culture, and in illustrating their influence on individuals' and communities' health and illness beliefs and practices. Self-assessment and an analysis of client–provider interactions are presented as learning experiences with implications for practice. After all, successful health promotion and illness intervention outcomes depend on our abilities to competently reach and work effectively with the diverse individuals and communities we serve.

DIVERSITY, ETHNICITY, AND CULTURE

Derived from the Latin *divertere*, meaning *to turn in opposite directions*, diversity is the condition of being different or having differences. No attempt is made here to imply a ranking, ordering, or prioritizing of differences; they simply exist. How we look at and deal with differences in human attributes can either build bridges or construct barriers between individuals in and across groups and communities. Rather than considering differences as sources of conflict, we should view them as part of the whole of social and individual identity. A celebration of differences can become commonplace when we understand that the principal strengths on which our country is built suggest a tolerance for individual uniqueness and a collective creativity.

Recognizing that each of us differs in what we consider functional in our lives, we must understand that those who act differently from the mainstream are not deficient in something or "disadvantaged"; they are rich in a different culture and are "other-advantaged" (Madrid, 1988). In daily practice, nurses provide care to patients and families who represent our global communities. Yet we know little about the basic cultures, beliefs, and values that shape our clients' health and healing beliefs and behaviors. As our clients and our health care settings become increasingly multicultural, care providers across all disciplines must understand the role culture plays in determining health and illness needs and behaviors, and strive to become culturally competent (AACN, 2013b; Douglas et al., 2011).

Asking clients to teach us about themselves will extend to others our sensitivities about being different and will empower others to share their own awareness. Taking the time to value both the differences and the commonalities across ethnic and cultural groups will provide us with valuable insights into the human experience and enable us to build bridges between providers and the growing numbers of diverse clients.

On the basis of the population trends discussed earlier (USCBNPP, 2012), a *new minority* is emerging. For the first time in American history, descendants of European whites will assume minority status by mid-century. In its purest form, the term *minority* implies a condition of difference based on enumerating an identifiable characteristic. Wirth (1945) suggested that a minority is "a group of people who, because of their physical or cultural characteristics, are singled out from others in the society in which they live, for differential and unequal treatment, and who therefore regard themselves as objects of collective discrimination" (p. 347). Health care providers need to make several important adjustments in response to this population shift while continuing to appreciate the special histories of all minority group members, past, present, and future. Regardless of how group memberships are described, all people want to have their ancestries and identities preserved and respected. All want to tell their stories about their unique struggles as well as their successes at overcoming barriers presented by change, exploitation, and prejudice (Kozub, 2013). Despite the fact that for many centuries European Americans comprised the majority population in the United States of America, little is known about the individual struggles they and their ancestors faced when prejudice and persecution drove them from their homelands. Some stories are surprisingly similar to those shared by persons of current minority status. In addition, we cannot lose sight of the fact that members of the new majority will carry with them their experiences of being minority. We still have a long way to go toward improving the delivery of health promotion and illness intervention services to all groups of Americans who are at great risk, whether they are members of our new or former minorities or majorities. To do this, we must understand that differences in health and healing beliefs between individuals, care providers, and care recipients are rooted in heritage, ethnicity, and culture (Stryer, Weinick, & Clancy, 2002; Thomas, Fine, & Ibrahim, 2004). This understanding is the basis for building common ground on which partnerships for positive health outcomes are constructed.

Whether ethnicity is associated with minority or majority populations, ethnic groups are composed of people who share a unique cultural background and social heritage that is passed from one generation to another. Ethnicity should be understood as a social differentiation that engenders in us a sense of self-awareness and exclusivity, a sense of belonging. Our ethnicity gives us membership in a distinct group and differentiates us from those in other groups. Our distinction is often based on such cultural criteria as a common ancestry; shared history; a commonplace of origin; language; dress; food preferences; and participation in rituals, networks, clubs, or activities (Ford & Kelly, 2005; Holzberg, 1982). For example, when members of an Italian American family gather at a wedding, the nature of the celebration expresses the ethnic culture in many ways. The ceremony and the formalities of receiving witnesses and guests are unique to each group and are representative of "the way things are done." At the celebration that follows the exchanging of vows, the guests may feast on antipasto, linguini, chicken marsala, and cappuccino. Soon after, the accordion player might strike up the tarantella, an Italian folk song. Young and old alike may grasp hands and promenade as they laugh and sing. Late in the evening, the elders may share stories about "the old country" with excitement and pride. Although members of this group may have emigrated at different times and may have been born in America, they share common bonds based on native language, history, and values. The passing of these beliefs, values, knowledge, and practices takes place through the rituals of sharing and participating in cultural events and celebrations.

It may be helpful to think of your own ethnic culture and ponder the following questions as you proceed through this chapter. With what group(s) do you identify and why? What are your common bonds? What cultural rituals do you celebrate and with whom? What are the purposes and meanings of your gatherings and celebrations? What types of things are shared and learned when people get together? What types of foods are prepared for the event? Are there dances, special rites, or ceremonies? Each of us can probably identify several shared beliefs, values, and practices that make us members of unique collectives, and many of us strive to preserve our rich cultures and histories by passing them on to each successive generation. Foods, languages, and other bonds of common ancestry are the cultural aspects of ethnicity that serve to offer consistency and structure to life, and provide individuals with abilities to interpret life events as significant and meaningful (Kim-ju & Liem, 2003; Trickett, 2009).

In health and illness, an ethnic group's shared beliefs, symbols, and customs serve as common reference points that members use to judge the appropriateness of their decisions and actions (Kleinman, Eisenberg, & Good, 2006). However, attention must be given to variations within and between generations that are sometimes attributed to acculturation, socioeconomic status, and education. All health care providers should take care not to generalize beliefs and practices to every member of an ethnic group or culture. Although ethnicity captures the larger cultural component of human experiences, we must not permit our awareness of a culture to erode its members' individual identities and dignity (Lopez-Class, Castro, & Ramirez, 2011; Saha, Beach, & Cooper, 2008; Tucker, Arthur, Roncoroni, Wall, & Sanchez, 2013).

CULTURE, HEALTH AND ILLNESS, AND NURSING

Ethnic culture is the medium through which a person's beliefs, standards, and norms for health and illness behaviors are structured, learned, shared, practiced, and judged. Cultural beliefs give meaning to health and illness experiences by providing the individual with culturally acceptable causes for illness, rules for symptom expression, interactional norms, help-seeking strategies, and determining desired outcomes (Kleinman, 1980; Street & Haidet, 2010). For example, when you awake before school with dryness in your throat and cramps in your stomach, several beliefs about what could be wrong and how you should act in response to what is wrong are set into action. What is causing this to happen to me? What can I do about it? Should I stay home from school? Whom should I call to help me? What will people think if I stay home today? The answers to these questions and the actions you take are learned and are influenced by the experiences you have had with your family and the larger ethnic aggregate. In some cultures, a special home remedy tea can be taken for specific complaints of dry throat and cramps, and going to work or school is an expectation. Other cultural groups may expect you to be visited by a healer, stay home from work or school, and tell no one else about your problem.

Noted psychiatrist and anthropologist Arthur Kleinman studied members of many diverse ethnic groups to gain an understanding of the links between cultural beliefs and health and illness behaviors and actions (Kleinman, 1988; Kleinman et al., 2006). The findings of his studies are especially helpful in guiding community practitioners who interact with clients in their homes and various types of community institutions. Like other researchers, he found that cultural beliefs based in shared meanings, values, and norms are the basic guidelines people use for recognizing that something is wrong, interpreting what it might be, and organizing a plan of appropriate actions (Kleinman, 1986). For example, before action is taken in response to a problem, individuals and family members must first agree that the symptoms represent a problem. Next, there is an examination of all possible and probable causes, which may range from behaviors and foods to violations of cultural norms. Once a cause has been identified, a plan of action is made and appropriate treatment is determined. In addition, how we act when we are "ill" is determined by our ethnic culture. Some cultures have specific norms for sick role behavior, whereas other cultures suggest that you continue to carry out your everyday role to the best of your abilities. In this overall illness recognition and management process, cultural beliefs influence the reasons the client formulates to explain the illness, the language, and terms used for communicating the health problem, the choice of whom one talks to about the problem, the range of acceptable healing alternatives, how choices are made, and expectations for treatment outcomes (Drew, 1997; Higginbottom et al., 2011; Katz & Alegría, 2009).

For those of us in the nursing profession, culturally sensitive health care continues to be a central focus of a holistic and humanistic philosophy that guides our practice (AACN, 2013b; Douglas et al., 2011). The healing goals of culturally sensitive care can be achieved only through conscious efforts at gaining knowledge of different groups' ways of explaining, understanding, and treating health problems. Strategies presented in this chapter are intended to assist practitioners with eliciting from clients their cultural models for health, illness, help seeking, and healing.

CULTURAL HEALTH CARE SYSTEMS

Basic to successful interactions between clients and providers is the understanding that we are all different from one another, with different ethnic and cultural backgrounds, and, therefore, different health and illness beliefs and practices. There's that word again: "different." But despite our differences, we come together at a mutually agreed on place to achieve a common goal: to maintain or regain health. The dilemma presented here is that health means different things to each of us; we recognize it and measure changes in it differently, act in diverse ways when faced with these changes, and seek different methods for achieving healing outcomes. The settings where we meet and interact with each other may take on different veneers and titles, but they are all what Kleinman (1980) calls *cultural health care systems*. The simple fact that culture influences health and illness beliefs and behaviors serves as a constant reminder to us that wherever clients and providers interact, there is a system, and it is influenced by the beliefs, values, norms, and standards that each of us brings to it. Cultural health care systems are made up of individuals experiencing and treating illness and the social institutions where interactions between clients and providers take place (Kleinman, 1980, 1986).

Sectors of Cultural Health Care Systems

Each cultural health care system can have several recognized sectors. The three sectors Kleinman's model addresses are referred to as popular, folk, and professional. Typically, the popular sector is composed of ordinary people, families, groups, social networks, and communities. The lay practitioners and healers comprise the folk sector, whereas the professional sector is composed of the licensed health professionals (Kleinman, 1980). Let us look at these sectors in some detail.

Popular

The popular sector of cultural health care systems is made up of informal healing relationships that occur within one's own social network. Although the family is at the nucleus of this sector, health care can take place between people linked by kinship, friendship, residence, occupation, or religion (Helman, 2000). In the United States, there are as many versions of the popular sector as there are ethnic cultures. In neighborhoods where many ethnic groups have settled, popular sectors of health care systems are found to have several different ways of managing health, illness, and healing.

In the popular sector, the process of defining oneself as ill begins with a self-diagnosis confirmed by significant others based on the implicit standards of what it means to be well (Angel & Thiots, 1987; Helman, 2000). Consequently, a person is defined as ill when there is agreement between self-perceptions of impairment and the perceptions of those around him (Weiss, 1988). The social, ethnic, and cultural values, on which the illness judgment is based, focus on the experience of discomfort, failure to function as expected, and a change in physical appearance. Whether a symptom is recognized as significant or normal is also influenced by the occurrence, persistence, and prevalence of the symptoms among group members (Drew, 1997; Kronish, Leventhal, & Horowitz, 2012).

Once a symptom has been recognized as significant, decisions about appropriate healing actions must be made. These decisions are also usually based on beliefs, standards, and norms passed along from previous generations. For example, the affected individual makes decisions about seeing a physician for a health problem, as opposed to taking care of the symptoms at home, in collaboration with family and the social network. If the symptom is commonly observed in other members of the family or community and home remedies have successfully treated the problem, then going to the physician is not a priority. Within this sector, both the care recipient and the network counselors share similar assumptions about the observed symptoms and recommended healing strategies. Therefore, misunderstandings are rare, and the healer's credentials are based on experience rather than professional education and licensure (Fox, 2005; Green, Carrillo, & Betancourt, 2002; Komaric, Bedford, & van Driel, 2012).

Folk

The folk sector of cultural health care systems includes the interaction between a client and sacred and secular healers. Most healers share the same basic cultural values and beliefs as their constituents. In many cases, family members and others in the social network work alongside the client and the healer to discover and treat the problem. Sources of holistic health problems are believed to include relationships the client has with other people, with the natural environment, and with supernatural forces (Helman, 2000).

Treatment rituals and strategies are prescribed to correct disequilibrium and to promote healing. Healers have little formal training, although some have served an apprenticeship with another, more accomplished healer. Most are believed to receive healing powers through family position, inheritance, signs, revelations, or gifts (Lewis, 1988).

Within the folk sector, illnesses are defined as syndromes from which members of a group suffer and for which their culture provides a cause, a diagnosis, preventive measures, and regimens of healing (Weller et al., 2002). It is very important that beliefs about causes of illnesses be compatible with selected treatments. In some cases, family and folk healers may be the only people who can effectively recommend or perform healing rituals. For example, some Hispanics believe that *susto* results from a traumatic experience or that sickness is a punishment from God. *Susto*, or fright, is an emotional response to a traumatic experience and is recognized as an illness that involves the loss of one's spirit from the body. Symptoms include crying, loss of appetite, listlessness, insomnia, nightmares, and withdrawal. *Susto* requires treatment by a *curandero* whose healing rituals attempt to get the individual's spirit back into the body. Sometimes, complementary and supportive treatment from a psychiatrist is sought (Alegria et al., 2010; Trotter, 2001). Working with clients and families to learn acceptable forms of healing for these problems is imperative.

Professional

The professional sector of cultural health care systems is made up of organized health professionals who are formally educated and legally sanctioned (Kleinman, 1980). Unlike in the popular and folk sectors, the clients and the providers in the professional sector typically differ in their social and cultural values, beliefs, and assumptions. Based on these differences, and taking into account the unfamiliar surroundings and rules of the institutions where care is given in the professional sector, the client–provider relationship may be one of mistrust, suspicion, and conflict.

Although many collaborative, complementary, and alternative models of healing are gaining popularity, practices in the professional sector remain dominated by a biomedical disease and treatment orientation. A biomedical orientation suggests that disease is a physiologic and psychological abnormality. This view is exclusive of and counter to the popular, holistic view of illness as a meaningful experience perceived and constructed in sociocultural context (Katz & Alegría, 2009; Komaric et al., 2012; Racher & Annis, 2007). Some of us have prepared a home remedy for a sore throat or have applied a poultice to relieve a headache or a persistent cough. These are examples of actions taken, in the popular sector, in response to symptoms that are interpreted as part of a meaningful illness experience. In the professional sector, these same symptoms may be viewed as significant threats to health.

Decision Making Within the Sectors

People who become ill make choices about whom to consult in the popular, professional, or folk sectors of the cultural health care system. Overwhelming evidence suggests that those choices are influenced by the individual's subjective definition of the illness, its meaning, and its expected course (Street & Haidet, 2010; Unger & Schwartz, 2012). Attitudes toward different types of providers and decisions about whom one should seek for help vary according to how the symptom is interpreted and what it means to that person as a significant life event.

Forming these decisions is also a function of shared, family, and culture-based learning (Fabrega, 1974; Mechanic, 1992). Remember back to your childhood and a significant episode of not feeling well.

- Who decided what was wrong with you?
- What were the interpretations of your symptoms?

- Who made the decision about what to do for you?
- With whom did this person consult?
- Did the meanings of your symptoms and who was consulted have anything to do with the selected treatments?
- What were the expected outcomes from your treatments?
- How were those outcomes evaluated?

Just as important as examining your own health, illness, and healing beliefs and practices is investigating the significance of these factors and processes in your clients' illnesses.

In developing a help-seeking pattern, most people establish a therapeutic network, which may include informal relationships with people and providers from some or all of the three sectors of cultural health care systems (Helman, 2000; Kleinman, 1980). Different types of providers, including family members and folk healers, may be used concurrently or in sequence, depending on the client's perception of the cause of the problem, course of the illness event, and desired healing outcomes. Typically, people make their help-seeking choices on the basis of prior learning, symptom significance, compatibility between the philosophies of the sectors, and evaluation of the treatment outcome. It seems logical that clients, in the process of seeking help, may involve a network of potential consultants ranging from informal structures in the nuclear family to select laypeople and professionals.

Conflict Among Sectors

Given our diverse cultural backgrounds, we should not be surprised to find that research across many health-related disciplines provides evidence that barriers, conflicts, and misunderstandings among the system's sectors are, in part, related to the differences in cultural beliefs about illness causation and management. Although we may never have viewed conflicts through Kleinman's (1980) perspective before, we have all encountered conflicts between providers and clients. We may have even been the clients! Have you ever gone to the physician only to find that he or she recommended a treatment that was not what you expected? Have you ever found that a medication prescribed by the physician is something that you would rather not take? None of us is a stranger to these types of conflicts. Even after students in undergraduate and graduate nursing programs are offered a greater knowledge of ethnicity and culture, the conflicts in beliefs and practices between sectors and resultant barriers to effective health care remain unresolved. The lack of progress in reducing barriers can be linked to professional providers' relative inattention to the popular sector of cultural health care systems. Have you ever heard a professional provider say, "This client is difficult" or "This client is noncompliant with his medicines and he won't follow his diet?" Perhaps you have made such comments yourself without thinking that what has been prescribed or recommended may not be compatible with the client's beliefs about treatment and healing. The problem could be more basic than a mere treatment conflict; perhaps the client and provider have incongruent beliefs about what is wrong and what caused the symptom of illness. In the popular or folk sector, illness is sometimes thought to be a somatization of a client's uneasiness with a stressful relationship, the natural environment, or supernatural forces. This is an example of how cultural beliefs about the cause and management of an illness provide the client with a foundation for interpreting the illness experience as meaningful.

Because belief systems in the popular and folk sectors have often been termed as *unorthodox*, *lay*, *subjective*, or *nonscientific* (Kleinman, 1980), and have been associated with non-Western societies, a client's preference for such healing practices may have been dismissed by some professional health care professionals. This dismissal is problematic because if recommended treatments do not fit the perceived cause, then the client may not follow suggested protocols.

If these problems are to be resolved, we need to understand and accommodate the ideologies and practices of diverse individuals. Professional providers must consider the significance of the illness interpretations and meanings for clients, thus facilitating a more comfortable and secure client–provider relationship. We must focus on the popular sector if working relationships are to have successful outcomes. Conflicts, misunderstandings, and barriers to effective health care will be reduced only by commitment to gain knowledge about the popular sector, where health beliefs and health practices are activated (Kleinman, 1980) and where 70% to 90% of all illness episodes are recognized and treated (Zola, 1972). The nursing profession's commitment to health and holism and its capacity to understand complex sociocultural responses to real and potential health problems make it the most logical choice for a professional segment to act as a client advocate in facilitating interactions between the sectors. Appropriate advocacy must be based on the ability to understand the popular sector's realities and to translate and negotiate between the system's sectors with the goal of reducing barriers to culturally sensitive care. In doing so, nursing will lead the charge for cultural competence among providers and will model the application of those attributes for health care institutions.

Without a doubt, differences are sources of conflict and misunderstanding in client–provider relationships (Kleinman, 1986). A detailed understanding of cultural health care systems will provide us with many reasons for the existence and resolution of real and potential barriers between providers and laypeople in the caregiving process. Beyond a basic understanding of the ingredients for conflict, this paradigm of differences should be used by providers, partners, and communities as a guide for becoming culturally competent.

THE CULTURALLY COMPETENT PROVIDER

Cultural competence implies an awareness of, sensitivity to, and knowledge of the meaning of culture and its role in shaping human behavior (Kleinman & Benson, 2006). If culture, broadly defined, is socially transmitted beliefs, values, ways of knowing, and patterns of behavior characteristic of a designated population group, then cultural competence is the ability to express an awareness of one's own culture, to recognize the differences between oneself and others, and to adapt behaviors to appreciate and accommodate those differences (Drew, 1997; Saha et al., 2008). Culture includes more than race and ethnicity and may include a person's gender, religion, socioeconomic status, sexual orientation, age, environment, family background, and life experiences.

Cultural competence depends on the development of an attitude of acceptance of others among health care providers. It is a process that begins with one's willingness to learn about cultural issues, proceeds with the commitment to incorporate the importance of culture at all levels of care, and is put into operation by making adaptations in services to meet culturally unique needs. Although some practitioners may have specific knowledge of the languages, values, and customs of other cultures, the most challenging tasks are understanding the dynamics of difference in the helping process and adapting practice skills to fit the client's cultural context.

Developing an awareness and acceptance of cultural differences is required as a first step in the process of becoming a culturally competent individual (Alegria et al., 2010; Douglas et al., 2011). Many ethnic minorities have beliefs and practices about health, illness, and treatment that differ significantly from the Western, scientific medical paradigm around which the U.S. health care delivery system is structured (Fox, 2005; Good & Good, 1981; Kirmayer, Groleau, Looper, & Dao, 2004). However, negatively labeling people because the provider believes them to differ from him or her and the mainstream is unacceptable. Differences must be explored and understood so barriers to seeking health care can be reduced. Understanding differences begins with an awareness that they exist and continues with a willingness to accept them. In the sections that follow, there are suggestions for exercises to enhance your awareness of your own culture.

Assessing Our Cultural Awareness

A major component of cultural competence is an acknowledgment and awareness of one's own culture and a willingness to explore one's own feelings and biases. Each person is responsible for building an awareness of how culture influences his or her own ways of thinking and making decisions. Included in this awareness must be an acknowledgment of how day-to-day behaviors reflect cultural norms and values perpetuated by our families and larger social networks. To develop this awareness, we must ask ourselves several questions that will direct our exploration of our cultural heritage and how our daily interactions are influenced by that culture. Sample questions include the following:

- To what ethnic group, socioeconomic class, religion, age group, and community do I belong?
- What about my ethnic group, socioeconomic class, religion, age, or community do I wish I could change and why?
- What experiences have I had with people different from me? What were those experiences like and how did I feel about them?
- What is there about me that may cause me to be rejected by members of other cultures or ethnic groups?
- What qualities do I have that will help me establish positive interpersonal interactions with people from other cultural groups?

One strategy used in teaching diversity awareness to health professions students is a cultural assessment project that serves as a purposeful self-examination and an exercise in appreciating differences. The project asks you to begin by identifying your own cultural beliefs and values about health and illness, education and vocation, foods, religion, and role expectations. (You can do this now as you read this section.) Once identified, think through your responses, and make notes about how you remember being taught about some of those values, practices, expectations, habits, and traditions. Ask yourself:

- Where and how was knowledge about my culture and heritage passed on to me?
- Who are the people in my network responsible for influencing and shaping the lives of the young people?

Proceed with this project by seeking out someone known to you but who has a background, heritage, or ethnicity different from your own. Ask that person's permission for an interview, and ask them the same things you asked yourself in establishing your basic cultural richness. When you have the data you set out to compare with your own, sit down, and analyze what sociocultural similarities and differences the two of you have.

This exercise is particularly beneficial to the beginner who has not ventured into self-awareness projects from a cultural beliefs and values perspective. Having analyzed similarities and differences, proceed with your analysis, and focus on predicting potential areas of conflict between the two views as well as the positive, congruent strengths. These may be as simple as food preferences and celebrated holidays or as complex as preferred vocations, generational hierarchies, and healing rituals. You may complete the practice assignment by asking the following question: *What potential strengths in similarities between us should I build on to begin interactions with this client?*

As this cultural assessment project points out, all interacting parties bring with them unique histories, communication styles, and learned expectations. Together, these contribute to potential misunderstandings and misinterpretations that manifest the dynamics of difference. Therefore, strategies of relating with clients must include eliciting information about their health and illness practices, as well as basic ethnic and cultural norms. Specific knowledge about the culture is necessary for the relationship to be structured within the helping framework. Bringing down barriers and facilitating the negotiation of individualized plans of care will support positive health outcomes for all clients. The ultimate goal in planning collaborative approaches to illness treatment and healing is to preserve the dignity of the client and to foster health promotion and healing programs that are likely to meet with adherence because they support rather than offend the client.

Eliciting Health and Illness Beliefs

We have explored the idea that cultural health beliefs are the major determinants of a person's recognition and management of an illness experience. Although these beliefs exist independently of and prior to a given episode of illness, they are activated when one has to cope with and explain a particular experience or situation (Kleinman, 1980). Therefore, as practitioners, we should expect that it is appropriate to elicit cultural health beliefs when (and not before) an illness experience becomes a reality. According to several researchers, time and experience with an illness are necessary for the client to work the set of beliefs into a functioning set of reasons for the illness, directions for sick role behavior, and options for achieving healing (Good & Good, 1981; Helman, 2000; Kirmayer et al., 2004). Understanding ethnic interpretations of health and illness enables the practitioner to further clarify the sources of beliefs from which clients formulate their illness realities.

This process begins with eliciting the client's subjective explanations for the cause, duration, and characteristics of symptoms. Further discussion with the client should include exploring the client's expectations for acceptable treatments, outcomes of the treatment, and the substance of the client–provider interaction. Kleinman's (1980) original set of questions can be adapted to ask clients about their perspectives on health and illness experiences. Attention to the answers to these questions increases the cultural competence of the provider:

- What do you think caused your problem?
- Why do you think it started when it did?
- How long do you think it will last?
- What have you done about your problem?
- With whom did you discuss your problem?
- What kind of help and from whom would you like to receive help for your problem?
- How will you know when your problem is getting better?

Additional questions formulated by this author for purposes of conducting explanatory model research include:

- What do you call your problem?
- What worries you most about having this problem?
- How did you come to know that you were having a problem?

Finding answers to these questions may take time and will take a conscious effort to collect and use. However, the process is well worth the time and commitment as we gain a greater understanding and respect for all clients' health beliefs and practices. This understanding can lead to both improved client–provider relationships and treatment outcomes. An analysis of the answers to these questions, and much introspection will enable health care providers to understand the complexities of cross-cultural interactions.

Adapting Skills

Providers must develop critical skills so that cultural assessments can be elicited and appropriate sociocultural care can be delivered in conjunction with prescribed treatment interventions. Delivering culturally competent care implies a contextual understanding that treating the illness and understanding what it means to the individual are as important as working to resolve the disease process. Although nurses study communication strategies as part of their educational preparation, the cognitive skills necessary to understand another's cultural beliefs and backgrounds need cultivation, refinement, and practice (AACN, 2013a).

Sound physical and psychosocial assessment skills, sensitive interviewing skills, active listening, neutral body language, and self-awareness are the basic attributes required of culturally competent providers. Several of these attributes can be built using the contents of this chapter, but it is expected that the practitioner will seek out continuing education that will expand the skills necessary for thorough data collection. For example, physical assessment of people of a different race may be a learning need for some, whereas spending more time in cultural self-assessment and analysis of potential conflicts between providers and their clients may be a priority for others.

Active listening, which is a learned skill that requires a lot of practice, is a necessary component of sensitive interviewing. It is helpful if you can audiotape a "client" interview that employs role-playing so you and a colleague can critique your style. Use the following questions to evaluate your progress toward becoming a skilled interviewer:

- Am I using slang or jargon that is only understood by other professionals?
- Are the questions I ask presented so rapidly in sequence that the client has no time to think and organize a response?
- Do I paraphrase a question so many times that it has lost its original intent?
- Are the questions I ask so long that the focus is diluted beyond recognition?

Sometimes the reasons questions seem to go unanswered are related to interviewing skills, styles, and competencies. For example, are you comfortable with pauses, or do you have the need to always hear a speaking voice, even if it is your own? Are you asking appropriate follow-up questions that will probe a client's response to an earlier question? It is important for you to demonstrate that you value what the client is saying. Active listening and planning appropriate responses are a sure way of accomplishing the task.

You must also learn how to present yourself with neutral body language during interactions with clients. Not everyone likes being touched or having someone else in their personal space. Although we may think touch is important in healing, remember it may not be culturally appropriate to the clients we serve.

In addition to physical assessment data, eliciting patient and family explanations of health status and illness realities helps providers take the patient's perspective seriously in organizing clinical care strategies. In turn, the provider's effective communication style assists patients and families in making more useful judgments about when to enter into treatment, with which practitioners, for what treatments, and at what ratio of cost and benefit (Kleinman, 1988). It is imperative to approach health teaching and self-care training with the attitude that providers and patients are collaborators and are working toward the same goals of positive outcomes for the patient and the family. Negotiation among patients and providers over conflicts in explanation, interpretation, and understanding can reduce barriers to effective care and instill in the patient the provider's respect for alternative viewpoints and preferences. These strategies work together to close the gap between the patient and the provider and are necessary to increase access to care and improve health for our entire nation.

THE CULTURALLY COMPETENT AGENCY

Cultural awareness, sensitivity, and competence are necessary attributes for all health care providers and for the delivery systems of which they are a part (AACN, 2013b; Association of American Medical Colleges [AAMC], 2005; Chun, Yamada, Huh, Hew, & Tasaka, 2010;

Kumagai & Lypson, 2009; Reyes et al., 2013). It makes no sense to have culturally competent practitioners in settings that are culturally ignorant. In services to individuals, families, and communities, culturally competent systems of care must acknowledge and incorporate the importance of culture, appreciate the dynamics of difference, and make a commitment to adapt services to meet unique needs. Culturally competent programs and services respect their clients' and staff members' cultural beliefs, and include in their mission statements goals to maintain and improve the self-esteem and the cultural identity of employees and clients. The driving forces behind culturally competent service delivery are knowing and understanding the people that you serve. It means appreciating the importance of culture and avoiding prejudices and biases. It also means that you and your organization understand and work to change the sociopolitical influences that create barriers to quality care.

Several types of movements toward agency-level cultural competence have been reported in the literature. When success is measured by community acceptance and use, some agencies are recognized as more successful than others (Tucker, Nghiem, Marsiske, & Robinson, 2013). Generic outreach models may be rejected by ethnic minority groups because the services are often the same ones offered to mainstream groups. This approach serves to maintain rather than remove barriers. A more meaningful and successful approach to agency cultural competence is mainstream support of local programs and services that employ and use staff who have similar cultural backgrounds to those for whom the services are intended (Tucker, Nghiem, et al., 2013). This approach means that multilingual and multicultural services should be offered in some neighborhoods and communities. A needs assessment must be employed to identify the types of services and the systems of service delivery that are most acceptable and efficient.

For many existing agencies and delivery systems, structures, services, and competencies must be modified or created to be consistent and compatible with the cultures they encounter in their client populations. Culturally competent services, systems, agencies, and practitioners possess the capacity to respond to the unique needs of populations whose cultures differ from dominant or mainstream America.

Awareness that racial, ethnic, and minority groups have different needs, have been underserved, or have underutilized available services has created an interest in agency cultural competence. Assessing the types of services identified as wanted and needed by target populations is crucial to the reception and use of services by people with culturally diverse backgrounds. Agencies striving for cultural competence must be able to accept the values of the community's ethnic cultures, and develop and refine services and skills for working with the local population and each other (Reich & Reich, 2006).

Summary

Educators and providers must remember that ethnicity provides a sense of belonging to people in a pluralistic society—a celebration of differences in identity, strength, and survival. An understanding of ethnic culture is necessary for coping with and appreciating differences. Research supports the roles of cultural heritage and identity in influencing people's behaviors and attitudes and the perpetuation of ethnicity throughout generations. Rather than eradication of differences, stimulation of conflict, and goals for sameness, cooperation with and respect for others with different heritages must be the focus of future practice and research. Cultural competence is an imperative for meeting HP 2020 goals for health promotion and improving access to quality care. It empowers individuals and providers alike to develop and nurture healing partnerships in health care that are aimed at successful health outcomes for all Americans. Many of the skills providers need are in place and available for enrichment through awareness, specialty and continuing education, and careful listening to what our clients teach us.

Critical Thinking Questions

1. The clinical director of the outpatient clinic where you work is often heard complaining about the unit secretary "who just doesn't seem to understand or speak English very well." Sometimes you notice other nurses laughing at the secretary's accent and native dress. You want to help others change their behaviors. What will you do? Be specific and use the hints in this chapter to make and carry out a plan.

2. You are invited to the wedding of a very close friend whom you have not seen in many years. He is marrying the love of his life, a Japanese woman he met while working in Project Hope. He calls you a few weeks before the wedding and asks you to escort the parents of his bride-to-be so they will feel "at home." He tells you that this is their first trip to the United States and they do not speak English. How will you prepare for this special assignment?

REFERENCES

Alegria, M., Atkins, M., Farmer, E., Slaton, E., & Stelk, W. (2010). One size does not fit all: Taking diversity, culture and context seriously. *Administration and Policy in Mental Health and Mental Health Services Research, 37*(1–2), 48–60.

American Association of Colleges of Nursing. (2013a). *Cultural competency in nursing education.* Retrieved October 25, 2013, from http://www.aacn.nche.edu/education-resources/cultural-competency

American Association of Colleges of Nursing. (2013b). *Enhancing diversity in the nursing workforce.* Retrieved August 25, 2013, from https://www.aacn.nche.edu/media-relations/fact-sheets/enhancing-diversity

Angel, R., & Thiots, P. (1987). The impact of culture on the cognitive structure of illness. *Culture, Medicine, and Psychiatry, 2,* 465–494.

Association of American Medical Colleges. (2005). *Cultural competence education for medical students.* Retrieved October 23, 2013, from https://www.aamc.org/download/54338/data/culturalcomped.pdf

Betancourt, J. R., Green, A. R., Carrillo, J. E., & Park, E. R. (2005). Cultural competence and health care disparities: Key perspectives and trends. *Health Affairs, 24*(2), 499–505.

Chun, M. B. J., Yamada, A. M., Huh, J., Hew, C., & Tasaka, S. (2010, March). Using the cross-cultural care survey to assess cultural competency in graduate medical education. *Journal of Graduate Medical Education, 2*(1), 96–101.

Condon, V. M., Morgan, C. J., Miller, E. W., Mamier, I., Zimmerman, G. J., & Mazhar, W. (2013). A program to enhance recruitment and retention of disadvantaged and ethnically diverse baccalaureate nursing students. *Journal of Transcultural Nursing, 24*(4), 397–407.

Douglas, M. K., Pierce, J. U., Rosenkoetter, M., Pacquiao, D., Callister, L. C., Hattar-Pollara, M., . . . Purnell, L. (2011). Standards of practice for culturally competent nursing care: 2011 update. *Journal of Transcultural Nursing, 22*(4), 317–333.

Drew, J. C. (1997). The ethnocultural context of healing. In P. Kritek (Ed.), *Reflections in healing.* New York, NY: National League for Nursing.

Engebretson, J., Mahoney, J., & Carlson, E. D. (2008). Cultural competence in the era of evidence-based practice. *Journal of Professional Nursing, 24*(3), 172–178.

Fabrega, H. (1974). *Disease and social behavior: An interdisciplinary perspective.* Cambridge, MA: MIT Press.

Ford, M. E., & Kelly, P. A. (2005). Conceptualizing and categorizing race and ethnicity in health services research. *Health Services Research, 40,* 1658–1675.

Fox, R. C. (2005). Becoming a physician: Cultural competence and the culture of medicine. *New England Journal of Medicine, 353*(13), 1316–1319.

Good, B., & Good, M. J. (1981). The meaning of symptoms: A cultural hermeneutic model for cultural practice. In L. Eisenberg & A. Kleinman (Eds.), *The relevance of social science for medicine.* Boston, MA: Reidel.

Green, A. R., Carrillo, J. E., & Betancourt, J. R. (2002). Why the disease-based model of medicine fails our patients. *Western Journal of Medicine, 176,* 141–143.

Helman, C. (2000). *Culture, health, and illness: An introduction for health professionals* (4th ed.). Oxford, England: Butterworth-Heinemann.

Higginbottom, G. M. A., Richter, M. S., Mogale, R. S., Ortiz, L., Young, S., & Mollel, O. (2011). Identification of nursing assessment models/tools validated in clinical practice for use with diverse ethno-cultural groups: An integrative review of the literature. *BMC Nursing, 10*(16), 1–11.

Holzberg, C. S. (1982). Ethnicity and aging: Anthropological perspectives on more than just the minority elderly. *The Gerontologist, 22*(3), 249–257.

Katz, A. M., & Alegría, M. (2009). The clinical encounter as local moral world: Shifts of assumptions and transformation in relational context. *Social Science & Medicine, 68*(7), 1238–1246.

Kim-ju, G. M., & Liem, R. (2003). Ethnic self-awareness as a function of ethnic group status, group composition, and ethnic identity orientation. *Cultural Diversity & Ethnic Minority Psychology, 9*(3), 289–302.

Kirmayer, L. J., Groleau, D., Looper, K. J., & Dao, M. D. (2004). Explaining medically unexplained symptoms. *Canadian Journal of Psychiatry, 49,* 663–672.

Kleinman, A. (1980). *Patients and healers in the context of culture.* Berkeley: University of California Press.

Kleinman, A. (1986). Concepts and a model for the comparison of medical systems as cultural systems. In C. Currer & M. Stacy (Eds.), *Concepts of health, illness, & disease: A comparative perspective.* New York, NY: Berg.

Kleinman, A. (1988). *The illness narratives: Suffering, healing, and the human condition.* New York, NY: Basic Books.

Kleinman, A., & Benson, P. (2006). Anthropology in the clinic: The problem of cultural competency and how to fix it. *Public Library of Science Medicine, 3*(10), 1673–1675.

Kleinman, A., Eisenberg, L., & Good, B. (2006). Culture, illness, and care: Clinical lessons from anthropologic and cross-cultural research. *Focus: The Journal of Lifelong Learning in Psychiatry, 4*(1), 140–149.

Komaric, N., Bedford, S., & van Driel, M. L. (2012). Two sides of the coin: Patient and provider perceptions of health care delivery to patients from culturally and linguistically diverse backgrounds. *BMC Health Services Research, 12*(322), 1–14.

Kozub, M. L. (2013). Through the eyes of the other using event analysis to build cultural competence. *Journal of Transcultural Nursing, 24*(3), 313–318.

Kronish, I. M., Leventhal, H., & Horowitz, C. R. (2012). Understanding minority patients' beliefs about hypertension to reduce gaps in communication between patients and clinicians. *Journal of Clinical Hypertension, 14*(1), 38–44.

Kumagai, A. K., & Lypson, M. L. (2009). Beyond cultural competence: Critical consciousness, social justice, and multicultural education. *Academic Medicine, 84*(6), 782–787.

Lewis, M. C. (1988). Attribution and illness. *Journal of Psychosocial Nursing, 26*(4), 14–21.

Loftin, C., Newman, S. D., Gilden, G., Bond, M. L., & Dumas, B. P. (2013). Moving toward greater diversity: A review of interventions to increase diversity in nursing education. *Journal of Transcultural Nursing, 24*(4), 387–396.

Lopez-Class, M., Castro, F. G., & Ramirez, A. G. (2011). Conceptions of acculturation: A review and statement of critical issues. *Social Science & Medicine, 72*(9), 1555–1562.

Madrid, A. (1988). Diversity and its discontents. *Black Issues in Higher Education, 5*(4), 10–18.

Mechanic, D. (1992). Health and illness behavior and patient-practitioner relationships. *Social Science & Medicine, 34*(12), 1345–1350.

Racher, F. E., & Annis, R. C. (2007). Respecting culture and honoring diversity in community practice. *Research and Theory for Nursing Practice, 21*(4), 255–270.

Reich, S. M., & Reich, J. A. (2006). Cultural competence in interdisciplinary collaborations: A method for respecting diversity in research partnerships. *American Journal of Community Psychology, 38*(1–2), 51–62.

Renzaho, A. M. N., Romios, P., Crock, C., & Sunderland, A. L. (2013). The effectiveness of cultural competence programs in ethnic minority patient-centered health care—A systematic review of the literature. *International Journal for Quality in Health Care, 25*(3), 261–269.

Reyes, H., Hadley, L., & Davenport, D. (2013). A comparative analysis of cultural competence in beginning and graduating nursing students. *International Scholarly Research Network: Nursing, 2013,* 1–5.

Saha, S., Beach, M. C., & Cooper, L. A. (2008). Patient centeredness, cultural competence and healthcare quality. *Journal of the National Medical Association, 100*(11), 1275–1285.

Siegel, C. E., Haugland, G., Laska, E. M., Reid-Rose, L. M., Tang, D. I., Wanderling, J. A., . . . Case, B. G. (2011). The Nathan Kline Institute cultural competency assessment scale: Psychometrics and implications for disparity reduction. *Administration and Policy in Mental Health and Mental Health Services Research, 38*(2), 120–130.

Street, R. L., & Haidet, P. (2010). How well do doctors know their patients? Factors affecting physician understanding of patients' health beliefs. *Journal of General Internal Medicine, 26*(1), 21–27.

Stryer, D. B., Weinick, R. M., & Clancy, C. M. (2002). Reducing racial and ethnic disparities in health care. *Health Services Research, 37*(5), xv–xxvi.

Thomas, S. B., Fine, M. J., & Ibrahim, S. A. (2004). Health disparities: The importance of culture and health communications. *American Journal of Public Health, 94*(12), 2050.

Trickett, E. J. (2009). Community psychology: Individuals and interventions in community context. *Annual Review of Psychology, 60,* 395–419.

Trotter, R. T. (2001). Curanderismo: A picture of Mexican-American folk healing. *Journal of Alternative & Complementary Medicine, 7*(2), 129–131.

Tucker, C. M., Arthur, T. M., Roncoroni, J., Wall, W., & Sanchez, J. (2013, August 13). Patient-centered, culturally sensitive health care. *American Journal of Lifestyle Medicine.* Advanced online publication. doi:10.1177/1559827613498065

Tucker, C. M., Nghiem, K. N., Marsiske, M., & Robinson, A. C. (2013). Validation of a patient-centered culturally sensitive health care provider inventory using a national sample of adult patients. *Patient Education and Counseling, 91*(3), 344–349.

Unger, J. B., & Schwartz, S. J. (2012). Conceptual considerations in studies of cultural influences on health behaviors. *Preventive Medicine, 55*(5), 353–355.

U.S. Census Bureau National Population Projections. (2012). *Methodology and assumptions for the 2012 national projections.* Retrieved November 6, 2013, from http://www.census.gov/population/projections/files/methodology/methodstatement12.pdf

U.S. Department of Health and Human Services, Office of Disease Prevention and Health Promotion. (2013). *Healthy people 2020*. Washington, DC: Author. Retrieved September 22, 2013, from http://healthypeople .gov/2020/

U.S. Department of Health and Human Services, Office of Minority Health. (2010). Introduction. In *National partnership for action to end health disparities: The national plan for action draft as of February 17, 2010* (Chap. 1). Retrieved October 22, 2013, from http://healthypeople.gov/2020/about/DisparitiesAbout

Weiss, M. G. (1988). Cultural models of diarrheal illness: Conceptual framework and review. *Social Science & Medicine, 27*(1), 5–16.

Weller, S. C., Baer, R. D., de Alba Garcia, J. G., Glazer, M., Trotter, R., Pachter, L., & Klein, R. E. (2002). Regional variation in Latino descriptions of *susto*. *Culture, Medicine & Psychiatry, 26*(4), 449–472.

Wirth, L. (1945). The problem of minority groups. In R. Linton (Ed.), *The science of man in the world crisis*. New York, NY: Columbia University Press.

Zola, I. K. (1972). Culture and symptoms: An analysis of patients' presenting complaints. *American Sociological Review, 5*, 141–155.

CHAPTER 8

Partnering With Communities for Healthy Public Policy

Julia Henderson Gist

LEARNING OBJECTIVES

This chapter focuses on the importance of healthy public policies for healthy communities.

After studying this chapter, you should be able to:

1. Discuss the different types of policy.

2. Describe the process of health policy development and the interface of politics.

3. Explain how community health nurses can contribute to health policy.

4. Apply the steps of policy development.

5. Partner with community groups to form healthy public policy.

Introduction

Nurses work with communities to promote population health. To promote the health of the community, health policy development is required. This chapter discusses the process of health policy development and why policy development is a part of the role of a community health nurse. Examples of nurses who have worked with communities to influence and develop policy are reviewed. Additionally, information is given on how to become part of the policy development process in a community and how politics is part of the policy development process. Finally, we use concepts of health policy development to analyze community health issues and derive an action plan.

POLICY COMES IN DIFFERENT FORMS

Policy is defined as a plan or course of action, as of a government, political party, or business, intended to influence and determine decisions, actions, and other matters (*American Heritage Dictionary*, 2000). Other authors describe policy as "the principles that govern action directed towards given ends" (Titmus, 1974, p. 23) and "a consciously chosen course of action (or inaction) directed toward some end" (Kalisch & Kalisch, 1982, p. 61). The development of policy includes the choices that a society, organization, or group makes regarding their goals and priorities, including how they will allocate their resources. The development and use of policies gives the entity a goal or a plan of action. The policy formed should reflect the values, beliefs, and attitudes of those who are designing the policy.

Policy is often explained further by describing its various types. The types we describe in this chapter are public policy, social policy, institutional policy, organizational policy, and health policy. When describing the different types of policy, we often find that a policy may fit several different types depending on the perspective of the person describing it. For example, public policy regarding assault laws may become part of health policy as we make laws for victims' rights to health care compensation following intentional injury.

Public policy applies to all members of a society and includes prescribed sanctions for failure to comply, such as fines for driving while intoxicated or fines for factories that do not comply with emission regulations. Public policy is formulated by governmental bodies and frequently restricts personal choice to improve public welfare, such as fines for unsafe driving. Additional examples of public policy include seat belt laws for both children and adults, and legislation that regulates where and to whom tobacco products may be sold and the fines or penalties that apply with failure to comply.

Policy that promotes the welfare of the public is termed *social welfare policy*. Examples of social welfare policy include child labor laws and income assistance, such as Social Security. Social welfare policy tends to focus on the nation's minorities and vulnerable populations. Aid to Families with Dependent Children (AFDC) as well as Temporary Assistance for Needy Families (TANF) and Supplemental Security Income (SSI) are examples of public welfare programs. Further information is offered about TANF in Table 8.1.

TABLE 8.1 Examples of Legislated Health Services

Programs	Benefits	Eligibility
Medicare	Health insurance program	65 years or older; people <65 years with certain disabilities; end-stage renal disease or Lou Gehrig disease
Medicaid	Health care Insurance assistance Nursing home coverage	Based on income and family size. Low-income US nationals, citizens, or permanent residents; pregnant women; have a child(ren) with a disability, or are responsible for children under age 19; people with disabilities; and some seniors aged 65 years and older
State Children's Health Insurance Program (SCHIP)	Doctor visits Immunizations Hospitalizations Emergency room visits	Children <19 years of age from families who earn too much to qualify for Medicaid but who meet SCHIP eligibility and are not covered by other insurance; US citizen or legal immigrant
Temporary Assistance to Needy Families (TANF)	Financial and medical assistance to needy dependent children and parents or relatives with whom they are living	People who are pregnant or responsible for a child <19 years of age; a US national, citizen, legal alien, or permanent resident; have a low or very low income, and are either underemployed, unemployed, or about to become unemployed
Women, Infants, and Children (WIC)	Supplemental foods, nutrition education, and referrals to health care	Pregnant, breast-feeding, and postpartum women; infants; and children up to age 5 who meet a low-income standard and are determined to be at nutritional risk

Source: U.S. Department of Labor. (2013). *Benefits.gov: Your path to government benefits*. Retrieved September 1, 2013, from www.benefits.gov

Institutional policy governs work sites. Institutional policies are based on the institution's mission and goals, and they determine how the institution will function and relate to employees. Institutional policies state when the work shifts begin and end, the location and rules of smoking environments for employees and clients, and criteria for paid sick leave and vacation time.

Organizational policy is formed and applies to groups that have similar interests or special interests, such as professional associations. An example of organizational policy is a state nurses' association or a specialty nursing organization that determines governing rules for membership, such as designated credentialing or registration.

Health policy includes the laws to promote the health of citizens. Often health policy is considered a part of public policy when it is directly related to legislated health care services and reimbursement (Mason, Leavitt, & Chaffee, 2007), such as Medicare and Medicaid. Health policy is established in many ways, including legislation, rules and regulations, and institutional mission and goals. Health policies determine what services are paid for and by whom, who is eligible to receive care, and who qualifies for financial assistance. Examples of health programs that are guided by health policy are described in Table 8.1.

Policy can be made in any organizational system and at many levels, including community agencies, state organizations, and national and international groups. Health policy may also be characterized by the level (i.e., community, state, national, or international) at which the policy development occurs. For example, health care policy decisions made on a community level, such as a new health clinic for low-income families, is funded with budget allocations from local city and county governments. State funding for health care policies may also focus on the provision of health care as well as policies related to the licensure of health care professionals and the regulation of health care institutions. At both state and local levels, policies may be formulated in legislation or emanate from regulations that control health-related behavior by citizens, such as state laws and local ordinances that limit smoking in public places. National health policy focuses on issues of concern to all citizens, such as legislation and regulations that focus on patient safety in hospitals and ensure access to public health care.

If policy reflects the needs of the public, then the public must assist in the development of the policy. How can community health nurses assist citizens to be part of health policy formulation? Community health nurses who work with community residents have a unique perspective for health policy decision making because of their nursing knowledge, their role as an advocate for community health, and their understanding of the political process. We begin with a brief historical overview of how nurses have partnered with communities and populations of need to form healthy public policy.

NURSES INVOLVED WITH POLICY: SOME EXEMPLARS

Florence Nightingale was active in setting policy to implement organizational changes, including hand washing and cleanliness procedures in the military hospitals in which she practiced during the Crimean War (Palmer, 1977). Nightingale believed that once she determined a course of action to be beneficial to the patients, it was then her responsibility to make sure that the policy continued to be followed. Even after Nightingale's health declined and she could not practice nursing, she worked from her bed to see that health care policies were implemented throughout the United Kingdom. Nightingale (1873) wrote, "Every great reformer began by being a solitary dissenter … But in every case it was a positive dissent; ending not in a protest, but in a great reform" (p. 26). Nightingale believed not only in being a part of the policy process, but also in being a participant in a positive process.

Another pioneer nurse in public health policy making was Lillian Wald, who practiced in the early 20th century in the tenements of New York City. She worked tirelessly to improve the health of some of the poorest residents who were often immigrants. She created cooperative relationships with organizations to provide her clients with needed items and services. Wald kept track of various incidents in her community and would relate the incidents when they were needed to influence and educate the public to understand their responsibility to the underserved community (Buhler-Wilkerson, 1993). Working with government and health officials, Wald led policy reform to improve living conditions, form child labor laws, and establish clinics for the residents. These reforms led to the establishment of the Henry Street Nurses' Settlement, for which Wald sought and received financing from private individuals. Various services were provided by the Settlement, including a milk station, a convalescent center, county homes, first aid stations, maternity services, home visits, kindergartens, job training, and recreational activities. This establishment was the beginning of what is now known as public health nursing.

Margaret Sanger was another nurse who saw policies that needed to be changed, and worked to improve the life of her community residents. Sanger sought to increase the use and availability of birth control measures, such as condoms and spermicides. Sanger's dedication to changing contraception policies began when she connected her mother's premature death to having experienced 18 pregnancies. Sanger helped to change laws that prohibited education about, use of, and sending information through the mail about contraception (Wardell, 1980).

Today, community health nursing is guided by the American Nurses Association (ANA) *Code of Ethics for Nurses with Interpretive Statements* (ANA, 2001) and the ANA Social Policy Statement (ANA, 2010). Both of these documents include sections on nurses' responsibility to the public and threats to the health and safety of the community. The ANA Code of Ethics also specifically states that nurses "participate in institutional and legislative efforts to promote health and meet national health objectives … support initiatives that address barriers to health such as poverty, homelessness, unsafe living conditions, abuse and violence, and lack of access to health services" (ANA, 2001, provision 8.2).

More recently, Healthy People 2020 directs providers of care, including community health nurses, to work toward the achievement of four overarching goals: to eliminate preventable disease, disability, injury, and premature death; to achieve health equity, eliminate disparities, and improve the health of all groups; to create social and physical environments that promote good health for all; and to promote healthy development and healthy behaviors across every stage of life (U.S. Department of Health and Human Services, 2009). Health care providers are encouraged to work with communities to implement health programs to further the health of the community and to use the Healthy People goals to set an agenda for community health improvements. Setting an agenda for health improvements involves using knowledge, expertise, and experience to work with local organizations and officials to enact health policies and set goals for the individual communities.

Florence Nightingale, Lillian Wald, and Margaret Sanger addressed community issues for community health. Today, our challenge is to work with community residents to identify the health issues of concern and collaborate to form an action plan.

POLICY OR POLITICS?

How is policy affected by politics? How does politics shape policy? *Politics* is defined as "the process of influencing the allocation of scarce resources" (Mason et al., 2007, p. 5). However, politics is a word that has assumed a meaning much broader and much less neutral than the definition. When a discussion of politics occurs, often the context determines the meaning. A person's perception of politics will depend on his or her experiences and knowledge of politics. Politics occur within all organizations, whether they are for-profit businesses, not-for-profit service agencies, social gatherings, faith communities, health care settings, or governmental agencies. The manner in which politics operate, positively or negatively, in an organization will depend on the rules that have been established as acceptable within that organization, whether the goals are important to the participants, and whether one person is in a position to change the rules of the organization (Mason et al., 2007).

The community health nurse lobbies for the allocation of resources and shapes policies by analyzing the impact of the policy on community health. Lobbying for resources and analyzing the impact of policy on health defines politics. The community health nurse is a politician for health. Politics is sometimes portrayed negatively when it appears that the politicians will do whatever is necessary to achieve their goals. Now is a good time to review Chapter 5 and consider the connection between politics and ethical quandaries. Consider the following potential ethical quandary. Schools in a geographic area with a high tax base fund a full-time school nurse for each public school. Schools in the same geographic area with a low tax base cannot afford a nurse for any of the schools. Should the taxpayers living in the geographic area with school nurses share their revenue to budget school nurses for schools without a nurse? Defend your answer. Describe how you could bring citizens together to discuss the issue. What health data would you want to gather about the students (in both the schools with and without a nurse) before the meeting? What would be the goal of the meeting?

POLICY MAKING IN ACTION

Policy making occurs in many settings and among many people. Any system involving people will necessitate policy making. Policy-making systems include governmental organizations, such as state, county, and city public health departments; federal and state legislatures; offices of the governor and mayor; as well as local and state regulatory agencies, such as public utilities, housing, and zoning. Additionally, private, not-for-profit organizations, such as faith communities, the American Red Cross, the Shriners, United Way, and the Lion's Club are also policy-making systems.

The Process

The basic building blocks of nursing, the steps of the nursing process, are similar to the process used in policy making. Please refer to Table 8.2 as we discuss this process.

Step 1: Problem Recognition and Definition

Policy making begins with recognizing and defining the problem of interest to the policy makers. We can use as an example a frequently encountered problem in urban community health—paved walkways (i.e., sidewalks) in disrepair. Broken or uneven paved walkways are a danger to all pedestrians. For example, pedestrians may be forced to walk around broken paved walkways and into the street, putting them at increased risk for a motor vehicle accident. The community health nurse may become aware of the problem of inadequate

TABLE 8.2 Steps of the Nursing Process and Policy-Making Process

	The Nursing Process	The Policy-Making Process
Step 1	Assessment	Problem recognition and definition
Step 2	Diagnosis	Policy formulation
Step 3	Planning	Policy adoption
Step 4	Implementation	Budgeting and policy implementation
Step 5	Evaluation	Policy evaluation

paved walkways through observation; conversations with community members and business owners; and reports from local police, hospital, or emergency aid workers who file accident reports. The community health nurse would confirm the problem by gathering information on the number of accidents that have occurred to different age groups. Next, the community health nurse would compare the number of accidents on inadequately paved walkways with the number of accidents on adequately paved walkways.

Step 2: Policy Formulation

Once the problem has been clearly defined, the policy maker (i.e., the community health nurse) determines what type of policy is required and who has jurisdiction over the problem. A policy would be proposed to maintain safe paved walkways. Or in nursing process terms, a diagnosis is made. Returning to the example of the paved walkways, the community health nurse would determine which agency and persons were responsible for the construction and maintenance of the paved walkways. Paved walkways on public property are usually the responsibility of public (i.e., city) government. Therefore, the appropriate place to begin a discussion about the need for safe paved walkways is city government, often city council members. Now is a good time to stop and learn who the city government representatives are where you live. What are their names? When were they elected? Where are their offices? How can you contact government representatives to discuss community problems affecting health and public safety, such as paved walkways in disrepair and the related information on accidents?

Continuing with Step 2, policy formulation, a group of concerned community members, including the community health nurse, must write a proposal to be presented to the responsible city government officials. The proposal is usually a brief statement about the problem and the need for action (i.e., a policy) to correct the problem. The goal of the proposal is to have the walkway issue placed on the agenda for consideration by city government policy makers when a meeting is convened. To bring the issue of inadequately maintained paved walkways to the attention of the authorities, increased public awareness is necessary. The community health nurse and interested citizens can increase public awareness by writing letters to the editor of the local newspaper regarding the lack of safe walkways and associated accidents. Detailing incidents of persons injured as a result of the walkway condition and presenting the information to local faith-based, service, and civic organizations as well as at public forums is an excellent way to inform the public about the problem.

Now is a good time to take a break, get a beverage, and review today's newspaper. What issues affecting the public's health are discussed in the newspaper? What further information would you need to gather to document the extent of one of these problems? How would you identify the responsible agency? What strategies do you suggest to increase public awareness about the problem?

Step 3: Policy Adoption

The third step of the policy-making process, which coincides with planning in the nursing process, is the adoption of the policy by the appropriate agency. Once a policy proposal has been presented to responsible officials and the policy has been adopted, governing rules and regulations are formulated to administer it. For example, the department responsible for paved walkways will be specified, along with a schedule for routinely assessing the condition of walkways and completing necessary maintenance. It is important for the community health nurse and interested community residents to be present during the discussion of the policy proposal by the public officials. The nurse and citizens must always request an opportunity to testify as to the importance of safe walkways and be prepared to offer the names of specific walkways needing immediate repair. Finances will need to be allocated to begin the fourth step, the process of implementation.

Step 4: Budgeting and Policy Implementation

Following approval from the appropriate agency and allocation of a budget, the policy can be implemented. For the paved walkway example, implementation is the completion of paved walkway repairs. Frequently during Step 4, public education programs are necessary to increase awareness of the new policy, especially if the new policy requires a change in citizen behavior, such as seat belt use or no smoking in public places.

Step 5: Policy Evaluation

After the policy has been implemented, the final step is evaluation of the new policy of paved walkway repair and maintenance. When the goals of the policy—routine walkway maintenance and repair—are being met, then the policy for safe walkways is effective. However, if the evaluation determines that paved walkway maintenance and repair is not completed, then the public policy process would begin again. The community health nurse must continue to collect data on the occurrence of accidents on pedestrian walkways. Accident data can help determine the efficacy of the new walkway policy. If accidents and injuries continue to occur at paved walkways, then the community nurse would collect data to determine the association of the injury with the condition of the walkway. The data may indicate that the cause of the pedestrian accidents is not associated with the condition of the walkway, but rather with the lack of paved walkways. If the problem is lack of paved walkways as opposed to our first problem of paved walkways in disrepair, then the community health nurse begins the policy-making process anew with the goal being a policy for the construction of new paved walkways.

Policy versus Program

You may be asking, "What is the difference between a 'program,' funded by local government, to repair paved walkways and a 'policy,' formed and funded by local government, to repair walkways?" Programs are usually a set of actions to achieve a goal, such as a program to build paved walkways around all schools in an area. In contrast, policy is a set of principles, frequently formally agreed on, such as those that govern the construction and routine maintenance of walkways. Frequently, paved walkways are required to be built for all new construction as part of a city building code; however, the maintenance and repair of the walkways is not formulated into a policy or code. Therefore, a community may confront the need for additional public policy regarding the maintenance of paved walkways. Let's discuss another public policy action that began with community action.

An additional policy that has followed the policy-making process and has impacted the health and well-being of children is that of mandatory child safety seat laws. The first step of the policy-making process, problem recognition, began when the incidence of children being killed or severely injured in motor vehicle accidents was associated with the injured or deceased children being unrestrained on vehicle impact. Citizens (i.e., policy makers) gathered data, consulted experts, and formulated a policy to address the issue. The policy was then presented to the appropriate governing body, which in this case was the state legislature. The requirement of child safety seats was discussed, debated, and approved by majority vote. A date for implementation was determined. Once the policy was implemented, the policy makers continued to measure the effectiveness of the policy and determine whether fewer deaths and injuries to children occurred following the policy. The answer has been yes, but the policy makers continue to adjust the policy to make children safer, such as including older children in the child restraint law.

IMPORTANT HEALTH POLICY ISSUES FOR ALL COMMUNITIES

Over the past several decades, three areas of greatest concern in health care have been (1) access to care; (2) cost of care; and (3) quality of care. These concerns have taken center stage in national health care and are issues of great concern on the community level. There has been much debate over the financing of health care and the health care delivery system in the United States. Some Americans contend they have the right (access) to the best care (quality) at the lowest cost (cost) regardless of their level of income. These issues continue to be at the forefront of nursing and health care policy discussions.

In 2007, the ANA legislative initiatives included the issues of access, cost, and quality at a level at which action can be implemented (ANA, 2007). For instance, access to care now includes access to health coverage, health plans, and Medicare reform. Cost of care includes advanced practice nurse coverage, health plans, Medicaid cost containment, medical errors, medical malpractice liability/tort reform, and Medicare reform/prescription drugs. Finally, quality of care now includes adequate and appropriate nurse staffing, mandatory overtime, safe health care reporting, "whistle-blowing" protection for nurses, and safe patient handling. It is now the role of the community health nurse to be aware of these issues, to learn how they affect the community, and to partner with the community to become a united voice for the citizens.

In 2010, the Affordable Care Act (ACA) was passed by the U.S. Congress. This legislation will bring about the largest change in American health care since the implementation of Medicare and Medicaid in 1965. The goal of the ACA is to put consumers in charge of their health care and to provide them with the stability and flexibility needed to make informed health care decisions. Most sections of the ACA will be implemented in 2014, with a few having been implemented earlier and a few delayed while waiting on clarification. The main benefits to consumers are fewer limits on coverage, more affordable health plans, financial help to purchase insurance, and Medicaid expansion. Some additional more specific benefits are adult children can remain on a parent's insurance plan until age 26, and insurance providers provide coverage for preventive services such as well child visits, blood pressure and cancer screening, and flu shots (Health Care Reform, 2013).

During the same time period that the ACA was being debated and then passed, the Institute of Medicine and the Robert Wood Johnson Foundation began a process to produce a report and prepare a blueprint for the future of nursing. The 2010 report, titled "The Future of Nursing: Leading Change, Advancing Health," includes four main points: (1) nurses should practice to the full extent of their education, (2) nurses should achieve higher education through seamless academic progression, (3) nurses should be full partners with physicians and other health care providers in redesigning U.S. health care, and (4) effective workforce planning and policy making require improved data gathering and information infrastructure (Institute of Medicine, 2010). This report is being utilized by many nursing organizations as nursing professionals establish their role in the current health care environment. Community health nurses continue to be vital links for community members in obtaining health care services and advocates in the areas of health promotion and disease prevention.

HOW CAN A NURSE AFFECT HEALTHY PUBLIC POLICY?

Nurses can and do influence health policy. Box 8.1 lists steps a community health nurse can take to advance policy making, and each action is discussed below.

- **Learn the legislative process**. To influence and initiate changes in the health care system, the nurse needs to know about the legislative process. Nurses can learn about the

> **Box 8.1   What Can a Nurse Do to Influence Health Policy?**
>
> 1. Learn the legislative process.
> 2. Stay informed on current issues.
> 3. Identify government representatives.
> 4. Be an active constituent.
> 5. Speak out.

legislative process by visiting websites of local, state, and federal governments. Many of these websites exist to educate the public on the legislative process and to inform constituents on how to be more involved. Information may also be obtained from government internet sites that inform and educate citizens on how to participate in local/city government by serving on boards or committees.

- **Stay informed on current issues**. It is important that community health nurses stay informed on issues that are important to the profession of nursing, to the community members we serve, and to the community at large. Without remaining current on the issues, it is impossible to know what information to collect, with whom to share the information, and when to speak out. Reading the local newspaper with attention to local community issues is an excellent way to stay informed.
- **Identify government representatives**. Most government websites have links to enable constituents to identify their representatives and provide addresses and phone numbers for contacting representatives.
- **Be an active constituent**. Nurses can be active members of a constituency by writing letters, making visits, or calling representatives. Nurses as professionals may also choose to provide nursing expertise as policies and programs are being designed and to work with coalitions who have similar interests in the issues.
- **Speak out**. Community health nurses can also be advocates for the people with whom they work. Being an advocate involves speaking for those who cannot speak for themselves. An additional role of a community health nurse is to be knowledgeable of new programs, evaluate whether targeted groups are being served as proposed, and keep policy makers aware of progress or lack of progress toward goals.

Finally, remember that successful policy making depends on you. To be a part of a successful policy-making process and healthy policy formation, stay focused on the needs of the citizens. Listen attentively. Personal relationships are the currency by which things happen. Be persistent. Show that you are concerned and will remain involved. Be prepared with data to demonstrate the effect of the problem on community health. Be positive. People are drawn to positive people. Positivity is a low-cost investment that has a high return. Be patient with the policy-making process, whether it occurs through a legislative body or a smaller organization. Time to reflect on the policy is part of the process, so patience is vital. Exhibit passion for the health issue. Your commitment will make a memorable impression on the community and policy makers. Lastly, be professional in every way and in everything you do. A lack of professionalism will always be remembered long after the issue is forgotten.

APPLYING YOUR NEW KNOWLEDGE IN HEALTHY PUBLIC POLICY

To apply your new knowledge in forming healthy public policy, please complete the following scenario. You read and hear news reports documenting an increase in the number of children drowning in your city. You ask, "What can I do?" Remembering the steps of the policy-making process, you begin with data collection. You need to know the actual number of children drowned this year compared with previous years. Has the number of deaths increased or decreased? Learn what the death rate from drowning is for children younger than 5 years this year compared with that in the last 5 years. Establish the death rate from drowning for children older than 5 years and younger than 18 years this year compared with that for previous years. (Now is a good time to review the calculation of rates and age-specific rates in Chapter 3.) What are the circumstances surrounding the deaths, such as time of day, day of the week? What are the specific ages and genders of the children who drown? Were the children unattended at the time of drowning? How many children drown in public pools? How many in private pools? What type of policy regulates pools in your city? Is there a policy for fences around pools? If yes, how high must the fence be? Must the fence be locked? Are lifeguards required at public pools? What about alarms for trespassers after pool operation hours? Are there regulations about having private pools in your city? Are there penalties for not complying with the policy? How often are the policies reviewed?

The next step would be to decide if there is a problem and if a new or revised policy is needed. If a problem exists, then it would be necessary to determine who has jurisdiction for the problem. Is it a local issue or a state issue? This distinction may depend on the location of the drownings and who has the authorization to implement and enforce the policies.

After determining that there are an increased number of children drowning or being injured at pools, and determining who has jurisdiction for the problem, a policy would be formulated to address the identified issue. To address the problem, the policy might institute regulations on fencing of pools, minimum height of fences, closure and locking of gates, penalties for noncompliance, and determination of who monitors compliance. Included in the policy proposal might also be a request for funding to educate the public on the dangers associated with pools and pool safety. Public awareness could be increased through school education, workplace meetings, highway billboards, or mailings. The policy proposal would then be presented to the appropriate legislative group. When a policy proposal is presented to a governing council, a presentation by the community health nurse and citizens in support of the policy is very helpful. Personal accounts of a family that lost a child to drowning are powerful testimony. You may also solicit support from other health care providers and request that they offer expert testimony on the issue of pool safety and child drowning. If the policy is approved, then financial resources must be allocated for the implementation of the policy. Setting a date for implementation is the next step. Included in the policy is the importance of public education on the health problem of children drowning and the new policy. After the policy has been implemented, the community health nurse needs to review the statistics on child drowning at pools each year to compare with previous years and to learn if the new pool policy is effective in decreasing the number of children drowning. This example is intended to encourage you to examine your local newspaper frequently and consider opportunities for you to act to form healthy public policy.

Summary

We have discussed the different types of policy and spent considerable time describing the process of healthy policy development, including the role of politics. We have stressed the importance of the community health nurse and community residents forming a partnership to enact healthy public policy, and we have described the specific steps of the policy development process. You are now ready to begin the dynamic process of partnering with community groups for healthy public policy.

Critical Thinking Questions

1. Discuss the different types of policy, offering examples of each.

2. Describe the personal attributes that contribute to successful policy making, and explain how a community health nurse could use each attribute toward improving health care for a community.

3. What actions can you as a community health nurse take to enact healthy public policy for each of the problems listed below? For each problem, list a plan of action according to the five steps in the policy-making process.
   a. No potable water supply in a segment of your rural county.
   b. No emergency plan for the evacuation of older community residents during an anticipated weather disaster, such as flooding.
   c. No paved bike paths in your community.

REFERENCES

The American heritage* dictionary of the English language (4th ed.). (2000). Boston, MA: Houghton Mifflin.

American Nurses Association. (2001). Code of ethics for nurses with interpretive statements. Retrieved September 1, 2013, from http://www.nursingworld.org/MainMenuCategories/EthicsStandards/CodeofEthicsforNurses

American Nurses Association. (2007). Nursing's legislative and regulatory initiatives for the 110th Congress. Silver Spring, MD: American Nurses Association, Department of Government Affairs.

American Nurses Association. (2010). Social policy statement (3rd ed.). Silver Spring, MD: American Nurses Publishing.

Buhler-Wilkerson, K. (1993). Bringing care to the people: Lillian Wald's legacy to public health nursing. American Journal of Public Health, 83(12), 1778–1786.

Health Care Reform. (2013, September 2). Retrieved from http://www.webmd.com/health-insurance/insurance-basics/affordable-care-act-provisions

Institute of Medicine. (2010). The future of nursing: Leading change, advancing health. Washington, DC: National Academy of Sciences.

Kalisch, B. J., & Kalisch, P. A. (1982). Politics of nursing. Philadelphia, PA: J.B. Lippincott.

Mason, D. J., Leavitt, J. K., & Chaffee, M. W. (2007). Policy & politics in nursing and health care (5th ed.). St. Louis, MO: Saunders.

Nightingale, F. (1873, July). A sub-note of interrogation: What will our religion be in 1999? Fraser's Magazine, 25–36.

Palmer, I. S. (1977). Florence Nightingale: Reformer, reactionary, researcher. Nursing Research, 26(2), 84–89.

Titmus, R. M. (1974). Social policy: An introduction. New York, NY: Pantheon.

U.S. Department of Health and Human Services. (2009). Healthy people 2020: The road ahead. Retrieved April 10, 2010, from http://www.healthypeople.gov/hp2020/

Wardell, D. (1980). Margaret Sanger: Birth control's successful revolutionary. American Journal of Public Health, 70(7), 736–742.

FURTHER READINGS

American Nurses Association. (2013, September 2). Retrieved from http://www.nursingworld.org/MainMenu-Categories/ANAPoliticalPower.aspx

Bell, J., & Standish, M. (2005). Communities and health policy: A pathway for change. Health Affairs, 24(2), 339–342.

Kaiser Foundation. (2013, September 2). The YouToons get ready for Obamacare. Retrieved from YouTube: http://www.youtube.com/watch?v=JZkk6ueZt-U&feature=youtu.b

National League for Nursing. (2013, September 2). Public policy. Retrieved from http://www.nln.org/publicpolicy/publicpolicytoolkit.htm

Thomas, S., Billington, A., & Getliffe, K. (2004). Improving continence services—A case study in policy influence. Journal of Nursing Management, 12, 252–257.

Toofany, S. (2005). Nurses and health policy. Nursing Management, 12(3), 26–30.

CHAPTER 9

Informatics and Community Health Nursing

Teresa J. Walsh

LEARNING OBJECTIVES

This chapter introduces you to the process of using and applying electronic information resources to promote the practice of community health nursing.

After studying this chapter, you should be able to:

1. Explain the process of using and applying electronic resources.

2. Locate, evaluate, and use electronic sources of health information.

3. Apply various search strategies to locate and retrieve electronic information.

Introduction

Informatics describes the science of information. Community health nurses use a variety of information to make health decisions and are expected to use informatics in practice to reduce errors; to obtain, evaluate, and manage information; in decision making; and in communication (Institute of Medicine [IOM], 2003). However, before we can use information, we must decide what information we need; obtain and evaluate the information; and then organize, synthesize, and communicate the information. Nurses who use informatics can better implement changes in health care. For example, new ways of retrieving, tracking, and storing patient information using computer technology demonstrate how informatics can support practice. Community health nurses focus on identifying sources of information on which to base health care decisions to improve the health status of aggregates and the community as a whole. The process of gathering information electronically to apply to community health nursing practice is the focus of this chapter.

Before we begin, you will need to familiarize yourself with commonly used terms associated with electronic information. Please refer to Box 9.1 for commonly used words and abbreviations. We begin with a historical overview of health information retrieval.

Box 9.1 Selected Vocabulary of Electronic Information

Bibliographic database: An electronic database available on the internet that organizes a collection of publications providing information about the title, author, source of the data, and a brief summary (i.e., abstract) of the document. Most bibliographic databases offer limited or full text of documents. These databases are often focused on one type of information such as health care and medical research or publications from the social sciences.

Blog: This term is a combination of two terms, *web* and *log*, thus blog. A blog is like an online diary, offering chronological sharing opportunities, usually on a specific subject.

Boolean searching: Using terms *AND*, *OR*, and *NOT* in the search string. These terms assist the user in increasing the precision of the search.

Directory: A list of websites found on the internet that have been organized by a hierarchy determined by the author of the directory.

FAQ: Frequently asked questions, a list often compiled as a help feature on websites or search engines to assist the new user.

Favorites: Similar to bookmarking, this is a feature used in Internet Explorer to create a list of websites you can return to later for further review.

Home page: The first screen or view of a website. The home page may have a welcome and links to more information about the site and Help pages to assist the new user.

HTML: Hypertext markup language is a format for creating documents for browser viewing. Text in the document is formatted with specific coding called "tags" to communicate with the browser program.

Hyperlink: Also known as a link, a hyperlink is a word or phrase or even icon or picture that the browser reads and uses to access another resource. The link may take the user to another website or another part of the website. *You* will know you have accessed a link when your cursor changes from a pointer to a hand when it is moved over the link.

Internet: A worldwide collection of networks in communication using special protocols.

ISP: Internet Service Providers (ISPs) provide access to the internet for a fee. *You* may access your ISP by using a telephone dial-up service, a cable network, or a wireless service provider.

Keyword: A descriptive term that can be used to search documents. When you use basic keyword searching, you are commanding the program to identify every document that has the word (your keyword) anywhere in the document. Keyword searching is useful to identify large amounts of information on a topic.

Mashup: When two or more sources of data are combined to create an online tool, often using mapping features.

Menu bar: Located at the top of your computer screen when you access your browser, the menu bar has a series of pull-down menus with commands to allow you to navigate your computer, the internet, or a website.

Search engine: A tool that uses computer programs to search the internet for websites and indexes those sites by keywords. You can access the search engine and search the indexed sites using keywords to describe your needed information. Each search engine uses a specific type of indexing, so different information sources could be produced searching different search engines with the same keyword.

Search string: The words and commands you enter into a search box to identify your desired information. Single word searching is keyword searching; adding Boolean terms or quotes around a phrase can increase the precision of the information yielded from the search engine.

URL: Uniform resource locator is the term for an internet address and is shown on your browser in the locator bar. The URL provides clues about the origin of the website, whether a commercial (.com) or an educational (.edu) site.

Web browser: Specific programs are needed to view websites on the internet. Your Internet Service Provider (ISP) will have a browser for you to view the internet. Most common browsers include Internet Explorer (IE), Mozilla Firefox, and others.

Wiki: An online collaborative writing opportunity often used in learning environments to allow multiple users to add to a growing document or site. Community agencies might use such a tool to develop a member site.

World Wide Web: The WWW is part of the internet supporting use of information exchange, including pictures, sounds, and movies, using what is known as Graphical User Interface (GUI).

Source: Hartman, K., & Ackermann, E. (2010). *Searching & researching on the Internet & the World Wide Web* (5th ed.). Sherwood, OR: Franklin, Beedle & Associates.

EVOLUTION OF HEALTH INFORMATION RETRIEVAL

Resources for use in community health nursing practice have evolved appreciably since Lemuel Shattuck first recommended the collection of vital statistics on community members in his 1850 report on public health in Boston (Shattuck, 1880), or when Florence Nightingale, in 1860, first published *Notes on Nursing: What It Is and What It Is Not* (Nightingale, 1860). These early publications stated the need for exact observation and recording of information such as the age, gender, cause of death, and number of infections experienced by a community over a period of time. Florence Nightingale stressed the importance of collecting and organizing health data. For example, her charts showed the decreased mortality in the military hospital at Scutari during the Crimean War, following nursing interventions to improve hygiene.

Now is a great time to get a beverage and look at some electronic information. A chart showing decreasing military deaths as a result of nursing interventions is available at http://www.florence-nightingale-avenging-angel.co.uk/Coxcomb.htm from the British website *Florence Nightingale: Avenging Angel*.

FORMAL ACCESS TO ELECTRONIC LITERATURE ON HEALTH

In America, the first collection of regularly published medical and health information was available in *Index Medicus*, first published in 1879 by the forerunner of the U.S. National Library of Medicine (NLM, 2012). As the NLM grew during the 1900s, formal cataloging of information led to publication of a list of titles owned and published for the medical community. In 1964, this computerized list became known as *Medical Literature and Analysis Retrieval Systems* or MEDLARS (NLM, 2011). In 1971, MEDLARS was computerized to provide access to medical literature. In 1997, MEDLARS Online (MEDLINE©) became available on the World Wide Web (WWW) (NLM, 2013). Today, MEDLINE is available electronically at the NLM website http://www.nlm.nih.gov/pubmed offering access to over 23 million documents, including articles with publication dates from earliest to the present. This database is available at no charge and can be accessed online. A tutorial to help you learn to use MEDLINE/PubMed can be accessed at the following site: http://www.nlm.nih.gov/bsd/disted/pubmed.html or from the homepage.

Another important electronic database available to support informed community health nursing decisions is the Cumulative Index for Nursing and Allied Health Literature (CINAHL©). CINAHL was initiated by a group of hospital librarians keeping index cards of articles helpful for the hospital's nurses. Today, CINAHL is a bibliographic electronic database offering some full-text access, usually available through medical or academic libraries. The most recent nursing and health care literature published is indexed in CINAHL, which is a valid and reliable source of information for community health nurses planning programming for aggregates in their community practice.

CINAHL is keyword searchable, meaning you can list primary words describing your topic of interest, such as "pregnancy" or "asthma." You can also search CINAHL using specific author names. Abstracts—short, descriptive paragraphs that provide summaries of articles—can assist you in choosing which full-text articles will be most helpful. Full-text publications and conference materials are also available in CINAHL, and you may limit your search to only those articles available in full text. However, for thorough searching, limiting a search to full-text articles is not an effective approach as it eliminates many valid publications not available electronically as full text.

Additional electronic databases of interest to community health nurses may be accessed from academic or public libraries with the assistance of reference librarians. For example, Psychology Information (PsycINFO©) from the American Psychological Association can help locate articles reporting information in psychology or social science. Education Resources Information Center (ERIC©) is an electronic database with many publications relating to teaching and education. These databases are excellent resources for community health nurses.

Electronic databases will help you determine the best strategies for evidence-based community health nursing practice. For example, what types of motivational programs have been most effective to increase exercise participation among community seniors? What strategies have proved effective to improve nutrition among adolescents making food choices from school vending machines? It is always advisable to learn what is published on a topic, such as exercise fitness and older persons or food choices and adolescents, before developing a health program. Always use at least two or three databases to complete a brief electronic review of a topic. The review will provide you with an overview of the current knowledge about the topic. The MEDLINE and CINAHL electronic databases are excellent, organizing a great deal of the current nursing and health care literature along with proceedings from formal conferences and meetings. Additional databases can be considered with the guidance of a reference librarian.

Now is a good time to review your agency or school library website. What electronic databases are available to you? Is CINAHL available? Is MEDLINE available? Locate searching tips and tutorials for each database from your library website or from the databases. How are the tutorials different? Search for information about informatics in both CINAHL and MEDLINE, using the keyword *informatics*. Did you find similar citations? What was different in CINAHL? Why do you think there was a difference?

GOVERNMENT SOURCES FOR HEALTH INFORMATION AVAILABLE ELECTRONICALLY

United States Census Bureau

As presented in Chapter 3, community demographic information is available electronically from the U.S. Census Bureau (n.d.). A national census is completed every 10 years, by household, to establish information on the population of the United States. Census data are compiled and available electronically at http://www.census.gov. The Census Bureau also completes many annual surveys that are helpful to community health nurses. You can access the census website and choose from a variety of survey findings, in chart or table form, to learn more about your city, county, and state. Annual surveys include economic information in narrative, chart, and table format.

Information available from the census website can facilitate community health planning, program development, and program evaluation. You can access the census data using a city, county, or state name, or using street addresses, census tract numbers, or zip codes. Census information can be compared with previous census data to identify changes in age, gender, and ethnic characteristics of a population. Census data enable the community health nurse to learn about the many characteristics of a community and to identify trends or patterns.

To begin using the census website, take advantage of the electronic tutorial available at http://factfinder2.census.gov/legacy/quickstart.html. Once you have explored the tutorial, practice your new skill of accessing census data by locating the city or area where you live. At the census website, in the box provided, select your state. You will be given choices regarding how you want to view the information for your home address: by county, by census tract, or by city. View the population chart; are there more males than females? Are there more males than females among persons over age 65? What are the ethnic characteristics? What ethnic group is the largest? Do these data reflect what you have witnessed in your community?

Access your census tract demographic data for the most recent census survey (2010), turning to geography and exploring the data first by county. Enter your census tract again and look for the population charts. What are the gender proportions? How do the gender proportions for the earlier decade compare with those for the later decade? What about the numbers of children under age 5 and the number of persons over age 65? Trends in population distribution can be noted by reviewing the census surveys. How can this information assist with health program planning?

Do you need a break from the computer screen? If so, I suggest you take a walk in your neighborhood and bring your census tract. Do you notice any differences from the information you reviewed from latest census data and what you witness? Are the ethnic, gender, and racial characteristics of the census tract similar to or different from the characteristics you learned from the census data? How has your census tract changed and how has it remained the same? How can you explain the changes? What implications are there for the changes in your census tract over the decades for community health programs?

The Centers for Disease Control and Prevention

The Centers for Disease Control and Prevention (CDC) is a government agency within the Department of Health and Human Services. The CDC electronically organizes health information that can be accessed at http://www.cdc.gov. Topics on the CDC website include prevalence of communicable diseases, such as influenza; updates for travelers, including tips for airline or cruise ship travel; and immunization information. Immunization requirements for all age groups are listed on the website, and an immunization record chart can be created by clicking on *Immunization Schedules* and following the guide. The CDC website also provides information on *Workplace Safety and Health* and lists resources for activities for health promotion programs at the work site and topics for workplace safety and health.

Under the CDC, the National Center for Health Statistics (NCHS) offers another source of health information called *FastStats*. Disease information, vital statistics, and health insurance facts can be accessed on this website found at http://www.cdc.gov/nchs/fastats.

Now is an excellent time to practice using NCHS data. Visit the NCHS website at http://www.cdc.gov/nchs/, choose two topics, and explore information available on the topics. As you place your cursor on different topics, you will see the pointer change to a hand, indicating a link to another source of information. Once you click on a link, you can access another website or web page on the internet. Click on the FastStats, and then click on Asthma, for example, to learn what information is provided. In addition to statistics describing the annual occurrence of asthma in the population, there are links to organizations and agencies that provide support for persons with asthma. Try exploring another condition listed on the "A to Z" list. What did you learn? How can this website assist community health nurses or community residents? Consider how you might share your retrieval of government health information skills with interested community groups.

Additional sources of government-managed health information available electronically through the CDC include *Morbidity and Mortality Weekly Report* (MMWR), available at http://www.cdc.gov/mmwr/; *Emerging Infectious Disease Journal*, available at http://www.cdc.gov/ncidod/eid; and *Preventing Chronic Disease Journal*, available at http://www.cdc.gov/pcd/. Each of these resources provides important health information and can assist you to identify, confirm, and track health problems. Their information is also helpful when planning for programming in communities. *Healthfinder* at www.healthfinder.gov is also offered online by government sources to provide reliable information on health topics impacting community health.

DIRLINE Directory of Health Organizations

The NLM offers a database called DIRLINE that provides access to organizations focusing on health. To identify resources available for a particular condition, such as diabetes or heart disease, begin your search at http://dirline.nlm.nih.gov/. DIRLINE is especially easy to use. Place the name of a disease or condition into the search box and click search. Information from this search will be returned in order of relevance. The DIRLINE search engine will identify documents or websites from organizations that contain the word or words you entered. Documents are listed according to how often the search term appears in the document. For practice, search for arthritis in DIRLINE. How many records were returned? If you link to each record, you will find information about the organization, contact specifics, and an abstract that summarizes available information. Now search for a condition that interests you.

Local Government Websites

State and city government websites are excellent sources of information. State websites have health information such as vital statistics, mental health services, and housing assistance. State and county Departments of Health compile information on the health events of the community, such as births, deaths, and marriages. They also maintain records on infectious disease occurrence, such as incidence of diseases, and reports of hospital activity, such as the number of admissions and discharges. City websites provide local information, including geographic locations of city services, such as fire departments, animal control services, and city planning.

Many larger cities have websites, usually sponsored by nonprofit organizations, such as the United Way. These websites contain listings of community health resources, such as clinic locations, services, and eligibility criteria. These electronic sites may have mapping programs to allow creation of a geographic map for a specific area that notes the location of all health and social service agencies. Public libraries frequently create web pages that organize lists of local resources. City and community agency websites may also compile information about the community, including the history of the community. Each of these websites may provide electronic access to a variety of information sources. Electronic websites provide convenient access to a large amount of data to confirm or refute what you witness in your community.

To locate your city or state website, use a general search engine such as Google or Yahoo. Search engines can search and index websites and information on the internet, and provide you with a list of websites pertinent to your topic. To locate the website for your city and state, type the city and state name in the search box of the search engine. If you wish to access only the state website, place only the name of the state in the search box.

To search for your city website, use a search engine such as Google. Place the name of your city and state in the search box on the Google website and click *Go* or press Enter on your keyboard. If you live in Chicago, Illinois, one website that will be returned by the search engine is the City of Chicago website (http://www.cityofchicago.org/city/en.html). You are most likely to see the headlines from the daily newspaper as well as a photograph of the Mayor and an accompanying message. Websites and homepages change often, so do not expect to find the same information each time you access a website. Links are available to specific information for residents, businesses, visitors, and tourists. Links also are often different colors than the surrounding text or are underlined. At the City of Chicago website, what information did you find under Health & Wellness? Did you find the locations for the public health clinics? Now access the website for your hometown. Can you find the location of a hospital for children? Are there services for senior citizens? What other information would be important to you if you were new to your city? Now go to the website for your county. Can you find the location of county health clinics? Dental clinics? Services for senior citizens? Are there maps to locate the geographic location of health services?

NONGOVERNMENT SOURCES OF HEALTH INFORMATION AVAILABLE ELECTRONICALLY

Many nongovernment organizations in the United States offer services and support for a variety of health conditions. For example, the March of Dimes and the American Cancer Society are organizations that provide educational materials about specific conditions within their mission. To explore one of these websites, go to the March of Dimes at http://www.marchofdimes.com/. The first page on this website is the home page, which gives you an overview of what is available. You may wish to explore general information about healthy pregnancies or choose to sign up for an electronic newsletter. Discussion groups are available for pregnant women to share information of interest. The website offers access to a section for *Professionals* or *Researchers*; place your cursor on these words to follow the links. As you link to additional websites and web pages, notice additional newsletters are offered as well as fact sheets of information. Continuing education programs are also available. Explore the list of continuing education programs and consider what might be helpful to a community health nurse working with pregnant teenagers at the local high school. Is there a continuing education course available? What other resources at this site might be helpful?

Visit the American Cancer Society, or another nongovernment organization of your choice, and learn what types of health information are available.

STRATEGIES FOR SUCCESSFUL SEARCHING FOR ELECTRONIC INFORMATION

All search engines offer help pages or tutorials to make searches more effective. For successful searching, first determine the terms that will identify the information you need. You may wish to start with general terms such as violence or use phrase searching, placing quotations around the words in phrase form, such as "violence against women," to increase the precision of your searching.

Boolean Searching

Boolean searching, a mathematical system used in computers, will increase the precision of a search. Boolean terms are word commands, including AND, OR, and NOT. When used in the search string, these terms instruct the search engine how to retrieve information indexed by the keywords chosen. For example, a community health nurse searching for information about the existence of crime in a particular community might enter the search string "*crime AND Mytown, Texas.*" The search engine would return all information indexed that pertains to crime as indexed in Mytown, Texas. Searching crime alone would return volumes of information on crime everywhere. Searching the location name would return volumes of information on the city or town. The Boolean word AND instructs the search engine to return only resources that have both terms in the documents, resulting in more effective searching.

The OR word enlarges the search yield by identifying all information focused on both terms searched. If a topic is referred to by more than one term, the OR word can be useful to identify information. When searching a topic such as smoking and adolescents, for example, the search string might be "*adolescents OR teenagers*" *AND smoking* to search for information about smoking that relates to this aggregate. What would be another term you might use in this search string? Using the term *tobacco use* in your search string would also be helpful to find information. Would you search hospitals for this information? Would you search the public school websites?

The NOT word can be used to limit yields when searching by identifying what you do not want. Limit setting is a tool to increase the precision of searches. If you need to learn about resources in your community that are provided by the private sector, the NOT operator might be used to remove government agencies from the returned list of websites. To do this you would add "*NOT.gov*" to the search string. Sites with URLs ending in ".gov" would be eliminated from your search results. Tutorials on searching are available on the internet and from most public library websites, and constitute time well spent before searching online. Now is a good time to review how to find a searching tutorial or a search engine.

Search Engines

Although a variety of search engines are available on the internet, they change frequently. Search engines change names or disappear altogether. Public library websites are good sources for identifying useful search engines, as is the internet site Search Engine Watch (http://www.searchenginewatch.com). This site monitors the development of search engines, organizes information using technical descriptions of search engine programming, and provides a list and descriptions of current search engines. General search engines also create their own directories and often allow open browsing in their subject-headed directories. Using these directories may help identify the terms to include in your search string.

Review the Search Engine Watch website at http://www.searchenginewatch.com and choose one search engine reviewed. Type the URL of the search engine into the locator bar on your computer screen, and press the enter key. When the website appears, find and read the help page, "about" page, or Frequently Asked Questions (FAQ) page to learn the special abilities and search commands useful for the search engine. Search for education information for your hometown. Use both the AND and the OR words to identify resources for descriptive information and indexed websites. The NOT word might be useful if the search engine is identifying information not needed for your topic.

Directories

A directory is a subject catalog available on the internet. Like a telephone directory, it is organized, often alphabetically, and provides access to a list (i.e., the index) of websites on the internet. Directories provide access to websites like an electronic database provides access to articles or documents. The Yahoo Directory is available at dir.yahoo.com and is searchable by subjects. Clicking on Health under the Directory list offers many increasingly narrowed topics from which to link for review. In addition to topics, websites are offered linking you to online sources of information, including government organizations and administrations offering wide sources of health information and resources.

To practice using a directory, access the Yahoo Directory at http://dir.yahoo.com and review the list of subjects. As the school nurse, you may have been tasked with learning more about the topic of bullying and ways to mediate bullying in schools. Choose the "K-12" link under education to start this search. Reviewing the many additional categories offered, choose the "Issues" link, opening a list offering bullying. How many websites are indexed? Read the brief paragraph describing the websites and choose one to explore by placing your cursor on the colored URL for that website at the end of the summary description. How would a community health nurse use this information? Remember, this directory will provide a list of websites to explore on topics that will link to more resources. This directory is an excellent start for you as you learn about accessing online sources for specific topics.

REFERENCING AND EVALUATING SOURCES OF ELECTRONIC INFORMATION

Once information has been located through your searches, you may wish to use the bookmarking function on your browser to mark websites for revisiting. In some browsers, the bookmarking function is termed *favorites* and is accomplished by clicking on the "favorites" command or icon on the menu bar. Other browsers may title bookmarking differently, and some browsers use only an icon, such as a heart. Practice organizing a document or a table to save your information for future use. Gathering electronic health information requires skills of searching, evaluating information, and saving the information to files or charts for future analysis.

It is also important to keep a reference list of electronic sources searched. Your final document must correctly cite all internet websites accessed. The correct citation for internet websites, according to the *American Psychological Association Manual*, 6th edition, provides the reader with the author, title of document, and date of retrieval if the source material may change over time (APA, 2010, p. 192). The website for the American Psychological Association format is http://www.apastyle.org/ and offers tutorials on this format; this is the most current source of format information for citation of internet or electronic information.

Finally, always evaluate the information you retrieve electronically as sources found online vary in their reliability and accuracy, even as nurses use these sources more often (Cader, 2013; Miller, Graves, Jones, & Sievert, 2010; Tierney, 2009). Consider the following criteria:

- *Author.* Who wrote the information? Does the author(s) have credentials to be a content expert? Does the website show institutional affiliation? Has the author written before on this topic or show other evidence of expertise?
- *Credibility and accuracy.* Is the information true, and can you confirm it with at least two other sources? Or is this information different from everything else you have found on the topic?
- *Currency.* When was this information last updated? Is it current information, or is more recent information available? Websites often have dates cited at the bottom of the first page to identify when the website was last updated. You will need to look for this date to know if the website is current.
- *Objectivity versus bias.* Information is used to inform the reader; sometimes, information is used to influence the reader. As you read information, be aware of potential bias exhibited by the author or website. Some information is produced to influence your opinions; likewise, some information may be omitted to influence your opinion.
- *Navigation.* Is the site easy to navigate? Are you lost constantly and unable to get back to the homepage, or is there so much flashing that you feel overwhelmed by the site? Or does the site make it clear how to find the information you need?

Summary

In this chapter, you have reviewed the development of representative electronic resources that offer demographic data, vital statistics, health data, and sources of health information useful to community health nurses. We reviewed and practiced basic skills of electronic searching, including how to access and locate electronic information, along with strategies for successful searching, and then evaluating information. Clients in the community are more informed each day and will expect the nurses they meet to be equally well informed. Informatics and the skill of electronic information retrieval can promote the partnership of communities and community health nursing practice.

Critical Thinking Questions

1. Compare the population demographics for your home town and two other towns of the same size from different regions of the country. Note the changes from the last decade to the present decade using census data. What are the health implications for changes you see?

2. Which electronic sources of information will be most important for the community health nurse using the latest research evidence to guide practice? Why?

3. Compare and contrast use of two reliable online sources of health information such as Healthfinder at www.healthfinder.gov and MedlinePlus at www.nlm.nih.gov/medlineplus. Each of these sites is a source of reliable health information published by governmental sources. Search for additional information on bullying on these two sites to locate useful information for the school nurse investigating this topic, noting the depth of information.

4. How could the electronic bookmarking function serve the community health nurse in practice? Why is this skill important to teach community residents?

REFERENCES

American Psychological Association. (2010). *Publication manual of the American Psychological Association* (6th ed.). Washington, DC: Author.

Cader, R. (2013). Judging nursing information on the World Wide Web. *CIN: Computers, Informatics, Nursing, 31*(2), 66–73.

Institute of Medicine. (2003). *Health professions education: A bridge to quality*. Retrieved from www.iom.edu/reports

Miller, L. C., Graves, R. S., Jones, B. B., & Sievert, M. C. (2010). Beyond Google: Finding and evaluating web-based information for community-based nursing practice. *International Journal of Nursing Education Scholarship, 24*, Article 31. doi:10.2202/1548–923X.1961

Nightingale, F. (1860). *Notes on nursing: What it is and what it is not*. New York, NY: D. Appleton.

Shattuck, L. (1880). *Report of the Sanitary Commission of Massachussetts, 1850*. Retrieved from Delta Omega Honorary Society in Public Health at http://deltaomega.org

Tierney, A. (2009). How do we judge reliability of information on the World Wide Web? Editor's choice. *Journal of Advanced Nursing, 65*(9), 1777.

U.S. Census Bureau. (n.d.). *U.S. census 2010*. Retrieved from http://www.census.gov

U.S. National Library of Medicine. (2011). *175 years: Our milestones*. Retrieved from http://apps.nlm.nih.gov/175/milestones.cfm

U.S. National Library of Medicine. (2012). *Index Medicus chronology*. Retrieved from www.nlm.nih.gov/services/indexmedicus.html

U.S. National Library of Medicine. (2013). *Fact sheet Medline*. Retrieved from http://www.nlm.nih.gov/pubs/factsheets/medline.html

Preventing and Managing Community Emergencies: Disasters and Infectious Diseases

Elnora P. Mendias and Deanna E. Grimes

LEARNING OBJECTIVES

This chapter introduces prevention and control of community health emergencies, incorporating principles from disaster preparedness and infectious diseases.

After studying this chapter, you should be able to:

1. Differentiate terminology applied to disaster preparedness.

2. Discuss a range of short-term and long-term negative effects of community disasters.

3. Describe principles of disaster preparedness.

4. Review principles related to the occurrence and transmission of infection and infectious diseases.

5. Apply the chain of transmission to describe approaches to control infectious disease.

6. Describe the legal responsibility for control of communicable diseases.

7. Identify nursing activities for community emergencies at primary, secondary, and tertiary levels of prevention.

Introduction

What are community emergencies? They are events large enough to have a major impact on community functioning. Because of the nature of these events, organized community efforts must be employed to prevent or control their impact. When such events exceed the

137

community's capacity to manage them, they are called disasters. Community emergencies may occur naturally, such as a hurricane, or may have a human etiology, such as an explosion or an inadvertent or deliberate release of a biologic agent. Community emergencies may occur spontaneously, such as an outbreak of the bird flu or a tornado, or may impact a community over a long period of time, as with the HIV/AIDS epidemic. Perhaps no other health issue has the potential to impact the total community—its people and all its systems, including the health care system—as do community health emergencies. Nor does any other health issue have the potential to impact nurses everywhere, irrespective of their practice setting, as do such emergencies. Therefore, nurses need to know essential information to enable them to respond to individual, family, and community needs related to these emergencies.

With its emphasis on partnerships, systems, and people as the core, the community-as-partner model can be appropriately applied to prevention and control of community health emergencies. Well-functioning community systems, with preparedness in mind, improve community lines of defense and resistance, thus decreasing the impact of negative environmental stressors and public reaction to the stressors. The principles implicit in the community-as-partner model, such as building partnerships among the people, health care providers, and relevant systems, are essential for prevention and control of community health emergencies.

Although community health emergencies may encompass many types of events, this chapter is divided into two sections for ease of presentation of content: prevention and control of community disasters, and prevention and control of infectious diseases. Nursing responsibilities and activities are incorporated in each section.

PREVENTING AND MANAGING DISASTERS

Disasters have occurred with tragic frequency throughout history. They have brought about injuries and deaths, environmental destruction, and disruptions in basic community services and systems. Depending on the type of event, a community can lose its ability to provide shelter, power and fuel, food and water, transportation, sanitation, education, communication, employment, recreation, governance, health care, and safety. Disasters can greatly affect a community's health and create immediate and long-term suffering and need. Disasters particularly affect vulnerable groups, including children and the elderly. Some disasters are potentially preventable; others cannot be prevented, but much can be done to ameliorate their effects.

Healthy People 2020 and Disaster Preparedness

Healthy People 2020 has identified a national preparedness goal: "Improve the Nation's ability to prevent, prepare for, respond to, and recover from a major health incident" (U.S. Department of Health and Human Services [DHHS], n.d., p. 1). *Healthy People 2020* has also identified a number of related objectives to address preparation, prevention, response, and recovery (see Box 10.1 for examples). Disasters may also affect other Healthy People 2020 health indicators and objectives.

Emergency preparedness activities or programs typically strengthen national or community capacity to deal with all emergencies, from initial response and recovery efforts to longer-term sustainable improvements (World Health Organization [WHO], 2007). National plans for emergency or disaster preparedness include collaboration between government and nongovernmental agencies or organizations, private sector groups, communities, and individuals aimed at enhancing preparation for, prevention of, response to, and recovery from health threats (DHHS, n.d.). Healthy People 2020 preparedness objectives are derived from national priorities denoted in the *National Health Security Strategy of the United States of America (NHSS)* (DHHS, n.d.).

> **Box 10.1 Examples of Healthy People 2020 Objectives for Disaster Preparedness**
>
> Develop and maintain the workforce needed for national health security.
>
> Ensure timely and effective communications.
>
> Ensure prevention or mitigation of environmental and other emerging threats to health.
>
> ---
>
> Source: USDHHS. (n.d.). *Healthy People 2020: Preparedness*. Retrieved from http://healthypeople.gov/2020/topicsobjectives2020/overview.aspx?topicid=34

Components of Community Disaster Management

As in other areas of community health practice, disaster management has its own unique terminology and classification schemes. We define terms and describe types of disasters and their impact on the community in this section.

Definition of Terms

Disasters are sudden or serious events of such a scale that there is considerable human, property, or environmental damage or loss, with resultant serious breakdowns or disruptions in community or societal functioning, and requiring exceptional efforts or outside resources for community management or recovery (Noji, 2005; Veenema & Woolsey, 2013; WHO, 2004). A *disaster* "is a function of the risk process. It results from the combination of hazards, conditions of vulnerability and insufficient capacity or measures to reduce the potential negative consequences of risk" (WHO, 2004, p. 3). *Hazards* are phenomena with "the potential to cause disruption or damage to people and their environment" (WHO, 2007, p. 7). *Risks* are the odds or possibilities that human lives or property will be lost or damaged, community economy or livelihood will be disturbed, or damage to the environment will occur as a result of natural or human-made hazards and vulnerabilities (WHO, 2007). *Vulnerabilities* are social, economic, physical, or environmental factors that increase individual or community susceptibility to the effects of hazards or that inhibit ability to expect, manage, or recover from a disaster (WHO, 2007). *Risk reduction* refers to actions intended to prevent or lessen the effects of hazards, including efforts to reduce vulnerability (WHO, 2007).

The terms *mass trauma* or *mass casualty incidents* (MCIs) are often employed to indicate events resulting in the deaths, injuries, disabilities, or emotional distress of many persons (AMA, 2004a, 2005). An MCI typically produces "more casualties than a customary response assignment can handle" (Thomas, n.d., p. 2). Examples of an MCI may include mass transit accidents, collapses of large buildings, exposures to hazardous chemicals, and other events of sufficient scale to involve numerous victims and to overwhelm the usual emergency response.

The terms *Weapons of Mass Destruction (WMD)* or W*eapons of Mass (or Multiple) Effect (WME)* are frequently used to describe circumstances that produce many casualties and influence health care or critical service access. Under US law (18 USC §2332a), WMDs are defined as explosive devices; weapons meant to produce serious human injury or death via poisons, toxic chemicals, or precursors; weapons using biological agents; or weapons producing radiation/radioactivity harmful to humans (The Federal Bureau of Investigations [FBI], n.d.) The mnemonic *CBRNE* is used to aid remembrance of WMD causes: **C**hemical agents, **B**iologic agents, **R**adiological agents, **N**uclear agents, and **E**xplosive agents (FBI, n.d.). WMD typically have a large impact on humans, property, or infrastructure (FBI, n.d.) and may also overwhelm customary emergency capacity to respond.

National preparedness plans in the United States rely on surge capacity to meet health care needs during disasters. *Surge capacity* is the ability of health care systems to quickly expand beyond customary services or capacity, in order to meet emergency needs, such as increased beds, personnel, supplies, etc. Although governments and public and private agencies at local, state, national, and international levels, as well as many individuals and communities, have attempted to increase emergency/disaster preparedness and response, persons experiencing or responding to these events are keenly aware that disasters and emergencies continue to overwhelm current response capacity. Nurses in all settings, then, must be prepared to encounter emergencies or disasters in their communities or larger arenas.

Types and Causes of Disasters

Disasters are frequently divided into two broad categories: *natural* (caused by environmental or natural forces) and *man-made* (caused by people). Examples of natural disasters include earthquakes; tornadoes, hurricanes, other storms; volcanoes; wildfires or other fires; land or mud slides; tsunamis; droughts; and heat waves (Federal Emergency Management Agency [FEMA], 2013d). Examples of man-made disasters include chemical spills or explosions, nuclear or radiologic disasters, acts of conflict or war, and terrorist acts (Veenema & Woolsey, 2013). Human-made disasters may be *accidental* or *unintentional*, or *deliberate* or purposive (Mendias & Grimes, 2011). Human-made disasters may have multiple causes, occur as a result of technological or industrial accidents, or follow a natural disaster (Veenema & Woolsey, 2013).

Health care organizations may experience emergencies related to interruption of normal function (building damage, power outages, interior flooding, etc.); overwhelming patient volume; or patients requiring specific injury care or treatment (triage, decontamination, isolation, or burn, surgical, or critical care, and so on). What poses a health care disaster, then, varies with needs and with available resources and capacities. For example, a plane crash with several severe injuries might be perceived as a health care disaster by a small or isolated facility. A large facility with a full-service emergency department and well-trained emergency personnel, or several smaller facilities working together, however, may have the capacity to handle many trauma victims at once. Or, while flooding or power outages can severely curtail or disrupt normal patient care in community health facilities, a health care disaster may be averted because other nearby resources expand services temporarily to handle increased needs.

Effects of Disasters on Communities

Several characteristics greatly influence whether a disaster can be predicted or prevented, or whether its effects can be controlled. In addition to critical characteristics such as the event's *onset, impact, and duration* (Veenema & Woolsey, 2013) are the event's location, *frequency, predictability, imminence* or *destructive capacity*. Further influencing disaster effects is human *potential to prevent or alleviate the effects of the event*. For instance, a gas line rupture and explosion may occur quickly and be unpredictable, but planning and activities that target prevention or minimization of such an event, such as regular inspections of pipelines and emergency response training and drills, can mitigate the effects of the event. Although hurricanes, tornadoes, and other powerful storms cannot be prevented, scientific advancements that permit prediction of a powerful storm's path may facilitate prestorm prevention and response, such as warning persons in the path to seek appropriate shelter or evacuating persons in low-lying areas before the event, as well as response and mitigation efforts during and after the storm, such as providing safe shelters, conducting quick postevent assessment, and offering emergency aid. An earthquake may be over in a few quick seconds, while a drought may affect an area for months or years; however, either may cause short- or long-term human, environmental, and economic harm or even trigger other emergencies or disasters, such as large fires or human starvation. Forest fires in heavily populated areas are more likely to result in deaths, injuries, and property damage than are fires in unpopulated or sparsely populated areas. Thus, these two types of fires are managed differently, with an eye to their potential for harm to humans, property, or the environment.

Examples of Community Disasters and Their Effects

It may take years for communities to recover from disasters, and some may never fully do so, unless they receive massive help. It is particularly challenging to recover to predisaster status when there are repeated disasters or complex disasters, where one disaster contributes to another. Several examples of disasters that have captured worldwide attention are presented here.

Fukushima, Japan, 2011

The 2011 East Japan earthquake and ensuing tsunami directly resulted in almost 16,000 deaths across Japan (Smith, 2013). While unexpected and not preventable in themselves, these disasters led to an event even more catastrophic and with greater impact, scope, and duration: the severe and extensive environmental contamination from radioactive material release by damaged Fukushima Dai-ichi nuclear power stations (Hayano et al., 2013; Tanaka, 2012). These have resulted in "seemingly infinite damage to the daily life of residents" (Tanaka, 2012, p. 471). In addition to the damage incurred directly because of the earthquake and tsunami, residents in the areas around the power plants encountered air and soil contaminated with radioactive cesium, capable of posing serious health risks for those who breathed or ingested it (Akiba, Tokonami, & Hosoda, 2013; Hayano et al., 2013; Tanaka, 2012).

Following the disasters, many persons in the Fukushima area evacuated voluntarily or because of government mandate. Japanese authorities and others undertook screening for exposure to radioactivity in power plant employees, first responders, and other residents and evacuees from Fukushima and nearby areas (Akiba, Tokonami, & Hosoda, 2013). While Japanese investigators have reported recent screenings indicating higher levels of radioactive cesium in some Fukushima senior citizens, they also indicated lower levels of radioactive cesium in nearby school children than initially estimated (Hayano et al., 2013). Owing to potential risks to human health, radiological experts are recommending meticulous scientific study of the radiation-related mortality and other health consequences in exposed plant workers, first responders, and clean-up personnel, as well as testing/screening of foods and continued screening and vigilance in persons exposed (Akiba et al., 2013; Hayano et al., 2013). Recently, an international team of experts has noted that the Japanese general population, as well as persons residing outside of Japan, has no or low risk for cancer as a result of the Fukushima nuclear accident (WHO, 2013).

Mainichi Shimbun (2013), a Japanese newspaper, recently surveyed 25 communities in Fukushima. Their report suggested that postdisaster mortality for Fukushima residents has been greater than the nearly 1,600 Fukushima deaths directly attributed to the earthquake and tsunami. The report ascribed causes of mortality to be stress-related, including exhaustion, fatigue, stress, worsening illness due to loss of medical care, and suicide. A spokesman for the International Federation of Red Cross and Red Crescent Societies (IFRC) was quoted as saying evacuees' displacement difficulties were exacerbated by evacuees not knowing when they would be able to return home, especially among older evacuees (*Mainichi Shimbun*, Stress induced deaths, 2013).

The full longer-term psychological and physical health effects of this 2011 environmental disaster may not be known for years. Moreover, when typhoons or other potential disasters pose threats to the area, the damaged power plants are still potentially vulnerable and require efforts to contain risks.

Aceh, Indonesia, 2004

The December 2004 Indian Ocean tsunami is among the most catastrophic natural disasters in recent memory. Although the earthquake that preceded the tsunami was recognized and the tsunami could have been *predicted*, the sudden *onset* of giant waves caught people unawares and unable to seek higher ground. The tsunami death toll was estimated at 250,000 persons in 13 affected countries (BBC NEWS Asia-Pacific, Indonesia's Aceh makes "remarkable" tsunami recovery, 2010). Many of the dead were cremated or buried without identification (CDC, 2005). In addition to immediate injury and loss of life and property, many countries in the region experienced devastation of their health systems, with potential long-term impacts on population morbidity and mortality. In Aceh, Indonesia, 53 of 244 health facilities were destroyed or severely damaged, and many health service employees were among the dead or missing. Moreover, the large numbers of persons displaced by the tsunami, flooding, crowding, and a vulnerable population further increased post-tsunami communicable disease risks (WHO, 2005). In addition, the economic structure of the area was severely compromised. Sources of income, such as fishing and tourism, were devastated. Recovery was predicted to take years.

The tsunami and Aceh have largely faded from the international news. However, various sources have claimed the region has made remarkable recovery in physical rebuilding since the tsunami (BBC NEWS Asia-Pacific, Indonesia's Aceh, 2010; Ki-Moon, 2009), at least in some part to international efforts to aid recovery. Nevertheless, Aceh still faces many challenges in quality of life measures, such as life expectancy and poverty (Ki-Moon, 2009).

New Orleans, Louisiana, 2005

In 2005, although *predicted*, the *force* of Hurricane Katrina demolished many US communities in the southern Gulf of Mexico region, especially in the states of Louisiana, Mississippi, and Alabama. The storm is thought to have instigated evacuation of more than 4 million persons, brought about destruction of more than 100,000 homes and many thousands of businesses, and resulted in more than 1,200 deaths (Norwalk, 2007/2013). The storm left hundreds of thousands homeless and their communities in ruins. The hurricane's massive effects disrupted local economies, but effects were also felt around the country, including loss of businesses, increased insurance costs, and higher prices for gasoline and natural gas. Following the storm, in New Orleans, Louisiana, a nightmare unfolded. Although the hurricane had been predicted, levee breaches after the storm were *unexpected*, creating rapid flooding of more than 80% of the city. Thousands of residents were left stranded without power, food, potable water, sanitation services, or shelter. Many health hazards emerged as community systems failed. As the days of misery continued, many persons in storm-damaged areas felt bitter and abandoned by their government.

As of August, 2013, The U.S. Federal Emergency Management Agency (FEMA, 2013c) had provided about 19.6 billion dollars to help Louisiana residents affected by the two hurricanes, including 11.9 billion dollars in public assistance, more than 1.86 billion dollars to help rebuild Louisiana communities affected by the two hurricanes through its Hazard Mitigation Grant Program (HMGP), and 5.8 billion dollars to help Louisiana families and individuals with housing assistance and other assistance needs through its Individuals and Household Program (IHP) grants. FEMA provided temporary housing to 92,000 Louisiana households through 2012, when the last such unit was vacated (FEMA, 2013c).

In 2013, according to the Greater New Orleans Community Data Center (GNOCDC, 2013), 8 years after Hurricanes Katrina and Rita and 3 years after the Deep Water Horizon explosion and oil spill in the Gulf (another disaster affecting many Gulf Coast states), only about three quarters of its pre-Katrina 2000 population live in New Orleans. Reports indicate that New Orleans still has a high poverty rate (about 29% in the city, 19% for the greater metro area), unaffordable post-Katrina housing, and violent crime rates twice the national average (GNOCDC, 2013; Waller, 2013). Nevertheless, signs of recovery are present. New Orleans has survived the national economic downturn, experienced growth in knowledge-based businesses and maintained industry-related businesses, and reports its public schoolchildren are exceeding pre-Katrina state education standards (GNOCDC, 2013; Waller, 2013). Tourists are visiting in record numbers and spending in greater amounts (New Orleans Convention & Visitors Bureau, 2013), and the city has hosted major sports and other large events.

Community Planning for Disaster Preparedness

Historically, initial responsibility for planning and responding to US disasters has been the responsibility of individuals and local communities and governments. When these entities become overwhelmed, higher governmental authorities may intervene on request of local authorities. Planning for and responding to disasters must begin at the community level.

Multiple organizations may be involved in disaster planning and disaster management, including health care, law enforcement, emergency services and first aid, financial institutions, emergency shelters, faith-based groups, utility companies, and the postal service. Individuals, serving as volunteers, have also played important roles. Cooperation and coordination among the organizations, levels of government, and communities are essential for rapid and effective planning and response.

Among better-known national US disaster-relief organizations are the American Red Cross (ARC), the previously mentioned government agency, FEMA, and the U.S. Department of Homeland Security (DHS). The ARC is a nongovernment agency that provides assistance to humans affected by disaster nationally and globally (ARC, n.d.). The mission of FEMA, a federal agency now part of the DHS, is to "support our citizens and first responders to ensure that as a nation we work together to build, sustain and improve our capability to prepare for, protect against, respond to, recover from and mitigate all hazards" (FEMA, 2013a, p. 1). The DHS, as a result of the Homeland Security Act of 2002, was created via consolidation of multiple federal agencies into one organization, with the vision that it would "ensure a homeland that is safe, secure, and resilient against terrorism and other hazards" (U.S. DHS, n.d.-a, p. 1). The DHS has five missions for national homeland security: (1) prevention of terrorism and enhancement of US security, (2) security and management of US borders, (3) enforcement and administration of US immigration laws, (4) safeguarding and security of cyberspace, and (5) ensurance of US disaster resilience (U.S. DHS, n.d.-b, p. 1). The National Disaster Recovery Framework, a guide to recovery for disaster-affected states and other areas, is available at http://www.fema .gov/national-disaster-recovery-framework.

Additionally, nongovernmental agencies, such as the ARC, as well as local, state, and federal governments, have increased efforts to recruit and train health professionals and other volunteers to augment customary services after a disaster. You may wish to check with your local or state health departments or the Board of Nurse Examiners for opportunities to volunteer. Additional training is often provided to volunteers.

Stages/Phases of Disaster Planning

Disaster experts have described several *disaster stages* or *phases* for the planning process. Although different models have been used, one commonly described model has four stages: preparedness, response, recovery, and mitigation. We apply this four-stage model to describe an example community and nursing activities later in this chapter.

Agent-Specific and All-Hazards Approaches

Disaster planners may use either agent-specific or all-hazards approaches in developing their plans. The *agent-specific approach* usually addresses the most likely threats or hazards. An example of the agent-specific approach may be planning for flooding in communities in flood-prone areas, with emphasis on public warning systems, flood prevention efforts, determination of evacuation routes and procedures, public education, and shelter provision. Another example could be planning done by the owners of a chemical plant and the surrounding community to prepare for a specific chemical release, with emphasis on warning systems, protection through sheltering in place, care for the injured or affected, control of the scene and its hazards, and investigation of the incident.

Experts generally recommend an *all-hazards* approach to disaster preparedness (CDC, 2012; FEMA, 2012b), recognizing that people may encounter multiple types of hazards, depending on where they live, work, play, and travel. All-hazards preparedness planning involves identification of potential hazards, assessment of vulnerabilities, and determination of potential effects (FEMA, 2012b). All-hazards planning includes five hazard categories for which health professionals should be prepared:

1. *Natural* or *accidental man-made* disasters (e.g., a storm or fire)
2. *Traumatic* or *explosive* disasters: deliberate (e.g., a bomb) or accidental (e.g., a plane crash)
3. *Nuclear* (e.g., nuclear weapon detonation) or *radiation* disasters (e.g., a dirty bomb)
4. *Biologic* disasters: intentional release of pathogens or biologic agents to cause harm, also *termed bioterrorism (e.g., anthrax), or natural or unintentional exposures (e.g., severe* acute respiratory syndrome [SARS] or Avian flu outbreaks)
5. *Chemical* disasters: deliberate or accidental release of a harmful chemical (e.g., cyanide or chloride).

The U.S. DHS (2013) also recommends planning that strengthens critical infrastructure vital to national security, including reinforcement of cybersecurity. Examples include protection of power plants, roads and bridges, and public buildings.

Consider a small island community and its potential disaster causes from an all-hazards perspective. The island is vulnerable to storms and flooding (potential for natural disasters), with limited access and egress and with a substantial vulnerable population (including the elderly, children, undocumented persons, the immunocompromised, and the poor). The community has a port, railroads, and an airport, and it is located near major chemical facilities and a military base (potential for traumatic or explosive disasters). There is a nuclear power plant not far away, and the island also has large medical facilities (potential for radiologic/nuclear disasters). The port has had experiences with infectious diseases from around the world (potential for biologic disasters). Accidents at nearby chemical plants have resulted in unintentional releases of hazardous gases (potential for chemical disaster). The community's location—in a highly populated region, near a very large city and major business, industrial, financial, health, transportation, shipping, and technology centers—raises fears about intentional disasters.

In preparing for all of these potential disaster causes, an all-hazards response would include broad community collaborative planning and response, including multiple representatives of the community (law enforcement, education, local businesses, power resources, health systems, city government and other city leaders, transportation, communications, planners, service organizations, churches, other disaster organizations, members of the public, etc.). In addition, because of the large population in adjacent counties, and the large numbers of persons living in the region, collaboration with other nearby cities, counties, and the state would facilitate effective planning and preparing for any possible disaster. Multiple issues would need to be addressed, including evacuation, provisions for shelters or sheltering in place, control of infectious diseases, ensuring communication systems, emergency and routine health care, and recovery efforts.

Disaster Plans

Disaster plans should be simple, clear, realistic, flexible, and easy to implement, regardless of the nature and extent of the disaster or who must implement the plan. Disaster plans should be tested (disaster drills, equipment checks, etc.), updated regularly, and evaluated periodically and every time used by those implementing the plan. All health care workers should be able to locate and implement the disaster plan at their workplace. In addition to professional responsibilities, nurses should also consider personal preparations and develop and practice personal family disaster plans. Nurses should also encourage community members to develop and practice their own personal/family disaster plans (Box 10.2).

Box 10.2 **Personal Emergency Preparedness**

The American Red Cross has identified simple emergency preparedness steps:

1. Assemble an emergency supply kit.
2. Prepare and practice your personal/family emergency plan.
3. Get trained or ensure at least one household member is trained in CPR/AED and first aid.
4. Get involved in your community; know the most likely disasters and assist the community to prepare for these.

Source: American Red Cross. (n.d.). *Prepare your home and family*. Retrieved from http://www.redcross.org/prepare/location/home-family

---

Responding to a Disaster: The Disaster Paradigm

The Disaster Paradigm (AMA, 2004a, 2005) remains a useful model for recognizing and managing a disaster scene. Using the acronym *DISASTER*, this paradigm establishes eight priorities.

Detect

Is this event a disaster or an MCI? Is it potential terrorism? Is its cause known?

Some disasters or other public health emergencies, such as those on September 11, 2001, at the World Trade Center, may be quickly obvious. Others may be difficult to detect for many reasons, such as: (1) delayed reactions to a biologic or chemical agent; (2) prolonged incubation period for a biologic organism; or (3) nonspecific symptoms that may be easily misdiagnosed. In addition, there may be *multiple causes or agents*, either concomitantly or sequentially.

Incident Command

Should emergency response or emergency management be activated? Is an Incident Command System (ICS) needed? If so, who will be in charge of the scene (e.g., who will be the Incident Commander [IC])?

The ICS is a standardized all-hazards approach to handling emergencies that provides organizational structure and implementation or adaptation of response processes. The ICS facilitates integration of resources, coordination of private and public jurisdictions and groups, and common procedures (FEMA, 2013b). The ICS has been used for many years by disaster response groups or organizations, such as fire, police, and emergency management. The ICS is organized according to five primary functions: Command, Operations, Planning, Logistics, and Finance/Administration. The ICS may have a single incident commander or a unified command, with the latter most commonly occurring when the incident is multijurisdictional or involves multiple agencies (FEMA, 2013b). There is also an ICS system for hospitals and other health care facilities (FEMA, 2012a). Training for courses that meet National Incident Management System (NIMS) requirements are available in an online, self-paced format at http://training.fema.gov/IS/NIMS.aspx.

Scene Security and Safety

Is the scene safe and secure?

Generally, a disaster scene is best thought *unsafe until proven otherwise*. Disaster and emergency workers should consider scene safety before entering a disaster scene. If the scene is potentially unsafe for victims or rescuers, entry may be denied or care may be held or halted until the scene is safe. Scene priorities suggested by the AMA (2004b) include self-protection, followed by protection of health team members, the public, patients, and, lastly, the environment.

The scene must be secured so that only authorized persons leave and enter. If the event was caused deliberately, the scene and the evidence must be preserved.

Safety of responders to the scene is an important consideration. What, if any, *personal protective equipment (PPE)* is needed? The purpose of PPE is to protect people from exposure to a hazardous agent. Key considerations for effective PPE use include the type and amount of agent; how the agent was dispersed and in what setting (indoors or outdoors, large or small area, etc.); the scene activities needed; type of PPE required; and training for proper PPE usage.

Personnel at an emergency or disaster scene (and later at other care sites) must act to protect themselves before they can help others. This self-protection includes wearing PPE appropriate for the type of hazard. Health care workers should be familiar with universal precautions and may have had additional experience with PPE for specific biologic or radiologic agents (e.g., gowns, gloves, surgical or other masks, protective goggles, booties, lead aprons, etc.). The U.S. Environmental Protection Agency (EPA) provides excellent descriptions of PPE needed by personnel dealing with various hazards (http://www.epa.gov/). For health professionals in health care settings, the Occupational Safety and Health Administration (OSHA) (http://www.osha.gov/) identifies circumstances requiring health professional PPE usage, and the Centers for Disease Control and Prevention (CDC) recommends guidelines on PPE usage (http://www.cdc.gov/).

Assess Hazards

Are scene hazards known? What hazard(s) are or might be present? Could this event be an act of terrorism?

One must assess both obvious and less-apparent hazards and be aware that disasters can involve multiple or sequential hazards. For example, an explosion can result in a release of toxic gases and fire. Secondary explosive devices may have been planted at a bomb scene and may be set to detonate when the rescuers arrive.

Support

What personnel, equipment, or supplies may be needed?

Depending on the situation, support considerations include personnel, organizations or agencies to be involved, facilities to be used, vehicles, and supplies (AMA, 2004b). Assessment of support needs also includes whether local, state, or federal assistance is needed.

Triage and Treatment

What are the injuries? Is triage (sorting of patients to determine treatment and evacuation priorities, using a standardized method) needed? What treatments are needed?

Many nurses are familiar with the concept of *triage* used in hospital emergency areas. Although triage is best done by those with triage and emergency care training and experience, and many courses exist to provide necessary training, nurses should be familiar with disaster triage models. In an overwhelming mass casualty event or true disaster, the emphasis of triage may shift from meeting the most urgent *individual* need to meeting the needs of the *largest numbers* of victims to maximize the number of lives saved. Because a mass casualty may compromise health systems' or professionals' abilities to provide established care standards, the Agency for Health Care Quality (AHRQ) and the Office of the Assistant Secretary for Public Health Emergency Preparedness, U.S. Department of Health and Human Services (DHHS), convened an expert panel to develop standards of care for mass casualty events. The resulting document, "Altered Standards of Care in Mass Casualty Events," (AHRQ, 2005) was prepared and is available online at **http://archive.ahrq.gov/research/altstand/altstand.pdf.**

More recently, however, some have argued that altering standards of care during times of disaster is dangerous and not necessary (Schultz & Annas, 2012). In 2008, the American Nurses Association (ANA) published a guide, "Adapting Standards of Care under Extremes Conditions: Guidance for Professionals during Disasters, Pandemics, and Other Extreme Emergencies" (available online at http://nursingworld.org/MainMenuCategories/WorkplaceSafety/Healthy-Work-Environment/DPR/TheLawEthicsofDisasterResponse/AdaptingStandardsofCare.pdf). As Gebbie, Peterson, Subbarao, and White (2009) have noted, during times of emergencies, nurses and other providers should remain focused on three actions: maintenance of patient and health care worker safety; maintenance of patients' airway, breathing, and circulation; and establishment and maintenance of infection control. Thus, we echo Markenson (2013) and others in suggesting that nurses provide care in all circumstances, including disasters, to the nurses' best skill, preparation, circumstances, resources, and environment.

Although there is no universal disaster triage system, several are well known and used. One such system is the *Simple Triage and Rapid Treatment (START)* system. The START system uses a systematic approach (flow chart available at http://www.cert-la.com/triage/start.htm) based on three observations (**R**espiration, **P**erfusion, and **M**ental status [RPM]) to triage multiple victims into four categories of care: minor, delayed, immediate, and dead (CERT Los Angeles, 2013). Box 10.3 provides a description of the START categories, the colors typically used to indicate each category, and a brief description of each.

As the first step of the START process, rescuers instruct persons at the scene of the incident to move to a designated area away from the scene. Those able to move to the designated area are considered to need minor care, on the assumption that their care can be delayed. Rescuers then move systematically through persons unable to move, allotting 60 seconds or less per patient, performing assessments, and designating patients to a general category based on patients' treatment needs (CERT Los Angeles, 2013). The triage assignment is to locate patients in the immediate care priority, address airway or severe bleeding issues, apply an immediate tag, then move on to the next victim (CERT Los Angeles, 2013). An online CERT training course is available (http://www.citizencorps.gov/cert/training_mat.shtm). Triage continues until all are seen.

Triage should be an ongoing activity, because injured persons' status can change rapidly. Thus, advocates of the START method suggest persons with potential or suspected injuries be rechecked as often as resources and time permit (CERT Los Angeles, 2013). Online Community Emergency Response Team (CERT) courses, including START, are available from various sources and can be located using a search engine.

First aid and medical treatment for disaster victims depends on the type of emergency or disaster, scene safety, and resources needed and available. For instance, an explosion may result

---

Box 10.3   Simple Triage and Rapid Treatment (START) Tagging

Label	Color	Significance or Meaning
Minor	Green	Care may be delayed up to three hours
Delayed	Yellow	Urgent care, but can be delayed up to one hour
Immediate	Red	Life threatening, need immediate care
Dead	Black	No emergency care needed

Source: Community Emergency Response Team Unit, LAFD Disaster Preparedness Section. (2013). *Simple triage and rapid treatment (START)*. Retrieved from http://www.cert-la.com/triage/start.htm

in blunt trauma injuries, crush injuries, penetrating injuries, blast injuries, burns, psychological distress, and so on. If needs and resources indicate a need for triage, initial treatment at the site of the event will be directed at emergency care and stabilization for the most severe injuries, and first aid or supportive care for those whose care can be delayed. Later treatment may include restorative and rehabilitative care.

Evacuation and Transport of Victims and Casualties

How many persons need evacuation and transportation, in what order, and by what mode of transport?

Evacuation indicates removal of both injured and uninjured persons to a safe environment. In general, triage categories also dictate transportation priority. One common estimate of transportation needs in mass casualty situations is to have one ambulance for every five patients (CERT Los Angeles, 2013). In an emergency, school buses, city buses, boats, trailers, planes or helicopters, private cars, and other vehicles may become emergency transport.

Care should be taken to minimize exposure to hazardous agents and contamination of transportation sources and care sites with hazardous agents. Guidelines to reduce further exposure may vary, depending on the agent. For instance, if a hazardous chemical has been released, it is recommended that the triage or "safe area" be upwind and uphill or elevated.

Victims of some hazardous agents may also require decontamination before transport. *Decontamination* involves removal or inactivation of the toxin or agent. Proper decontamination prevents further harm or injury to the victim; minimizes the risk of exposure to rescue workers, other health care workers, other patients, and other persons in the community; and avoids or minimizes environmental contamination. Decontamination should be done by those properly trained and equipped. Multiple resources are available that identify when decontamination is needed and how it should be done. Among these resources are the Agency for Toxic Substances and Disease Registry (ATSDR) (http://www.atsdr.cdc.gov/) and the CDC (http://www.cdc.gov/).

Recovery

What are immediate needs? What are needs several days after the incident? What are long-term needs?

Recovery is defined as "the period during which the community strives to return to a 'normal' function level" (AMA, 2004b, p. 8-1). Immediately after a disaster or emergency, the focus is usually on saving lives. Most lives "are saved in the period immediately following the disaster, with fewer lives saved following the first day of the event" (AMA, 2004b, p. 8-1). Within several days, however, communities need to begin to be able to meet their customary needs. In the long term, the community may have multiple physical and mental health, economic, environmental, safety, transportation, communication, education, and other needs. However, disaster preparedness has a significant effect on reducing disaster stressors and assisting recovery.

Community and Nursing Activities for Disaster Preparedness

Many nursing skills needed in emergency or disaster situations are familiar to nurses, who have been performing them in the course of their normal duties in their routine work setting. Other skills, such as decontamination following a chemical release, may require specialized knowledge and training. Depending on the disaster and the setting, nurses may function dependently, independently, or interdependently as part of a response team. Although it is beyond the scope of this chapter to teach comprehensive community disaster or emergency preparedness, a number of excellent sources for additional learning have been described. Examples of activities to be performed by the community and nurse are described in Table 10.1.

TABLE 10.1 Stages of Disaster Response: Community and Nursing Roles

	Community Activities	Examples of Nursing Activities
Stage 1: Prevention (Deterrence and early warning)	• Plan and prepare before event is expected, with the aim to prevent • Analyze community vulnerabilities and implement preventive activities • Identify community resources and capacities • Implement effective community warning systems	• Organize and participate in community immunization activities • Participate in agency or community vulnerability assessments and strategies for improvement • Develop/implement prevention strategies for worksites, community sites, home
Stage 2: Preparedness (Continued prevention and preparation for disaster response)	• Implement community disaster education • Evaluate and update policies and procedures • Develop cooperative agreements • Plan drills and training	• Volunteer for emergency response teams • Locate/be able to respond to institutional emergency plans • Develop/update institutional/community emergency plans or protocols • Develop volunteer registry to respond to emergency needs
Stage 3: Response (Management and mitigation)	• Respond to the event (short and long term) • Assess community damages, injuries, or needs immediately • Mitigate potential hazards • Provide aid and assistance from within the community and request and secure other needed resources • Involve public health and other agencies for surveillance and hazard control	• Assist with emergency plan activation • Assist with resource mobilization • Assist with public education • Assist with establishment and maintenance of shelters • Provide nursing care (first aid, triage, immunizations, prophylaxis, treatment, etc.) • Assess public health needs of affected communities or populations • Implement disease surveillance, vector control, hygiene measures, safety measures for food and water, etc.
Stage 4: Recovery (Restoration, rebuilding, rehabilitation, and evaluation)	• Continue to manage and assess disaster effects • Monitor community systems and services • Evaluate community disaster response and implement needed changes	• Participate in continued surveillance activities • Participate in planning for and resuming normal health services • Participate in debriefing and evaluation activities • Advocate for disaster victims/survivors • Participate in policy development: support disaster preparedness activities

Competencies

Planning for, preventing, and responding to public health needs caused by disasters and emergencies have long been a role of community health nurses. Emergency preparedness competencies have been established by multiple organizations. Because these may be updated periodically, it is recommended that you become familiar with those applicable to you and periodically check for revisions.

Levels of Prevention

Emergency/disaster planning includes primary, secondary, and tertiary levels of prevention. For instance, evacuation before a major storm, provision of shelter to persons displaced by the storm, and assurance of a safe drinking water supply during and after the storm are examples of primary prevention (efforts to prevent harm or injury to persons in the affected community). Using the same storm analogy, screening for communicable diseases or anxiety reactions among shelter residents would be examples of secondary prevention (early identification and treatment of health problems). Caring for persons dying from storm-related effects, treating persons severely injured by the storm, and providing rehabilitation or psychological counseling services for persons with storm-related health problems would be examples of tertiary prevention.

PREVENTING AND MANAGING INFECTIOUS DISEASES

Despite amazing advances in public health and health care, such as the development of vaccines and improved sanitation, preventing and managing infectious diseases continue to be formidable challenges for health care systems everywhere. One contributor to the challenge is the rapid proliferation of drug-resistant organisms and diseases connected to antibiotic resistance (CDC, 2013a). Up-to-date information on drug resistance can be found at http://www.cdc.gov/drugresistance/diseases.htm. A second contributor is the emergence of new pathogens and new infectious diseases (CDC, 2013b). This is such an important issue that the CDC is now publishing a journal, *Emerging Infectious Diseases*, which is available at http://www.cdc.gov/ncidod/eid/. A third contributor to the challenge of preventing and managing infectious diseases arises from the recent threat that deadly pathogens will be used by terrorists (CDC, 2013d) with information available at http://www.bt.cdc.gov/bioterrorism/. These threats and challenges all have profound implications for nursing practice. Infectious disease control can no longer be limited to the jurisdiction of the public health department or the hospital infection control nurse. Every nurse, regardless of specialty area or practice setting, will be required to be knowledgeable about recognizing, preventing, and controlling infectious diseases. This section provides all nurses with the knowledge necessary to help prevent and control infectious diseases.

Healthy People 2020 and Infectious Diseases

One only needs to examine the Healthy People 2020 objectives to appreciate the magnitude of the infectious disease problem. Three of the 42 topic areas of Healthy People 2020 are devoted to infectious diseases. These topic areas include immunization and infectious diseases (31 objectives), sexually transmitted diseases (STDs) (10 objectives), and HIV/AIDS (18 objectives). The objectives for each category specify the target populations at risk for the condition and specific prevention and early treatment activities. Examples of the objectives are listed in Box 10.4. Baseline and target data for the objectives can be found on the U.S. Department of Health and Human Services (2013) Healthy People website www.healthypeople.gov/2020/topicsobjectives2020.

Principles of Infection and Infectious Disease Occurrence

Biologic and epidemiologic principles inherent in infection and infectious disease occurrence are reviewed, and major terms are defined in the following sections.

Multicausation

In a simpler time in medical and nursing history, science promulgated cause and effect theories of disease that relied on specifying one cause for each disease. Today, we recognize that all disease causation is complex and multicausal. Infectious diseases are the result of interaction among the *human host*, an *infectious agent*, and the *environment* that impacts the human host. This interaction is often pictured in a triangle of agent, host, and environment. The principle of multicausation emphasizes that an infectious agent alone is not sufficient to cause disease— the agent must be transmitted in the environment to a susceptible host.

Box 10.4 Healthy People 2020 Objectives

Topic Area – Immunization and Infectious Diseases (selected from 31 objectives)

IID-1 Reduce, eliminate or maintain elimination of cases of vaccine preventable diseases

IID-2 Reduce early onset group B streptococcal disease

IID-3 Reduce meningococcal disease

IID-4 Reduce invasive pneumococcal infections

IID-5 Reduce the number of courses of antibiotics for ear infections in young children

IID-6 Reduce the number of courses of antibiotics prescribed for the sole diagnosis of the common cold

IID-7 to IID-11 Achieve and maintain effective vaccination coverage levels for universally recommended vaccines among children and adolescents

IID-12 Increase the percentage of children and adults who are vaccinated annually against seasonal influenza

IID-13 Increase the percentage of adults who are vaccinated against pneumococcal disease

IID-14 Increase the percentage of adults who are vaccinated against zoster (shingles)

IID-15 Increase hepatitis B vaccine coverage among high-risk populations (hemodialysis patients, men who have sex with men, health care personnel and injection drug users)

IID-23 to IID-28 Reduce hepatitis A, hepatitis B and hepatitis C

IID-29 to IID-32 Reduce tuberculosis; increase treatment completion rate

Topic Area – Sexually Transmitted Diseases (selected from 10 objectives)

STD-1 Reduce the proportion of adolescents and young adults with Chlamydia trachomatis Infections

STD-5 Reduce the proportion of females aged 15 to 44 years who have ever required treatment for pelvic inflammatory disease (PID)

STD-6 Reduce gonorrhea rates

STD-7 Reduce sustained domestic transmission of primary and secondary syphilis

STD-8 Reduce congenital syphilis

STD-9 Reduce the proportion of females with human papillomavirus (HPV) infection

STD-10 Reduce the proportion of adults with genital herpes infection due to herpes simplex type 2

Topic Area – HIV (selected from 18 objectives)

HIV-1 to HIV-3 Reduce new HIV infection, transmission and diagnosis among adolescents and adults

HIV-4 to HIV-7 Reduce new cases of AIDS among all adolescents and adults

HIV-8 Reduce perinatally acquired HIV and AIDS

HIV-9 Increase the proportion of new HIV infections diagnosed before progression to AIDS

HIV-10 Increase the proportion of HIVinfected adolescents and adults who receive HIV care and treatment consistent with current standards

HIV-11 Increase the proportion of persons surviving more than 3 years after a diagnosis with AIDS

HIV-12 Reduce deaths from HIV infection

HIV-13 Increase the proportion of persons living with HIV who know their serostatus

HIV-14 Increase the proportion of adolescents and adults who have been tested for HIV in the past 12 months

HIV-15 Increase the proportion of adults with tuberculosis who have been tested for HIV

HIV-16 Increase the proportion of substance abuse treatment facilities that offer HIV/AIDS education, counseling, and support

HIV-17 Increase the proportion of sexually active persons who use condoms

HIV-18 Reduce the proportion of men who have sex with men who reported unprotected anal sex in the past 12 months

Source: U.S. Department of Health and Human Services. (2013). *Healthy People 2020: Immunizations and infectious diseases*. Retrieved from http://www.healthypeople.gov/2020/topicsobjectives2020/objectiveslist.aspx?topicId=23; U.S. Department of Health and Human Services. (2013). *Healthy People 2020: Sexually transmitted diseases*. Retrieved from http://www.healthypeople.gov/2020/topicsobjectives2020/objectiveslist.aspx?topicId=37; U.S. Department of Health and Human Services. (2013). *Healthy People 2020: HIV*. Retrieved from http://www.healthypeople.gov/2020/topicsobjectives2020/objectiveslist.aspx?topicId=22

Spectrum of Infection

Not all contact with an infectious agent leads to infection, and not all infection leads to an infectious disease. The processes, however, begin in the same way. An infectious agent may contaminate the skin or mucous membranes of a host, but not invade the host. The agent may also invade and multiply and produce a *subclinical (asymptomatic) infection* without producing overt symptomatic disease. The host may also respond with symptomatic infectious disease. *Infection*, then, is the entry and multiplication of an infectious agent in a host. *Infectious disease* and *communicable disease* (synonyms, according to Heymann, 2008) refer to the pathophysiologic responses of the host to the infectious agent, manifesting as an illness. Such a person, when diagnosed, would be considered a *case*. Once infectious agents replicate in the host, they can be transmitted from the host, irrespective of whether disease symptoms are or are not present. Some persons without any disease symptoms become *carriers* and continue to shed pathogens.

Stages of Infection

An infectious agent that has invaded its host and found conditions hospitable will replicate until it can be shed. This period of replication before shedding is called the latent period, or *latency*. The *communicable period* or communicability follows latency and begins with shedding of the agent. *Incubation period* refers to the time of invasion to the time when disease symptoms first appear. Frequently, the communicable period begins before symptoms are present. The ability to distinguish these stages of infection (Fig. 10.1) is important in controlling transmission.

Spectrum of Disease Occurrence

The principles reviewed to this point apply to individuals and their acquisition of infections and infectious diseases. Control of infectious diseases in a population requires identifying and monitoring the occurrence of new cases (*incidence*) in a population. Some infectious diseases are *endemic* and occur at a consistent, expected level in a geographic area. Such is the case with some STDs and with tuberculosis. *Outbreak* refers to the unexpected occurrence of an infectious disease in a limited geographic area during a limited period of time. Outbreaks of pertussis and salmonellosis are common. *Pandemic* defines the steady occurrence of disease over a large geographic area or worldwide, such as malaria in Africa. *Epidemic* refers to the

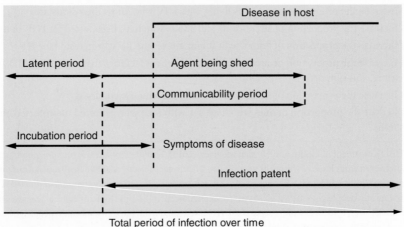

FIGURE 10.1   Stages of infection. (Adapted from Grimes, 1991, p. 19, with permission from Elsevier.)

unexpected increase of an infectious disease in a geographic area over an extended period of time. Epidemics are defined relative to the infectious agent and the history of the disease in the area. One case of smallpox anywhere will constitute an epidemic, whereas 1,000 new cases of gonorrhea will not be considered an epidemic in an area where cases of gonorrhea commonly exceed that number.

Chain of Transmission

Transmission is frequently conceptualized as a chain (Fig. 10.2) with six interconnected links. Each of the links (infectious agent, reservoir, portal of exit, mode of transmission, portal of entry, and host susceptibility) represents a different component that acts to produce transmission. The chain of transmission and its elements are summarized in Table 10.2.

Infectious Agents

Infectious agents are organisms capable of producing infection in a host. Because the process of transmission is different for every infectious agent, one might envision a different configuration of the chain and its links for every infectious agent. Infectious agents act differently, depending on their intrinsic properties and how they interact with their human host. For example, an agent's size, shape, chemical composition, growth requirements, and viability (ability to survive for extended periods of time) have an impact on transmission and the type of parasitic relationship it establishes with its host. Agents are classified as viruses, bacteria, fungi, protozoa, *Rickettsia*, helminths, and prions, based on their characteristics. Knowing the classification is helpful in understanding how specific agents are transmitted and produce disease. Also important is how the agent interacts with its host. What is its mode of action in the body? Does it kill cells, as does *Mycobacterium tuberculosis*, or does it interfere with circulation, as does the spirochete of syphilis? Or maybe it produces a toxin (*toxigenicity*), as does *Clostridium botulinum*, or stimulates an immune response in the host (*antigenicity*), as does the rubella virus. Other considerations for understanding the action of agents include their power to invade and infect large numbers of people (*infectivity*); their ability to produce disease in those infected with the agent (*pathogenicity*); and their ability to produce serious disease in their hosts (*virulence*). Applying the above concepts, the chickenpox virus has high infectivity, high pathogenicity, and very low virulence. On the other hand, *M. tuberculosis*

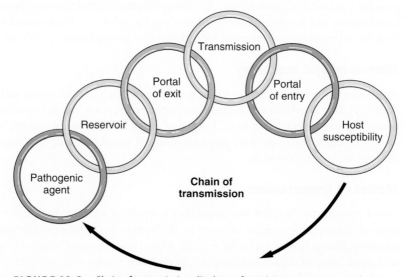

FIGURE 10.2   Chain of transmission. (Redrawn from Grimes, 1991, p. 21, with permission from Elsevier.)

TABLE 10.2 Chain of Transmission

Links of the Chain	Definition	Factors
Infectious agent	An organism (virus, *Rickettsia*, bacteria, fungus, protozoan, helminth, or prion) capable of producing infection or infectious disease	Properties of the agent: morphology, chemical composition, growth requirements, and viability Interaction with the host: mode of action, infectivity, pathogenicity, virulence, toxigenicity, antigenicity, and ability to adapt to the host
Reservoirs	The environment in which a pathogen lives and multiples	Humans, animals, arthropods, plants, soil, or any other organic substance
Portal of exit	Means by which an infectious agent is transported from the host	Respiratory secretions, vaginal secretions, semen, saliva, lesion exudates, blood, and feces
Mode of transmission	Method whereby the infectious agent is transmitted from one host (or reservoir) to another host	Direct: person-to-person Indirect: implies a vehicle of transmission (biologic or mechanical vector, common vehicles, or fomite) Airborne droplets
Portal of entry	Means by which an infectious agent enters a new host	Respiratory passages, mucous membranes, skin, percutaneous injection, ingestion, and through the placenta
Host susceptibility	The presence or lack of sufficient resistance to an infectious agent to avoid prevent contracting an infection or acquiring an infectious disease	Biologic and personal characteristics (e.g., gender, age, genetics), general health status, personal behaviors, anatomic and physiologic lines of defense, and immunity

has low infectivity, low pathogenicity, but high virulence if untreated. Smallpox is high on all three concepts. Last, how adaptable is an agent to its human host, and does the agent change (mutate) over time, as does HIV?

Reservoirs

The reservoir is the environment in which a pathogen lives and multiplies. Reservoirs can be humans, animals, arthropods, plants, soil, or any other organic substance. Some pathogens have more than one reservoir. Knowing the reservoir is important because in some cases transmission can be controlled by eliminating the reservoir. Understanding the reservoir of bird flu, for example, is important for any plans to prevent future pandemics in humans.

Portals of Exit and Entry

Agents are communicated from the human host through a *portal of exit* and invade through a *portal of entry*. Portals of exit include respiratory secretions, vaginal secretions, semen, saliva, lesion exudates, blood, and feces. Portals of entry frequently correspond with the portal of exit and include the respiratory passages, mucous membranes, open wounds, ingestion, and through the placenta or skin.

Modes of Transmission

Direct transmission implies the immediate transfer of an infectious agent from an infected host or reservoir to a portal of entry in the human host through physical contact such as touching, biting, kissing, or sexual contact. Direct projections of mucous secretions in the way of droplet spray to the conjunctiva; or mucous membranes of the eye, nose, or mouth during coughing, sneezing, and laughing is also considered direct transmission. Direct contact is responsible for the transmission of many communicable diseases, including scabies and STDs.

Indirect transmission is the spread of infection through a vehicle of transmission outside the host. Such vehicles may be contaminated fomites or vectors. *Fomites* can be any inanimate object, material, or substance that acts as a transport agent for a microbe (e.g., water, a telephone, or a contaminated tissue). Reproduction of the infectious agent may take place on or in the vehicle before the transmission of the pathogen. Substances such as food, water, and blood products can provide indirect transmission through ingestion and intravenous transfusions.

Vectors can be animals, insects, or arthropods, and they can transmit infection through biologic and mechanical routes. Biologic transmission occurs when the parasite grows or multiplies inside the animal, vector, or arthropod. Examples of diseases spread by this method of transmission include malaria, hemorrhagic fevers, and viral encephalitis. The mechanical route involves no multiplication or growth of the parasite or microbe within the animal or vector itself. Such is the case when a housefly carries gastrointestinal agents from raw sewage to uncovered food.

Fecal–oral transmission can be both direct and indirect. Examples of indirect transmission include water or food contaminated with fecal pathogens by way of raw sewage or unwashed hands. Unprotected oral–genital–anal sexual activity may result in direct transmission of fecal pathogens.

Airborne transmission mainly occurs through aerosols and droplet nuclei. The time frame in which an airborne particle can remain suspended and the size of the particle greatly influence the infectivity of the organism. Aerosols are extremely small solid or liquid particles that may contain fungal spores, viruses, and bacteria. Droplet nuclei, such as the spray from a sneeze, travel approximately 1 m, but usually not farther before the droplets fall to the ground. Within this distance, contaminated droplets may make direct contact with an open wound or with a mucous membrane (e.g., conjunctiva, nose, or mouth), or they may be inhaled into the lung. *M. tuberculosis* is transmitted through inhalation of contaminated droplets.

Host Susceptibility

Not all humans are equally *susceptible* or at risk for contracting an infection or developing infectious diseases. Biologic and personal characteristics play an important role in host resistance (defense against the infectious agent). Just as the young are more susceptible to diphtheria, older adults are at greater risk for bacterial pneumonia. General health status is important, as evidenced by the increased risk for gastrointestinal parasites experienced by children living in poverty. Personal behaviors certainly influence susceptibility, as does the presence of healthy lines of defense. One is reminded of the importance of the immune system and immunization status when observing the preponderance of infections experienced by the unimmunized and immune-compromised persons.

Breaking the Chain of Transmission

Breaking of one of the links in the chain of transmission is presented in Figure 10.2. Breaking just one link of the chain at its most vulnerable point is, in fact, what is done to control transmission of an infectious agent. Of course, where the chain is broken depends on all of the factors that have just been discussed—characteristics of the agent, its reservoir, portals of exit and entry, how the agent is transmitted, and susceptibility of the host.

Controlling the Agent

Controlling the agent is an area in which technology and medical science have been effective. Inactivating the agent is the principle behind disinfection, sterilization, and radiation of fomites that may harbor pathogens. Anti-infective drugs, such as antibiotics, antivirals, antiretrovirals, and antimalarials, all play an important part in controlling infectious diseases. These drugs not only permit recovery of the infected person, but also play a major role in preventing transmission of the pathogens. Recall that an important step in preventing transmission of tuberculosis and syphilis is to treat the infected person with antibiotics.

Eradicating the Nonhuman Reservoir

Common nonhuman reservoirs for pathogens in the environment include water, food, milk, animals, insects, and sewage. Treating these reservoirs or eliminating them, for example, by spraying for mosquitoes, are effective methods of preventing replication of pathogens and, thus, preventing transmission.

Controlling the Human Reservoir

Treating infected persons, whether they are symptomatic or not, is effective in preventing transmission of pathogens that can be transmitted directly to others. Another method of control is to quarantine, which means restricting the activities of those who have been exposed to an infectious agent during the incubation period. Quarantine was used effectively during the outbreak of SARS in 2003, when some hospitals required that their staff, which was exposed to SARS patients, remain at the hospital until proven symptom free at the end of the incubation period.

Controlling the Portals of Exit and Entry

Nurses and other health care providers break the transmission chain at the portal of exit by properly disposing of secretions, excretions, and exudates from infected persons. In addition, controlling portals of exit and entry may involve isolating sick persons from others and requiring that persons with tuberculosis wear a mask in public.

The portal of entry of pathogens can also be controlled in a variety of ways, including using barrier precautions (masks, gloves, condoms); avoiding unnecessary invasive procedures such as indwelling catheters; and protecting oneself from vectors, such as mosquitoes. Universal precaution guidelines are based on the observation that infected people may have no signs or symptoms or may not have any knowledge of their conditions; therefore, all people are assumed to be infectious, and health care workers treat them as such.

Improving Host Resistance and Immunity

Many factors, such as age, general health status, nutrition, and health behaviors, contribute to host resistance. Immunity, however, is an indispensable defense against infection. There are several different kinds of immunity, each providing resistance in different ways to different pathogens. *Natural immunity* is an innate resistance to a specific antigen or toxin. *Acquired immunity* is derived from actual exposure to the specific infectious agent, toxin, or appropriate vaccine. The two types of acquired immunity are *active* and *passive*. *Active immunity* is when the body produces its own antibodies against an antigen, either as a result of infection with the pathogen or introduction of the pathogen in a vaccine. *Passive immunity* is the temporary resistance that has been donated to the host through transfusions of plasma proteins, immunoglobulins, and antitoxins, or transplacentally from mother to neonate. Passive immunity lasts only as long as these substances remain in the bloodstream.

When properly administered according to established guidelines and protocols, vaccines provide acquired immunity in most cases; however, there are exceptions. *Primary vaccine failure* is the failure of a vaccine to stimulate any immune response and can be caused by improper storage that may render the vaccines ineffective, improper administration route, or exposure of light-sensitive vaccines to light. Some immunized persons never seroconvert, owing to either failure of their own immune system or some other unknown reason. *Secondary vaccine failure* is the waning of immunity following an initial immune response. This failure occurs in immune-suppressed patients whose immune memory is essentially destroyed.

Herd immunity refers to a state in which those not immune to an infectious agent will be safe if a certain proportion (generally considered to be 80%) of the population has been vaccinated or is otherwise immune. This effect applies only if those immune are distributed among the population. Without the presence of a susceptible population to infect, the organism will be unable to live because the vast majority of the population is immune. An example that demonstrates the principle of herd immunity appears in Figure 10.3.

Public Health Control of Infectious Diseases

Most human diseases can be classified as "personal health problems." Individuals with a personal health problem can be treated by the health care system one person at a time. In contrast, infectious diseases are categorized as public or "community" health problems. Because of their potential to spread and cause communitywide or worldwide emergencies, infectious diseases require organized, public efforts for their prevention and control.

Such organized, public efforts are under the jurisdiction of official public health agencies at the local, state, national, and international levels. Each of these units of government obtains its powers through a complex array of laws. An important concept to remember is that, in areas of health within a state, state laws usually prevail over federal law. The U.S. Constitution does not address health, and the Tenth Amendment reserves power to the states over all issues not addressed in the Constitution (Schneider, 2006). Historically, states have accepted this responsibility. For example, all states have laws addressing infectious disease control, such as which diseases must be reported and who has authority to implement quarantines. All states have boards of health and departments of health to implement and enforce state health laws.

The CDC is the public health entity at the national level responsible for infectious disease control. The CDC has the responsibility for monitoring infectious diseases and supporting local and state governments in control of outbreaks or epidemics, if such assistance is needed.

Although there are many aspects of public health control of infectious diseases, four are discussed here: reporting diseases, preventing diseases by vaccination, responding to an outbreak, and risk communication.

Defining and Reporting Infectious Diseases

Standardizing definitions of diseases is important for public health monitoring and surveillance at all levels of government. Diseases are defined and classified according to confirmed

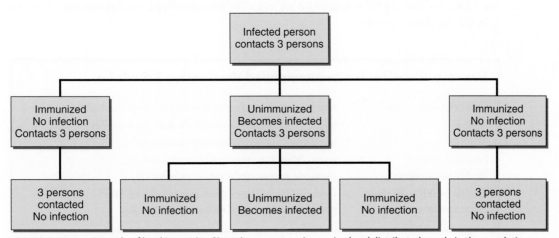

FIGURE 10.3   Example of herd immunity. Sixty six percent are immunized and distributed evenly in the population: 77% (10/13) are protected.

cases, probable cases, laboratory-confirmed cases, clinically compatible cases, epidemio-logically linked cases, genetic typing, and clinical case definition. Once defined, disease occurrence can be compared across time, populations, and geographic areas, and appropriate control efforts can be implemented.

Along with the Council of State and Territorial Epidemiologists, the CDC has designated notifiable infectious diseases, meaning that health care providers who encounter these diseases must report them to the local or regional health department. A list of notifiable diseases published by CDC (2013c) can be found at http://wwwn.cdc.gov/nndss. Because state health departments have the responsibility for monitoring and controlling communicable diseases within their respective states, they determine which diseases will be reported within their jurisdiction. While not all nationally notifiable diseases are reportable in every state or territory, some states have notifiable disease lists that are longer than the CDC's list. As a health professional, you are advised to check the websites of your state health department for specifics about reporting laws in your state. The processes for reporting also vary by state, and this information is generally available on the state health department's website. Generally, providers are encouraged to report cases of infectious diseases to their local or regional health departments, which will then report to the state and to the CDC.

The CDC publishes a weekly listing of notifiable diseases reported by region, state, and nation in *Morbidity and Mortality Weekly Report* (MMWR). MMWR can be found in medical libraries, at local health departments, at infection control departments in hospitals and medical centers, and on the internet at htpp://www.cdc.gov.

Preventing by Vaccination

As with other areas of health care, information and recommendations on immunizations and vaccine usage change regularly. Therefore, it is imperative that you seek the most current information on the CDC website and in its publications. Recommendations, policies, and procedures concerning international immunization practices are determined by the World Health Organization (WHO). National governance is provided by the American Academy of Pediatrics (AAP) Committee on Infectious Diseases and the U.S. Public Health Service Advisory Committee on Immunization Practices (ACIP). Occasionally, these agencies differ on their recommendations. Therefore, it is important to consider the population involved when implementing these recommendations and procedures.

Precautions must be taken when giving any immunization. The most recent recommendations regarding which immunizations to give; to whom they should be given; how they should be given; and how they are to be transported, stored, and administered can be obtained from the CDC. See Box 10.5 for important websites for recommended vaccination schedules for selected population groups.

Box 10.5 Websites for Recommended Vaccination Schedules

Children/adolescents	http://www.cdc.gov/vaccines/schedules/hcp/child-adolescent.html
Adults	http://www.cdc.gov/vaccines/schedules/hcp/adult.html
Travelers	http://wwwnc.cdc.gov/travel/destinations/list
Pregnant women	www.cdc.gov/vaccines/pubs/preg-guide.htm
Health care workers	www.cdc.gov/vaccines/spec-grps/hcw.htm
Specific health conditions	www.cdc.gov/vaccines/spec-grps/conditions.htm
Other special groups	www.cdc.gov/vaccines/spec-grps/default.htm

The CDC produces Vaccine Information Statements (VISs) that explain both the benefits and risks to vaccine recipients, their parents, or their legal representatives. Federal law requires that VISs be handed out before vaccinations are given. These statements can be downloaded from the CDC website at www.cdc.gov/vaccines/pubs/VIS/default.htm.

Legal documentation of vaccinations is important for future administration and follow-up of hypersensitivity reactions. The health care provider, often the nurse, is responsible for maintaining accurate records, including patient name, date(s) immunized, vaccine type, vaccine manufacturer, vaccine lot number, date of the VIS; and the name, title, and address of the person administering the vaccine (CDC, 2013f).

To monitor actual and potential vaccine-related problems, health care providers must report specific postvaccination "adverse events" to the Vaccine Adverse Event Reporting System (VAERS). Information and reporting forms are available in both the FDA Drug Bulletin and the Physicians' Desk Reference and through a 24-hour recorded telephone message at 1-800-822-7967. Information from the CDC (2013e) on VAERS is available at www.cdc.gov/vaccinesafety/Activities/vaers.html. The National Vaccine Injury Compensation Program reviews all VAERS reports.

The National Vaccine Injury Compensation Program became effective as a result of the National Childhood Vaccine Injury Act of 1986. This system provides assistance for individuals and families who experience a vaccine-related injury, including disability and death.

Responding to an Outbreak

An outbreak of an infectious disease requires organized community efforts to investigate and contain the outbreak as well as to provide care to infected persons. The investigation and containment are generally the responsibility of the local health department, interacting with the health care system that provides treatment to the ill. Systematic and overlapping steps for investigating and containing an outbreak have been identified (Heymann, 2008). These are summarized here:

1. Verify the diagnosis and establish a case definition. This requires recognition and reporting by a health care worker to the health department of the first and subsequent cases of an unusual condition. The report should include characteristics of the case that will aid in the investigation, such as history, physical exam findings, and results of laboratory tests.
2. Confirm the existence of an outbreak. Is the incidence of the infectious disease greater now and in this place than expected? This requires comparing recent new cases with incidence over an appropriate period of time for the area. Mapping the new cases by geographic area may help to confirm the areas where the outbreak is greatest.
3. Identify the characteristics of the affected persons. Record their case histories and identify new cases. Enumerate all cases and their distribution by person, place, and time (i.e., who are they, where are the cases located, when did they get ill. What do these persons have in common demographically, socially, and behaviorally?).
4. Define and investigate the population at risk. Did they eat in the same restaurant, attend the same sporting event, go to the same school, or travel on the same airplane? Once the population at risk is identified, the denominator is known and attack rates can be calculated.
5. Investigate the outbreak and formulate a hypothesis as to its chain of transmission. What was the causative agent, reservoir, mode of transmission, portal of exit, portal of entry, and host susceptibility?
6. Determine the most effective control measures based on the chain of transmission. Implement control measures.

Risk Communication

Local public health agencies have the official responsibility for communicating with the public during infectious disease outbreaks in their jurisdiction. Regional and/or state public health agencies may assume such responsibilities if the outbreak extends beyond the boundaries of a local agency. All health professionals who are knowledgeable and/or caring for victims of the outbreak may also be asked to communicate with the public about the event. Effective communication is essential to prevent widespread panic and to elicit support from the public to behave in a fashion that will help to contain the outbreak. Given the importance of conveying the message effectively and in a timely manner, public health professionals are emphasizing the principles of communicating risks to the public, also known as "risk communication."

Characteristics of an infectious disease outbreak create challenges for those responsible for communicating with the public, according to Kindhauser and Thompson (2008). First, infectious disease outbreaks are generally cloaked in uncertainty—uncertainty about the causal agent, about transmission, who is and is not at risk, effective preventive and treatment measures, etc. Facts may unfold incrementally, and yesterday's communication may prove to be wrong. Second, anxiety can be expected. It can have social, economic, and political consequences and lead to unproductive behaviors if ignored. Third, the outbreak may have a social, economic, and political impact beyond the immediate area where it occurred. An example of this in the United States was the detection of one cow with bovine spongiform encephalopathy (BSE), which was estimated to cost the US economy $2 billion in lost beef sales (Kindhauser & Thompson, 2008).

Given these specific challenges, Kindhauser and Thompson (2008) have identified five principles for effective risk communication: trust, early announcement, transparency, listening, and planning. These principles are summarized here as a resource for nurses who are frequently asked to provide information to professional and community groups before, during, and after an infectious disease outbreak.

Trust needs little explanation. It is important, however, to recall that trust or distrust is established long before an emergency event occurs. The public who trusts that the nurse or agency spokesperson will be honest about the event is more likely to hear the message and heed the advice. Announcing early is an important prerequisite to maintaining the public's trust as well as alerting the public to preventive measures. Good risk communicators do not wait until all of the facts are collected. They tell what is known as soon as it is known, admitting that they do not yet have complete information. This fulfills the "information vacuum" before it becomes filled with information from less-reliable sources.

Transparent communication is truthful and easy to understand. It reinforces trust. This principle is probably the most difficult to achieve. Health officials and professionals may withhold information because of the worry that they will be blamed or held accountable for the emergency. In addition, if resources, such as vaccines or ICU beds, are limited, the communicator may not want to acknowledge publicly who will or will not receive the resources. With the speed of communication today, the truth will eventually emerge, reinforcing the need for transparency from the onset of the emergency.

Nurses learn early that listening to the patient, the family, and the community is the first step in communicating. Nurses ask questions about what someone knows before trying to provide information to the person, and nurses avoid preaching. One-way communication with the public must be avoided during emergencies of any type. Good risk communicators monitor what people know and are saying during an emergency. They also monitor the press and, lately, the late night talk shows and the internet blogs. The intent of the monitoring is not to be judgmental, but rather to understand the public's perceptions so as to shape the message to that perception.

Communicating effectively with the public during any type of a community emergency is complex and, like all community health work, requires planning. All health care and public health agencies should designate and train knowledgeable persons to communicate with the public during an infectious disease outbreak. Nurses with the knowledge of the community may be the best risk communicators in such a situation.

Community and Nursing Activities for Preventing and Controlling Infectious Diseases

All practicing nurses have a role in primary, secondary, and tertiary prevention of infectious diseases, both for individuals and for the community as a whole. Table 10.3 provides examples of primary, secondary, and tertiary prevention strategies directed at individuals and populations for specific diseases.

TABLE 10.3 Examples of Prevention Activities for Control of Infectious Diseases at the Individual and Population Levels

Infectious Disease	Individual	Population
Primary Prevention		
Sexually transmitted disease (STD)	Teach safe sex practices	Place condom machines in accessible areas, in places where young adults congregate Immunize for human papillomavirus (HPV)
Diseases caused by blood-borne pathogens	Teach barrier precautions to all health care workers Teach injecting drug users about dangers of sharing needles	Provide an adequate supply of gloves and sharp containers available in patient care areas Initiate citywide Needle Exchange programs and Methadone programs
Vaccine-preventable diseases	Ensure that all children who come to the clinic have age-appropriate immunizations	Work with community groups to cosponsor immunization clinics where immunization rates are low
Hepatitis A, gastrointestinal infections	Teach safe food-handling practices at home	Require, as part of the licensing of restaurants, that food handlers take a course in safe food handling
Hepatitis A and B	Immunize against hepatitis B; immunize those at risk against hepatitis A Provide immune globulin after exposure to hepatitis A or B	Mandate that health care workers are immunized for hepatitis A and B
Secondary Prevention		
STDs	Screen and treat for all STDs	STD Partner Notification Program
Tuberculosis	Screen close contacts of persons with TB Treat persons with a recent skin test-conversion	Initiate a program of yearly testing of health care workers for TB Provide treatment to all recent converters free of charge at their workplace
HIV/AIDS	Provide testing and treatment for HIV in local clinics Ensure that patients adhere to antiretroviral therapy; monitor adherence	Initiate reporting of HIV cases by name to the local health department to facilitate surveillance of HIV in population
Meningitis	Immunize and provide chemoprophylaxis for persons exposed to meningitis	Provide immunization and chemoprophylaxis to all students in a school following an exposure
Tertiary Prevention		
Tuberculosis	Provide therapy for person with active TB Teach patients to take all doses of prescribed antibiotics and monitor adherence	Initiate a Directly Observed Therapy (DOT) program in the community shelters and jails Initiate community education campaigns about the problem of drug resistance associated with incomplete antibiotic use

Summary

In this chapter, we have confronted the challenges posed by two forms of community emergencies: disasters and infectious diseases. Though different, disasters and infectious diseases share characteristics. Both may impact the entire community; both require organized community efforts for prevention and control; and both will impact nurses wherever they practice. The knowledge base for preventing and managing community emergencies is evolving. Nurses are advised to continue to learn about and prepare themselves to live and practice safely and effectively when such emergencies occur.

Critical Thinking Questions

1. You have been asked to participate as a member of your worksite's All Hazards emergency preparedness team. What knowledge and skills do you bring to the team? What skills or knowledge would you need to improve? How would you improve your effectiveness as a team member?

2. As you are driving down a small country road on the way to a community festival, you come on the scene of an accident involving a tanker truck and a train. The truck is on its side, with liquid leaking from its tank. You cannot see the truck driver. Several railroad cars have derailed and are lying on their sides. You can see writing on the cars' sides, which seems to indicate there could be chemicals in the rail cars, though you cannot read the writing from your vantage point. No one else is visible at the scene, although you see people running down the track from the railroad engine toward the derailment site, and you also see another vehicle coming up from behind you. You know you are about 3 miles from the community. What should you do and in what order (what are the scene priorities)?

3. You are employed as a school nurse by Student Health Services at a local college. You are called to a dorm room to see a student who is extremely ill with symptoms that are consistent with meningococcal meningitis. After you send (or escort) the student to the local hospital emergency department for confirmatory diagnosis and treatment, you recognize the implication of the student's infection on the health of the college population.

   a. What multicausal factors for meningococcal meningitis are applicable to the college population? What risk factors are likely to be present in this population?

   b. What is the chain of transmission for meningococcal meningitis?

   c. What is the most effective way of breaking the chain of transmission?

   d. Where can you access information to answer the above questions?

   e. What is your responsibility for reporting this case of meningitis?

   f. How can you learn the requirements and procedures for reporting infectious diseases in your state?

   g. What are the primary, secondary, and tertiary prevention strategies related to meningococcal meningitis that you will implement now and in the future at the college? Which of these strategies are identified in the Healthy People 2010 objectives?

REFERENCES

Akiba, S., Tokonami, S., & Hosoda, M. (2013). Summary of discussions at the symposium focusing on problems resulting from the nuclear accident at the Fukushima Daiichi nuclear power plant [Editorial]. *Journal of Radiological Protection: Official Journal of the Society for Radiological Protections, 33*(1), E1, R1, E1–E7.

Altered Standards of Care in Mass Casualty Events. (2005). Prepared by Health Systems Research Inc. under Contract No. 290-04-0010. AHRQ Publication No. 05-0043. Rockville, MD: Agency for Healthcare Research and Quality. Retrieved from http://www.ahrq.gov/research/altstand/

American Medical Association. (2004a). *Basic disaster life support* (version 2.5). Chicago, IL: Author.

American Medical Association. (2004b). *Core disaster life support* (version 1.01). Chicago, IL: Author.

American Medical Association. (2005). *Management of public health emergencies: A resource for physicians and other community providers.* Washington, DC: Author.

American Red Cross. (n.d.). *About us.* Retrieved from http://www.redcross.org/about-us/mission

BBC NEWS Asia-Pacific. Indonesia's Aceh makes "remarkable" tsunami recovery. (2010, December 22). Retrieved from http://www.bbc.co.uk/news/world-asia-pacific-12056882

Centers for Disease Control and Prevention. (2005). Health concerns associated with disaster victim identifications after a tsunami—Thailand, December 26, 2004–March 31, 2005. *MMWR, 54,* 349–352. Retrieved from http://www.cdc.gov/mmwr/preview/mmwrhtml/mm5414a1.htm.

Centers for Disease Control and Prevention. (2012). *Preparedness for all hazards.* Retrieved from http://emergency.cdc.gov/hazards-all.asp

Centers for Disease Control and Prevention. (2013a). *Diseases connected to antibiotic resistance.* Retrieved from http://www.cdc.gov/drugresistance/diseases.htm

Centers for Disease Control and Prevention. (2013b). *Emerging Infectious Disease Journal.* Retrieved from http://www.cdc.gov/ncidod/eid.

Centers for Disease Control and Prevention. (2013c). *Nationally notifiable infectious diseases.* Retrieved from http://wwwn.cdc.gov/nndss

Centers for Disease Control and Prevention. (2013d). *Pathogens associated with bioterrorism.* Retrieved from http://www.bt.cdc.gov/bioterrorism/.

Centers for Disease Control and Prevention. (2013e). *Vaccine adverse event reporting system (VAERS).* Retrieved from http://www.cdc.gov/vaccinesafety/Activities/vaers.html

Centers for Disease Control and Prevention. (2013f). *Vaccine information statements (VIS).* Retrieved from http://www.cdc.gov/vaccines/pubs/VIS/default.htm

Community Emergency Response Team Unit, LAFD Disaster Preparedness Section. (2013). *Simple triage and rapid treatment (START).* Retrieved from http://www.cert-la.com/triage/start.htm

Federal Bureau of Investigations. (n.d.). *What are weapons of mass destruction?* Retrieved from http://www.fbi.gov/about-us/investigate/terrorism/wmd/wmd_faqs

Federal Emergency Management Agency. (2012a). *Course Overview – IS-100.HCB: Introduction to the incident command system (ICS100) for healthcare/hospitals.* Retrieved from http://training.fema.gov/EMIWeb/IS/courseOverview.aspx?code=IS-100.HCb

Federal Emergency Management Agency. (2012b). *Planning.* Retrieved from http://www.ready.gov/planning

Federal Emergency Management Agency. (2013a). *FEMA's mission statement.* Retrieved from http://www.fema.gov/media-library/assets/videos/80684

Federal Emergency Management Agency. (2013b). *Incident command system (ICS) overview.* Retrieved from http://www.fema.gov/incident-command-system

Federal Emergency Management Agency. (2013c). *Louisiana recovery: Eight years after Hurricanes Katrina and Rita.* Retrieved from http://www.fema.gov/news-release/2013/08/28/louisiana-recovery-eight-years-after-hurricanes-katrina-and-rita

Federal Emergency Management Agency. (2013d). *Natural disasters.* Retrieved from http://www.ready.gov/natural-disasters

Gebbie, K. M., Peterson, C. A., Subbarao, I., & White, K. M. (2009). Adapting standards of care under extreme conditions. *Disaster Medicine and Public Health Preparedness, 3,* 111–116. doi:10.1097/DMP.0b013e31819b95dc

Greater New Orleans Community Data Center. (2013). *Facts for features: Hurricane Katrina recovery.* Retrieved from https://gnocdc.s3.amazonaws.com/reports/GNOCDC_HurricaneKatrinaRecovery.pdf

Grimes, D. E. (1991). *Infectious diseases.* St. Louis, MO: Mosby Year Book.

Hayano, R. S., Tsubokura, M., Miyazaki, M., Satou, H., Sato, K., Masaki, S., & Sakuma, Y. (2013). Internal radiocesium contamination of adults and children in Fukushima 7 to 20 months after the Fukushima NPP accident as measured by extensive whole-body-counter surveys. *Proceedings of the Japan Academy Series B-Physical & Biological Science, 89,* 157–163. doi:10.2183.pjab.89.157

Heymann, D. L. (Ed.). (2008). *Control of communicable diseases manual* (19th ed.). Washington, DC: American Public Health Association.

Ki-Moon, B. (2009, April 24). *Remarks at tsunami lessons learned event.* UN News Center. Retrieved from http://www.un.org/apps/news/infocus/sgspeeches/print_full.asp?statID=476

Kindhauser, M. K., & Thompson, D. (2008). *Risk communication during a communicable disease out-break.* In D. L. Heymann (Ed.), *Control of communicable diseases manual* (pp. A20–A27). Washington, DC: American Public Health Association.

Mainichi Shimbun. (2013, September 9). Stress-induced deaths in Fukushima top those from 2011 natural disasters. *Mainichi Shimbun.* Retrieved from http://mainichi.jp/english/english/newsselect/news/20130909p2a00m0na009000c.html

Markenson, D. (2013). Hospital and emergency department preparedness. In T. G. Veneema (Ed.), *Disaster nursing and emergency preparedness for chemical, biological, and radiological terrorism and other hazards* (3rd ed., pp. 61–78). New York, NY: Springer.

Mendias, E. P., & Grimes, D. E. (2011). Preventing and managing community emergencies: Disasters and infectious diseases. In E. T. Anderson & J. McFarlane (Eds.), *Community as partner* (6th ed., pp. 141–168). Phildadelphia, PA: Wolters Kluwer/Lippincott Williams & Wilkins.

New Orleans Convention & Visitors Bureau. (2013). New Orleans achieves 9.01 million visitors in 2012, the highest visitor numbers in nearly 10 years. Retrieved October 24, 2013, from http://www.neworleanscvb.com/articles/index.cfm?action=view&articleID=7792&menuID=1602

Noji, E. K. (2005). *Public health disaster consequences of disasters*. Retrieved from http://www.pitt.edu/~super1/lecture/lec20351/index.htm

Norwalk, L. V. (2007/2013). *Post Katrina health care: Continuing concerns and immediate needs in the New Orleans region*. Retrieved October 24, 2013, from http://www.hhs.gov/asl/testify/2007/03/t20070313a.html

Schneider, M.-J. (2006). *Introduction to public health* (2nd ed.). Boston, MA: Jones and Bartlett.

Schultz, C. H., & Annas, G. J. (2012). Altering the standard of care in disasters—Unnecessary and dangerous. *Annals of Emergency Medicine, 59*, 191–195.

Smith, A. (2013, September 10). *Fukushima evacuation has killed more than earthquake and tsunami, survey says*. World News on NBC.com. Retrieved from http://worldnews.nbcnews.com/_news/2013/09/10/20420833-fukushima-evacuation-has-killed-more-than-earthquake-and-tsunami-survey-says

Tanaka, S. (2012). Accident at the Fukushima Dai-ichi nuclear power stations of TEPCO—Outline and lessons learned. *Proceedings of the Japan Academy Series B-Physical & Biological Sciences, 8*, 471–484. doi:10.2183/pjab.88.471

Thomas, J. (n.d.). *Mass casualty incident (MCI): An overview*. Retrieved from http://www.emsconedonline.com/pdfs/EMT-Mass%20Casualty%20Incident-an%20overview-Trauma.pdf

U.S. Department of Health and Human Services. (2013). *Healthy People 2020*. Retrieved from www.healthypeople.gov/2020/topicsobjectives2020

U.S. Department of Health and Human Services. (n.d.). *Healthy People 2020: Preparedness*. Retrieved from http://healthypeople.gov/2020/topicsobjectives2020/overview.aspx?topicid=34

U.S. Department of Homeland Security. (n.d.-a). *Our mission*. Retrieved from http://www.dhs.gov/our-mission

U.S. Department of Homeland Security. (n.d.-b). *Strategic plan for fiscal years (FY) 2012–2016*. Retrieved from http://www.dhs.gov/strategic-plan-fiscal-years-fy-2012-2016

U.S. Department of Homeland Security. (2013). *Strengthening cybersecurity for the nations' critical infrastructure*. Retrieved from http://www.dhs.gov/blog/2013/02/14/strengthening-cybersecurity-nation%E2%80%99s-critical-infrastructure

Veenema, T. G., & Woolsey, C. (2013). Essentials of disaster planning. In T. G. Veenema (Ed.), *Disaster nursing and emergency preparedness for chemical, biological, and radiological terrorism and other hazards* (3rd ed., pp. 1–20). New York, NY: Springer.

Waller, M. (2013). Hurricane Katrina eight years later, a statistical snapshot of the New Orleans area. *The Times Picayune*. Retrieved October 24, 2013, from http://impact.nola.com/katrina/print.html?entry=/2013/08/hurricane_katrina_eight_years.html

World Health Organization. (2004). *Living with risk: A global review of disaster reducation initiatives 2004 version–volume II annexes*. New York & Geneva: United Nations. Retrieved from http://www.unisdr.org/files/657_lwr21.pdf

World Health Organization. (2005). *Tsunami recovery process focuses on long-term development*. Retrieved from http://www.who.int/mediacentre/news/releases/2005/pr30_searo/en/print.html

World Health Organization. (2007). *Risk reduction and emergency preparedness: WHO six-year strategy for the health sector and community capacity development*. Retrieved from http://www.who.int/hac/techguidance/preparedness/emergency_preparedness_eng.pdf

World Health Organization. (2013). *Global report on Fukushima nuclear accident details health risks*. Retrieved from http://www.who.int/mediacentre/news/releases/2013/fukushima_report_20130228/en/#

The Process of Working With the Community

CHAPTER 11

Community Assessment: Using a Model for Practice

Elizabeth T. Anderson and Judith McFarlane

LEARNING OBJECTIVES

Part 1 of this book focused on the foundational concepts of community health, epidemiology, environment, culture, ethics, empowerment, health policy, informatics, bioterrorism, and emerging infectious diseases. Part 2 of this book focuses on the application of the nursing process in the community using a selected model. This chapter takes you through the process of assessing a community using a nursing model.

After studying this chapter, you should be able to:

1. Begin to use a community nursing model in practice.

2. Complete a community health assessment using a selected model.

Introduction

Community assessment is a process; it is the act of becoming acquainted with a community. The people in the community are partners and contribute throughout the process. Our nursing purpose in assessing a community is to identify factors (both positive and negative) that impinge on the health of the people to develop strategies for health promotion. As Hancock and Minkler point out, "Health professionals concerned with . . . community building have two reasons for implementing effective and comprehensive community health assessments: information is needed for change, and it is needed for empowerment" (Hancock & Minkler, 2005, p. 139). We will use the community-as-partner model (Fig. 11.1) as a framework for the assessment. (For a specific assessment guide for the workplace, see Appendix A.)

USING A NURSING MODEL TO GUIDE PRACTICE

Boundaries are needed to define areas of concern for nursing, and a conceptual "map" of the nursing process is a necessary guide for action. This is particularly true when the nursing practice focuses on the entire community. The community-as-partner model provides us with

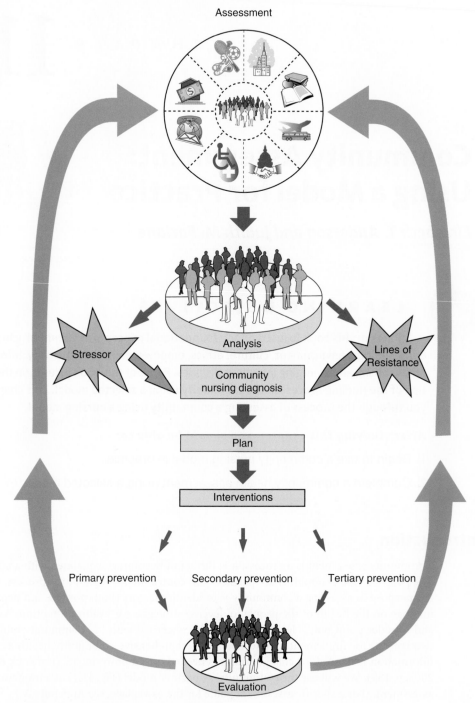

FIGURE 11.1 Community-as-partner model.

both the map and the boundaries and is used throughout this chapter and subsequent chapters to describe the nursing process applied to the community as a whole. The community-as-partner model is presented in the context of selected community models.

A model with which nurses identified for many years was the medical model (i.e., a disease-oriented, illness- and organ-focused approach to patients, with an emphasis on pathology).

However, reliance on the medical model excludes health promotion and the holistic focus that is central to nursing. In addition, important aspects of care, such as psychological, socio-cultural, and spiritual areas, were not included in the medical model. Thus, a nursing model should encompass all aspects of health care needs and incorporate long-range goals and planning.

Take Note

There are many other models applicable to practice in the community. Three, in particular, are used by community health nurses: Pender's health promotion model, the community participation and ethnographic model developed at the University of Virginia reported by Kulbock and others, and Green and Kreuter's PRECEDE–PROCEED model. You will find sources for these models listed in the Further Readings section at the end of this chapter.

Community-as-Partner Model

Based on Neuman's model of a total-person approach to viewing patient problems (1972), the *community-as-client model* was developed by the authors to illustrate the definition of public health nursing as the synthesis of public health and nursing. The model was renamed the *community-as-partner model* to emphasize the underlying philosophy of primary health care.

Neuman's total-person approach and, subsequently, the community-as-partner model are considered systems models. You are already familiar with several kinds of systems, for instance, body systems (endocrine, neuromuscular); social systems; and filing systems. Systems have a common purpose, interrelated parts, and boundaries. The whole system is considered greater than the sum of its parts, and there is emphasis on the interaction of those parts to make up the whole. An individual, group, or community can be considered an open system in that there is constant interaction with the environment through boundaries.

In addition to the systems theory, Neuman's model incorporates Selye's stress adaptation theory, *gestalt* theory from psychology, and field theories. For application to community work, stress adaptation has been included in the community-as-partner model.

Definitions of the four concepts that are central to nursing—person, environment, health, and nursing—provide a framework for the community-as-partner model. *Person* is a population or an aggregate. Everyone in a defined community (total population) or aggregate (the elderly, teens, nurses) represents the person. In effect, *environment* may be thought of as community (i.e., a network of people and their surroundings). The links between the people in the community may be where they live, the work they do, their ethnicity or race, the way they live, and any other factors that they have in common. *Health* in this model is seen as a "resource for everyday life, not the objective of living. [It is] a positive concept emphasizing social and personal resources, as well as physical capacities" (World Health Organization, 1986). *Nursing*, based on definitions of the other three concepts, is prevention. That is, all of nursing is considered preventive: primary prevention is aimed at reducing possible encounters with stressors or strengthening the lines of defense (e.g., sunscreen to prevent skin cancer; immunizations); secondary prevention occurs after a stressor crosses the line of defense and causes a reaction, and it is aimed at early detection to prevent further damage (e.g., breast self-examination); and tertiary prevention aims to maintain and restore a more-or-less healthy state (e.g., rehabilitation, meditation).

Take Note

The types of prevention may seem confusing, and sometimes they are! For instance, meditation, listed under tertiary prevention because it can be practiced after a major bodily insult (breast cancer followed by chemotherapy and radiation), can also be considered a form of primary prevention. Meditation diminishes the effects of stress overall and may actually strengthen the lines of defense.

Consider the community-as-partner model (Fig. 11.1). There are two central factors in this model: a focus on the *community* as partner (represented by the community assessment wheel at the top, which incorporates the community's people as the core) and the use of the *nursing process*. The model is described in some detail to assist you in understanding its parts; this will guide your practice in the community. Refer now to Figure 11.2, the community assessment wheel, for the following discussion.

The core of the assessment wheel represents the *people* who make up the community. Included in the core are the demographics of the population as well as their values, beliefs, and history. As residents of the community, the people are affected by and, in turn, influence the eight subsystems of the community. These subsystems are physical environment, education, safety and transportation, politics and government, health and social services, communication, economics, and recreation.

The solid line surrounding the community represents its *normal line of defense*, or the level of health the community has reached over time. The normal line of defense may include characteristics such as a high rate of immunity, low infant mortality, or middle-income level. The normal line of defense also includes usual patterns of coping, along with problem-solving capabilities; it represents the health of the community.

The *flexible line of defense*, depicted as a broken line around the community and its normal line of defense, is a buffer zone representing a dynamic level of health resulting from a temporary response to stressors. This temporary response may be neighborhood mobilization against an environmental stressor such as flooding or a social stressor such as an unwanted adult bookstore. The eight subsystems are divided by broken lines to remind us that they are not discrete and separate, but influence (and are influenced by) one another. (Remember: A principle of ecology is that everything is connected to everything else. This also applies to the community as a whole.) The eight divisions both define the major subsystems of a community and provide the community health nurse with a framework for assessment.

Take Note

Take a moment to examine the selection of subsystems that have been identified. Can you think of any that have been omitted? Think of the community where you live. What examples of each subsystem can you identify?

Within the community are *lines of resistance*, internal mechanisms that act to defend against stressors. An evening recreational program for young people implemented to decrease vandalism, and a freestanding, no-fee health clinic to diagnose and treat sexually transmitted diseases (STD) are examples of lines of resistance. Lines of resistance exist throughout each of the subsystems and represent the community's strengths.

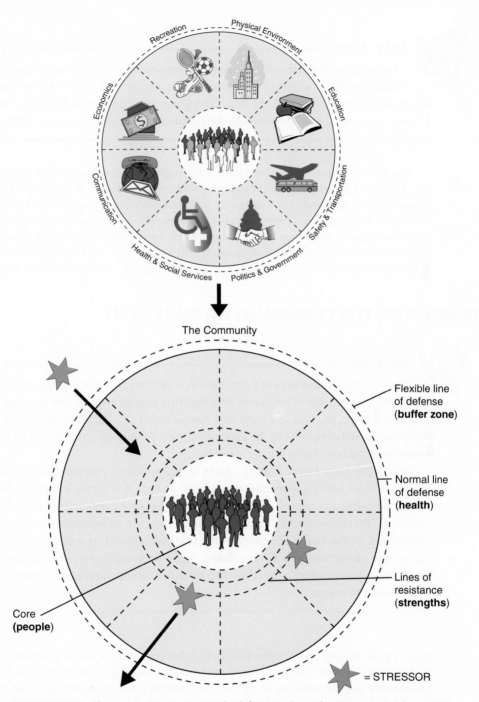

FIGURE 11.2   The community assessment wheel, featuring lines of resistance and defense within the community structure.

Stressors are tension-producing stimuli that have the potential of causing disequilibrium in the system. They may originate outside the community (e.g., air pollution from a nearby industry) or inside the community (e.g., the closing of a clinic). Stressors penetrate the flexible and normal lines of defense, resulting in disruption of the community. Inadequate, inaccessible, or unaffordable services are stressors on the health of the community.

Take Note ———————————————————————————————

The outcome of a stressor impinging on a community is not always negative. Often, it is positive. For example, in the face of a crisis, people may band together and develop a community group to deal with the crisis. This group may continue to function after the crisis is over—strengthening the community and continuing to contribute to its "health."

Stressors and lines of resistance (strengths) together become part of the community nursing diagnosis by giving rise to the *degree of reaction*. The degree of reaction is the amount of disequilibrium or disruption that results from stressors impinging on the community's lines of defense. For instance, if there is a case of measles (stressor) in an elementary school and the lines of resistance are strong (99% of students are up-to-date on immunizations), the degree of reaction (potential outbreak of measles) will be minimal. The degree of reaction may be reflected in mortality and morbidity rates, unemployment, or crime statistics, to name a few.

BEGINNING THE COMMUNITY ASSESSMENT

Take Note ———————————————————————————————

Community assessments are not done in a vacuum. You are probably already familiar with some aspects of the community by virtue of your involvement in caring for people who reside there, perhaps in a clinic or a nearby hospital. In addition, this is not a solo job; many people will contribute to the assessment, so try not to get discouraged by the seeming enormity of the task. Tackle it in increments.

Your community health nursing course time limitations may not permit each student to complete an entire community assessment. In fact, it is a rare instance when an individual completes a community assessment alone, because community assessment requires teamwork. Therefore, teams of students may be assigned to assess one or two community subsystems. At the end of the course, each team will present its assessment, and the total community assessment may be completed. A similar situation may arise in agencies when health care providers from a variety of disciplines are assigned one aspect (one subsystem) of a community to assess.

Begin by identifying your community. Recall that a system is a whole that functions because of the interdependence of its parts. A community, too, is a whole entity that functions because of the interdependence of its parts, or subsystems. The community assessment wheel (see Fig. 11.3) will be your overall framework, while the assessment is facilitated by using the model in survey form. The windshield survey shown in Table 11.1 was adapted from an earlier version that has been expanded to include each component of the community assessment wheel. Note that the guide has three parts: (1) the community core; (2) the community subsystems; and (3) community perceptions. In addition, there are columns for the listing of observations and data. From now on, we will refer to the survey as the windshield survey.

The community of Rosemont, comprising Census Tracts (CT) 4104 and 4107, will be used to illustrate the use of the model in conducting a community assessment (as well as subsequent analysis, diagnosis, planning, intervention, and evaluation). Although we have chosen an urban

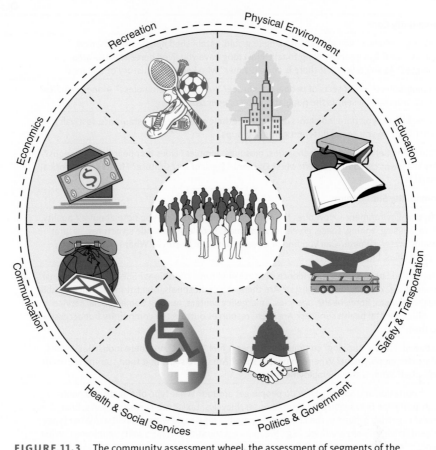

FIGURE 11.3   The community assessment wheel, the assessment of segments of the community-as-partner model.

community defined by census tracts, the guide can be used to assess any community regardless of size, location, resources, or population characteristics. It can also be used to assess a "community within a community," such as a school, an industry, or a business. Examples of these communities are included in Part 3 of this book. In addition, this guide can be used to assess an aggregate (i.e., a defined group within the community [e.g., teenagers, battered women, the elderly, or children under age 5]) by providing the context in which this group is found. The *process* of assessment, regardless of where it is applied, always remains the same.

 Take Note

Some students choose to format their assessment with observations and data reported in narrative form with data presented in tables. Others simply include their information directly in the table. As you will learn, there is no one way to collect and report data in the community. Do, however, agree with your team on a model-based format such as those illustrated here, and adhere to it.

Assessment is a skill that is refined through practice. Everyone feels awkward and unsure as he or she begins (remember the first time you took a blood pressure?); this is normal. The first step is always the most difficult.

TABLE 11.1 Windshield Survey*

	Observations	Data

I. Community Core

1. History—What can you glean by looking (e.g., old, established neighborhoods; new subdivision)? Ask people willing to talk: How long have you lived here? Has the area changed? As you talk, ask if there is an "old-timer" who knows the history of the area

2. Demographics—What sorts of people do you see? Young? Old? Homeless? Alone? Families? What races do you see? Is the population homogeneous?

3. Ethnicity—Do you note indicators of different ethnic groups (e.g., restaurants, festivals)? What signs do you see of different cultural groups?

4. Values and Beliefs—Are there churches, mosques, temples? Does it appear homogeneous? Are the lawns cared for? With flowers? Gardens? Signs of art? Culture? Heritage? Historical markers?

II. Community Subsystems

1. Physical Environment—How does the community look? What do you note about air quality, flora, housing, zoning, space, green areas, animals, people, man-made structures, natural beauty, water, climate? Can you find or develop a map of the area? What is the size (e.g., square miles, blocks)?

2. Health and Social Services—Evidence of acute or chronic conditions? Shelters? "Traditional" healers (e.g., *curanderos*, herbalists)? Are there clinics, hospitals, practitioners' offices, public health services, home health agencies, emergency centers, nursing homes, social service facilities, mental health services? Are there resources outside the community but accessible to them?

3. Economy—Is it a "thriving" community or does it feel "seedy?" Are there industries, stores, places for employment? Where do people shop? Are there signs that food stamps are used/accepted? What is the unemployment rate?

4. Transportation and Safety—How do people get around? What type of private and public transportation is available? Do you see buses, bicycles, taxis? Are there sidewalks, bike trails? Is getting around in the community possible for people with disabilities? What types of protective services are there (e.g., fire, police, sanitation)? Is air quality monitored? What types of crimes are committed? Do people feel safe?

5. Politics and Government—Are there signs of political activity (e.g., posters, meetings)? What party affiliation predominates? What is the governmental jurisdiction of the community (e.g., elected mayor, city council with single-member districts)? Are people involved in decision making in their local governmental unit?

6. Communication—Are there "common areas" where people gather? What newspapers do you see in the stands? Do people have TVs and radios? What do they watch/listen to? What are the formal and informal means of communication?

7. Education—Are there schools in the area? How do they look? Are there libraries? Is there a local board of education? How does it function? What is the reputation of the school(s)? What are major educational issues? What are the dropout rates? Are extracurricular activities available? Are they used? Is there a school health service? A school nurse?

8. Recreation—Where do children play? What are the major forms of recreation? Who participates? What facilities for recreation do you see?

III. Community Perceptions

1. The Residents—How do people feel about the community? What do they identify as its strengths? Problems? Ask several people from different groups (e.g., old, young, field worker, factory worker, professional, minister, housewife) and keep track of who gives what answer.

2. Your Perceptions—General statements about the "health" of this community.
What are its strengths?
What problems or potential problems can you identify?

Note: Supplement your impressions with information from the census, police records, school statistics, Chamber of Commerce data, health department reports, and so on to confirm or refute your conclusions. Tables, graphs, and maps are helpful and will aid in your analysis.

*This survey form was renamed "Learning about the Community on Foot" to underscore the necessity of walking around the community. Also, when one of the authors (Elizabeth T. Anderson) used it in rural Mexico, the area being assessed was not accessible by automobile. For ease of citation and referral, we will continue to use "windshield survey" as its title.

COMMUNITY CORE

We think of the core as something that is essential, basic, and enduring. The core of a community is its people—their history, characteristics, values, and beliefs. The first stage of assessing a community, then, is to learn about its people. In fact, partnering with people in the community is an integral part of working in the community. Table 11.2 lists the major components of the community core along with suggested locations and sources of information about each component. Because every community is different, information sources available about one community may not be available for another.

The History of Rosemont

The Rosemont property was originally deeded to a Miss Ima Smith, who received a land grant of 3,370 acres in 1827. For almost 100 years, the area remained as prairie, dotted with cattle ranches and small farms. In 1920, John Walker and William Bell formed a land corporation and began developing the Smith property. The first area that was improved and deed restricted was named Rosemont after a legendary town in Scotland. After development, Rosemont prospered and attracted newcomers to the area. Numerous prominent families made their homes in Rosemont, including a state governor, a Nobel laureate, and a president of the United States. However, during the economic depression of the 1930s and the years before and during World War II, a drastic decrease in building activities occurred. Many stately homes deteriorated and either became multifamily dwellings or were left to decay. Eventually, economic forces succeeded in breaking deed restrictions, and residential areas were forced to accept the introduction of industry and

TABLE 11.2 Community Core Data

Components	Sources of Information
History	Library, historic society Interview "old-timers," town leaders

Demographics
    Age and sex characteristics
    Racial distribution
    Ethnic distribution
	Census of population and housing
	Planning board (local, city, county, state)
	Chamber of Commerce
	City hall, city secretary, archives
	Observation

Household types by
    Family
    Nonfamily
    Group
	Census

Marital status by
    Single
    Separated
    Widowed
    Divorced
	Census

Vital statistics
    Births
    Deaths by
        Age
        Leading causes
	State department of health (distributed through city
	    and county health departments)

Values and beliefs	Personal contact
	Observation (see Table 11.1)
	    (To protect against stereotyping, avoid the library
	    for this portion of the assessment.)

Religion	Observation Telephone book

TABLE 11.3 Population Age and Sex Characteristics for CT4104, CT4107, City of Hampton, and Jefferson County

Age (years)	CT 4104			CT 4107			Hampton		Jefferson County	
	Males	Females	Total %	Males	Females	Total %	Number	Total %	Number	Total %
Under 5 years	333	326	9.6	29	11	0.5	110,835	7.0	170,332	7.6
5–19	1,080	892	28.6	217	176	5.8	373,572	23.7	512,992	22.8
20–29	329	358	10.1	439	237	10.0	123,922	7.8	225,290	10.0
30–34	356	393	10.8	1,769	820	38.3	463,235	29.3	644,788	28.6
35–54	753	873	23.7	1,583	645	33.0	305,508	19.4	435,943	19.3
55–64	200	333	7.8	199	163	5.4	105,152	6.7	141,935	6.3
65 and over	243	405	9.4	158	315	7.0	96,625	6.1	121,659	5.4
Total	3,294	3,580	100	4,391	2,366	100	1,454,927	100	2,027,639	100

Data from Census of Population and Housing, selected characteristics.

small businesses. As a result, property values plummeted, leaving quaint boutiques and antique shops to exist alongside an increasing number of nightclubs and nude modeling studios.

From 1950 to 1970, Rosemont witnessed the influx of a large population of young adults, commonly referred to as "hippies," who used the large, spacious homes for group living. This practice of communal living attracted drug addicts and runaways. Rosemont gradually assumed the reputation of tolerating "nontraditional" lifestyles—a factor that precipitated an influx of a large population of gay men.

Because of low property values and affordable rent during the mid- to late 1970s, large groups of Vietnamese and Mexican immigrants also settled in Rosemont. Simultaneously, established families and single professionals, weary of the lengthy commute from suburbia to the inner city, began returning to Rosemont—a trend that continues today. Today, old homes have been refurbished, businesses have been revitalized, and pride, once lost, has been reclaimed.

Demographics and Ethnicity

Tables 11.3 and 11.4 show age, sex, race, and ethnicity data for CT 4104 and CT 4107 as well as for the nearest city and county. Gathering data on city, county, state, and nation affords comparisons that may be important for the analysis. (The census lists only numbers of people; you must calculate percentages.) Tables 11.5 and 11.6 list data on family types and marital status. (We calculated the percentages.)

TABLE 11.4 Population Race and Ethnicity for CT 4104, CT 4107, City of Hampton, and Jefferson County

	CT 4104		CT 4107		Hampton		Jefferson County	
	Number	Total %	Number	Total %	Number	Total %	Number	Total %
White	852	12.4	5,871	88.5	970,489	61.5	1,562,091	69.4
Black	3,732	54.3	305	4.6	434,014	27.5	467,177	20.7
Asian/Pacific Islander	1,321	19.1	54	0.7	32,335	2.1	45,432	2
Hispanic	625	9.1	321	4.7	131,763	8.3	163,774	7.3
American Indian	242	3.5	38	0.6	3,203	0.2	4,923	0.2
Other	111	1.6	58	0.9	7,045	0.4	9,532	0.4
Total	6,874	100	6,757	100	1,578,849	100	2,252,929	100

Data from Census of Population and Housing, selected characteristics.

TABLE 11.5 Population Family Types for CT 4104 and CT 4107

| | CT 4104 | | CT 4107 | |
	Number	Total %	Number	Total %
Family	5,706	83	2,443	36.2
Nonfamily	1,168	17	4,103	60.7
Female-headed household	721	994		
Male-headed household		447	2,189	
Group quarters			211	3.1
TOTAL	6,874	100	6,757	100

Data from Census of Population and Housing, selected characteristics.

TABLE 11.6 Persons Age 15 and Over by Sex and Marital Status for CT 4104 and CT 4107

| | CT 4104 | | | CT 4107 | | |
Marital Status	Male	Female	Total %	Male	Female	Total %
Single	348	408	15.2	2,418	1,016	53.5
Married	1,510	1,498	60.1	796	768	24.4
Separated	120	245	7.2	113	72	2.8
Widowed	52	119	3.4	68	198	4.3
Divorced	294	407	14.1	572	397	15
TOTAL	2,324	2,677	100	3,967	2,451	100

Data from Census of Population and Housing, selected characteristics.

 Take Note

Figures in the tables do not reflect current data but are for illustration. Of course, for your assessment, be sure to use the latest figures and include the date within the citation. During the next step of the nursing process, analysis, you will need data about the other comparable entities, so collect all needed data now.

Vital Statistics

Table 11.7 lists birth and death statistics for CT 4104 and CT 4107 as well as for the city, county, and state. Using a similar format, Table 11.8 lists the leading causes of

TABLE 11.7 Selected Birth and Death Vital Statistics for CT 4104, CT 4107, City of Hampton, and Jefferson County

	CT 4104	CT 4107	Hampton	Jefferson County	State
Births	210	117	30,726	56,865	363,325
Deaths (rates)*					
Infant	7 (33)	2 (17)	372 (12)	698 (12.3)	2,064 (5.7)
Neonatal	5 (23)	2 (17)	245 (7.9)	471 (8.3)	1,226 (3.4)

*Rates are per 1,000 live births.
Data from State Vital Statistics, Department of Health.

TABLE 11.8 Deaths by Selected Causes for CT 4104, CT 4107, City of Hampton, and State of Texarkana

Cause of Death	CT 4104 Number	%	CT 4107 Number	%	Hampton Number	%	State Number	%	Rate*
Heart disease	16	22.2	10	23.8	3,186	33.4	42,968	28.7	211.2
Malignant neoplasms	17	23.6	11	26.1	2,078	21.8	33,298	22.2	163.7
Cerebrovascular diseases	6	8.3	2	4.7	690	7.3	10,721	7.2	52.7
Accidents	4	5.6	4	9.5	585	6.2	7,602	5.1	37.4
Chronic lower respiratory diseases	0	0	0	0	79	0.8	7,284	4.9	35.8
Diabetes mellitus	0	0	2	4.8	139	1.4	5,195	3.5	25.5
Diseases of early infancy	7	9.7	1	2.4	248	2.6	NI	NI	NI
Homicides	6	8.3	1	2.4	592	6.2	NI	NI	NI
Cirrhosis of liver	0	0	1	2.4	163	1.7	2,092[†]	1.4	10.3
Pneumonia	2	2.8	1	2.4	210	2.2	3,708	2.5	18.2
Suicides	3	4.2	1	2.4	195	2	2,093	1.4	10.3
Congenital anomalies	0	0	2	4.8	99	1	NI	NI	NI
Nephritis and nephrosis	0	0	0	0	13	0.1	NI	NI	NI
Tuberculosis	1	1.4	0	0	17	0.2	NI	NI	NI
All other causes	10	13.9	6	14.3	1,239	13	31,631	21.1	155.5

*Rates per 100,000 estimated population. (Note: It is always preferable to report rates because you can then make comparisons. However, if you do not know the population at risk [the denominator], it is not possible to calculate rates. The above mortality data for the census tracts and for the city of Hampton do not allow the calculation of rates.)
[†]Includes chronic liver disease for state.
NI, not included in "Leading Causes of Death" in state.
Data from Hampton Vital Statistics, city of Hampton health department, and from the State Department of Health.

death. Some of these mortality data in Table 11.8 do not allow the calculation of rates for that reason (see table footnote for more information). See Chapter 3 for help in calculating rates.

Values, Beliefs, and Religion

Included in the community core are the values, beliefs, and religious practices of the people. All ethnic and racial groups have values and beliefs that interact with each community system to influence the people's health. Review Chapter 7 for methods to help you understand the cultural elements of the community. Notice that Table 11.2 cautions against the exclusive use of the library for information about values, beliefs, and religious practices; the reason is that books and articles frequently offer broad generalizations to describe the practices of ethnic and racial groups (e.g., the lifestyles of urban African Americans) or discuss one practice of one ethnic group (such as breast-feeding practices of Mexican-born Hispanics). However, all types of media, including books, films, and music, can enrich your knowledge about different cultures. (An example is the movie "Gran Torino" in which the protagonist gets to know and appreciate his Hmong neighbors.)

To validate the published, secondary demographic data, use your survey to establish the presence and geographic location of different racial and ethnic groups.

It is during this phase—assessment of the physical system—that we enter the community to learn and experience the values, beliefs, and religious practices of the community.

COMMUNITY SUBSYSTEMS

Our partner, the Rosemont community, is located within the city of Hampton and is in Hampton's central business district. It is bounded by Way Drive on the west, Buff's Bayou on the north, Live Oak Boulevard on the south, and Hampton Street on the east. Figure 11.4 is a map of the Rosemont community. Using the windshield survey (see Table 11.1) as a guide, we step into the community.

Physical Environment

Just as the physical examination is a critical component of assessing an individual patient, so it is in the assessment of a community. And just as the five senses of the clinician are called into play in the physical examination of a patient, so, too, are they needed at the community level. Table 11.9 provides the components of the physical examination, both of an individual and of a community, and compares tools and sources of data for each.

Inspection

Rosemont Boulevard bisects the community and serves as a major north–south thoroughfare for residents traveling to or through the community. It is tree-lined and divided by a grassy median into sections. Many businesses, especially restaurants, are located along Rosemont

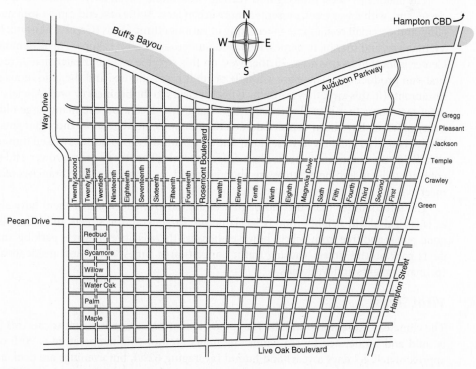

FIGURE 11.4   Rosemont community streets and boundaries.

TABLE 11.9 Physical Examination Components and Sources of Data

| Components | Sources of Data | |
	Individual	Community
Inspection	All senses Otoscope Ophthalmoscope	All senses Windshield survey Walk through community
Auscultation	Stethoscope	Listen to community sounds/residents

Vital signs	Thermometer
	Sphygmomanometer
		Observe climate, terrain, natural
		  boundaries, and resources
		"Life" signs such as notices of community
		  meetings; density

Systems review	Head-to-toe	Observe social systems, including
		  housing, businesses, churches, and
		  hangouts

Laboratory studies	Blood tests X-rays Scans, other tests	Almanac; census data Chamber of Commerce planning studies and surveys

Boulevard. Many of the restaurants are of the specialty health-promoting types that serve quiche, sprout sandwiches, and herbal teas. Other businesses along the boulevard include gas stations; office buildings; art-supply stores; a veterinarian; small art galleries; a nursery; one Mexican *barbacoa* stand in a grocery store; florists; a bank; a pharmacy; and various shops specializing in leather goods, books, and handcrafted items. (See the Economics section of this chapter for a summary of business units.)

The major east–west thoroughfare through Rosemont, Pecan Drive, is also lined with businesses and, with fewer trees, presents a more urban face. At the east end can be seen nude modeling studios; small restaurants specializing in various ethnic foods (Greek, Pakistani, Mexican, Vietnamese, and Indian, to name a few); and numerous small art shops. The Rosemont Health Center is located in this area. Further west on this street is a large theater that attracts many first-run productions. There are a couple of adult movie houses and the ubiquitous specialty restaurants (in this area, they are of the type that caters to the business or professional crowds—quiet tea rooms that play classical music). Along this street, too, are many large old houses, many of which have been converted into antique shops, flower shops, and other small stores. There is no large industry in Rosemont. The area behind the two business-filled thoroughfares that divide the community seems like a different world. The streets are narrower, and some are cobbled; old oak and pecan trees are abundant, and, in many areas, the branches of the trees meet over the streets to form protective canopies.

The streets other than the thoroughfares are narrow, and most of them have sidewalks, as is typical of old neighborhoods in Hampton. In general, the streets and sidewalks are in good repair and free from debris; however, because there is little off-street parking, many residents park on the streets, causing traffic congestion at times when most residents are home (primarily nights and weekends).

Vital Signs

The climate of Rosemont (and the Hampton Standard Metropolitan Statistical Area [SMSA]) is mild and moderated by sea winds. Summers are hot (the temperature is 90°F or higher approximately 87 days a year) and humid (averaging 62%), but evenings are cool, and there is rarely a hard freeze in the winter. Flora, both temperate and tropical, abounds—live oaks, hibiscus, and pines may grow in one block, for example.

The terrain is generally flat, with little variation in grade. It is 20 feet above sea level. The only naturally occurring water in the area is Buff's Bayou, a concrete-lined "river" that serves to carry off excess rain and drainage to reduce chances of flooding in Hampton. The bayou ends in the Hampton Ship Channel, which leads to the sea.

Rosemont is the third most densely populated area in Hampton, with 14.4 people per acre. An area in CT 4104 that contains the subsidized-housing complex is the most densely populated in all of Hampton, with 221 people per acre.

The variety of local stores reflects the diversity of interests in Rosemont. Posters advertising a meeting of the Gay Political Caucus share bulletin-board space with senior citizens' meetings; church announcements; educational programs at the community college's "Sundry School;" Vietnamese relocation services; the community's STD clinic; and a musical show by "El Barrio" from the Mexican–American area. Rosemont is a community of rich diversity, a microcosm of Hampton.

The churches of Rosemont also reflect its diversity—virtually all denominations are represented. From the large Methodist, Unitarian, and Presbyterian churches on its borders to the small storefront churches serving refugees, Rosemont contains resources for all major religious groups.

Systems

Most of Rosemont is developed; there is little space not in use. Four small neighborhood parks, a narrow strip along the bayou, and the land around the community college comprise the green space available to the community (Fig. 11.5), although most houses have well-kept lawns with trees and shrubs. Table 11.10 presents land use data for Rosemont.

The majority of houses in Rosemont are old, reflecting the early development of the area. Within certain sections, the houses resemble each other (e.g., all one-story, wood-frame houses with porches); however, there may also be great heterogeneity from one block to the next.

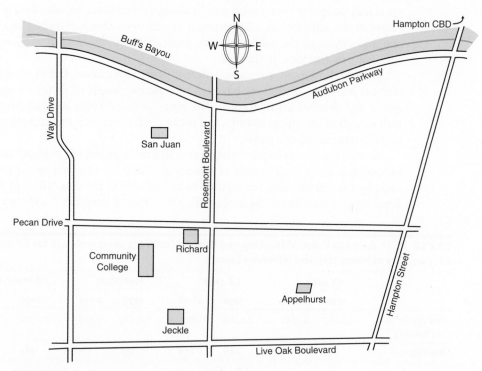

FIGURE 11.5 Rosemont community greens and parks.

TABLE 11.10 Rosemont Land Use

Land Use	CT 4104		CT 4107	
	Number of Acres	Total %	Number of Acres	Total %
Single-family dwellings	161.2	28.03	95.4	31.78
Multifamily dwellings	46.4	8.06	46.5	15.49
Commercial	210.2	36.55	61.2	20.39
Industrial	44.9	7.8	0.2	0.06
Public	6.8	1.18	11.1	3.69
Open	52.9	9.2	53.2	17.72
Water	6.3	1.09	4.7	1.56
Undeveloped	46.3	8.05	14.6	4.86
Right-of-way	0	0	13.2	4.39
Total acres	575	100	300.1	100

Data Book, Rosemont Community Development, city of Hampton, Planning Department.

In the northeast quadrant is a large subsidized-housing area of run-down apartments with broken windows and poorly kept streets, whereas in the southwest quadrant houses have been remodeled and well maintained. Also in the northeast is an area covering several blocks of what are called "shotgun houses" (the story is told that one can shoot a shotgun from the front door, and the shot will go out the back door); placed side by side, they are tiny and poorly maintained. See Table 11.11 for housing information.

During the day, most of the people seen on the streets move quickly and purposefully as though on business or an errand. Those who could be described as "strolling" are elderly people or young men, usually alone. Few children are seen during the day except in the schoolyards, which are not on the main thoroughfares. Dogs bark as one walks through the neighborhoods, and cats sun themselves in windows; however, few pets run loose in the area.

At night, Rosemont assumes a different flavor along Pecan Drive; all of the restaurants are open, and many have outdoor patios. Smells of fajitas, curry, exotic spices, and charbroiling fill the air. "The Strip," as Pecan Drive is called, comes alive with sounds of rap, disco, country, and rock music, along with the stroking of a sitar or quiet strumming of a guitar.

Most of the clients in these restaurants and nude modeling "studios," according to residents, come from outside of Rosemont. Many are attracted by the food, and some by the freewheeling sex reputed to be available in the area. Many of the residents express disdain for the Strip, calling it a "tourist attraction," and they believe

TABLE 11.11 Average Value of Housing and Rent ($) for Years 2000 and 2010 for CT 4104, CT 4107, City of Hampton, and Jefferson County

	CT 4104		CT 4107		Hampton		Jefferson County	
	1990	2000	1990	2000	1990	2000	1990	2000
Average value of housing	43,400	47,630	62,400	71,600	61,900	79,300	70,500	87,000
Average rent	284	476	346	650	337	575	489	590

Data from Census of Population and Housing, selected characteristics.

it is contributing to the deterioration of Rosemont. They state that "outsiders" and "cowboys" exploit and prey on unsuspecting tourists and that the unsavory reputation of the area is not the fault of the people who live there. An absence of zoning laws has facilitated the establishment of some of the less-than-desirable businesses in the area.

The physical examination of Rosemont reveals it to be a community of contrasts: churches and nude modeling studios; subsidized city housing units and restored homes from a more affluent time; old people and young; white and black (and all shades between); quiet tree-lined streets and busy thoroughfares; sedate tea rooms and garish adult movie theaters; families and singles; and the rich and poor.

Health and Social Services

One method of classifying health and social services is to differentiate between facilities located outside the community (extracommunity) and those within the community (intracommunity). Once the health and social service facilities are identified, group them into categories, perhaps by type of service offered (e.g., hospitals, clinics, extended care); by size; or by public versus private usage. Table 11.12 suggests a classification system as well as possible major components of each facility requiring assessment.

Extracommunity Health Facilities

Hospitals
Jefferson County has 50 hospitals with a total of 12,321 beds, 4,321 of which are in the Hampton Medical Center, a complex that includes all medical subspecialties as well as sophisticated diagnostic and treatment services. The medical center is located 7 miles from Rosemont. All patients admitted to the medical center must be referred by a physician; self-referral is not permitted. (Self-referral allows the individual to choose and acquire medical

TABLE 11.12 Health and Social Services

Component	Sources of Information
Health Services	
Extracommunity or intracommunity facilities	Chamber of Commerce
Once identified, group into categories (e.g., hospitals and clinics, home health care, extended-care facilities, public health services, emergency care).	Planning board (county, city) Phone directory Talk to residents
For each facility, collect data on 1. Services (fees, hours, and new services planned and those discontinued) 2. Resources (personnel, space, budget, and record system) 3. Characteristics of users (geographic distribution, demographic profile, and transportation source) 4. Statistics (number of persons served daily, weekly, and monthly) 5. Adequacy, accessibility, and acceptability of facility according to users and providers	Interview administrator or someone on the staff Facility annual report
Social Services	
Extracommunity or intracommunity facilities.	Chamber of Commerce
Once identified, group into categories (e.g., counseling and support, clothing, food, shelter, and special needs).	United Way directory Phone directory
For each facility, collect data on areas 1–5 listed above.	

care independently.) Although the existence of the medical center is common knowledge among Rosemont residents, few people know anyone who has sought or received care there. Numerous private hospitals are located in Jefferson County, most of which are in Hampton. All private hospitals require third-party reimbursement for services rendered. (Third-party reimbursement means payment for services by an entity other than the patient. For example, Medicare, Medicaid, insurance, and Workmen's Compensation are third-party reimbursers.) In addition to private hospitals, most communities use tax revenues to support at least one hospital for the general public. In Jefferson County, the public hospital is Jefferson Memorial.

Jefferson Memorial is a full-service facility located 5 miles south of Rosemont. Care units and clinics at Memorial include medical, surgical, pediatrics, maternity, gynecology, trauma and burns, psychiatry, and emergency rooms (ERs). People can self-refer to Jefferson Memorial. According to the director of the ER, 290 people are seen daily in the ER (approximately 100,000 people annually). Of these, some 40% are admitted. Follow-up care is provided by the Memorial's outpatient clinics. The Memorial is supported by city and county taxes as well as by fees collected for services. Health care provider fees, as well as treatments and diagnostic services, are in addition to the base fee. All fees are on a sliding scale according to income and family size. Rosemont residents use Memorial, but complain of lengthy waits of up to 8 hours and of having to undergo repeated assessments as they are moved from one health care provider to another.

Hospital personnel recognize the lengthy waiting period and fragmentation of care, but they cite budget constraints and a shortage of qualified providers as major obstacles to improving care. No services have been discontinued at Memorial, and no new services or staff positions are budgeted for the next 2 years.

Private Care Providers, Group Practices, and Specialty Clinics

A full selection of general medical and specialty care is available in Jefferson County through private practitioners, group practices, and specialty clinics. Payment is usually third-party reimbursement. Two health maintenance organizations (HMOs) are located in Jefferson County. Rosemont residents with adequate finances use a variety of private practitioners and specialty clinics. The residents usually self-refer after a favorable recommendation from a neighbor, friend, or work colleague.

Public Health Services: The Health Department

To monitor, maintain, and promote the public's health, each state has a state health department and accompanying regional, county, and sometimes city health departments. National, state, and local tax revenues are used to support public health services. There is a Hampton Health Department as well as a Jefferson County Health Department. Because Rosemont is within the city limits of Hampton, the services of the Hampton Health Department are assessed.

The Hampton Health Department offers all medical outpatient services through its seven satellite clinics. The Sunvalley Clinic, located 6 miles from Rosemont and the closest to the area, provides the following services:

- Immunizations
- Well and ill infant, child, adolescent, and adult care
- Antepartum/postpartum care
- Family planning
- Nutrition counseling
- Screening and testing for genetic and acquired conditions such as sickle-cell anemia, diabetes, and phenylketonuria (PKU)
- Dental assessment, cleaning, and restoration
- Mental health counseling and referral
- Health education

- Maternal and infant home visitation after early hospital discharge (defined as earlier than 48 hours after delivery)
- Child abuse, battered spouse, and abandoned person counseling and referral
- STD screening and follow-up (including HIV testing)

Additional services include a pharmacy, laboratory, and radiation department. Payment for most services is on a sliding scale; remaining services are free to all city residents. Free services include immunizations as well as screening and treatment for STDs. The majority of Rosemont residents who use the health department attend antepartum or postpartum clinics. The staff nurse in the maternity clinic estimates that of the 75 women seen in the prenatal clinic each week, 20 to 25 are Rosemont residents.

The major service-delivery problem cited by nurses in the maternity clinics is the long waiting period (frequently 8 to 10 weeks) between a woman's initial request for an appointment and the scheduled appointment date. Because many women wait until they are 6 or 7 months pregnant to request antepartum care, the first available appointment time may be after the woman's expected delivery date. Consequently, a large number of women from Rosemont deliver at Jefferson Memorial having received no antepartum care. The administrator of the Sunvalley Clinic felt additional education, support, and monitoring services for pregnant patients and new mothers to be a top service priority.

No services have been discontinued in the recent past. With regard to the question of services that are needed, the elderly were identified as a target group. Plans were under way to establish a nursing clinic for the elderly as well as a wellness program to be offered at day care for the elderly and at senior centers. There are presently more than 10 such facilities for seniors within the city of Hampton.

Numerous Rosemont residents use the health department services, especially the Sunvalley Clinic. Problems cited include lack of a direct bus connection to the clinic (three bus transfers are required) and "impersonal" service. Because patients are not assigned to a primary care provider, it is customary for them to see a different health care provider at each visit. Maternity patients have an additional concern. Each woman must make her own delivery arrangements, and frequently women who qualify for antepartum care at Sunvalley Clinic do not meet eligibility requirements for delivery at Jefferson Memorial. Consequently, women must search for a facility that will admit them for labor and delivery. All too often, they are forced to deliver at home, a situation documented by Sunvalley nurses and confirmed by several Rosemont residents.

Home Health Agencies

The Visiting Nurses Association (VNA) of Hampton is the largest home health agency in Jefferson County. Services of the VNA include home health care by registered nurses, physical and occupational therapists, speech therapists, social workers, and home health aides. The VNA accepts paying clients and third-party reimbursements. Paying clients are charged on a sliding scale according to income and family size. Patients who are unable to pay a fee can request financial assistance from several community social service agencies, such as the United Way.

Numerous other home health agencies are located in Hampton and Jefferson County. Although more limited in scope of service, all offer home health services and require fees or third-party reimbursement for payment.

Long-Term, Extended-Care, and Continuing-Care Facilities

There are two long-term facilities within 8 miles of Rosemont: the Pinewoods Rest Center and the Windsail Nursing Home. Each facility is classified as an intermediate-care facility and is licensed by the state health department. A profile of the services, resources, and characteristics of the residents for each facility is presented in Table 11.13. In addition, several hospitals offer extended-care services.

TABLE 11.13 Services, Resources, and Resident Characteristics at Pinewoods Rest Center and Windsail Nursing Home during the Preceding Year

	Pinewoods Rest Center	Windsail Nursing Home
Services	Convalescent nursing care; physical, occupational, and speech therapy	Convalescent nursing care
Full-time personnel	Six registered nurse (RNs), four licensed visiting nurses (LVNs), three nurse aides, one administrator	Three RNs, two LVNs, one nurse aide, one administrator
Licensed bed capacity	96	38
Patient days	33,524	12,965
Occupancy rate	0.96	0.93
Certified bed capacity*	96	38
Median age of residents	79	76
Average duration of stay	4 years	6 years

*Recommended occupancy rate for nursing home beds is 90%.
Data from Jefferson County Planning Council, Pinewoods Rest Center, and Windsail Nursing Home record books.

Emergency Services

The Poison Control Center provides information to individuals and health care providers on harmful substances and methods of assessment and treatment. The center provides educational materials and programs for schools and interested groups.

The Medical Emergency Ambulance Service (MEAS) is financed by Hampton city taxes, public donations, Jefferson County contributions, and organized fundraisers. The MEAS first-aid services are free and available 24 hours a day to all residents of Rosemont. (The MEAS operates in conjunction with the local fire stations. See the Safety and Transportation section of this chapter for a description of fire protection services.)

The MEAS closest to Rosemont has two ambulances; one is used daily, and the other serves as a backup. The MEAS averages 90 to 110 calls a month, with a response time of less than 8 minutes. (Table 11.14 presents specific reasons for ambulance service to people in Rosemont during the last 3-month period.) Calls are received through the central fire department and dispatched by radio to the nearest MEAS team. Each MEAS team consists of 25 people: 3 paramedics having completed 100 hours of class work and 200 hours of hospital experience, and

TABLE 11.14 Reasons for Medical Emergency Ambulance Service (MEAS) to Persons in Rosemont during the Preceding 3-Month Period

Reason	Total %
Cardiac-related problems and cerebrovascular accidents	25
Falls and household accidents	19
Respiratory problems	12
Dizziness and weakness	12
Lacerations	11
Fractures and dislocations	9
Abdominal pain	7
Mental–psychiatric disorders	5

Data from MEAS paramedic records.

22 emergency medical technicians (EMTs) with basic paramedic training and additional experience in intravenous therapy and intubation. Both paramedics and EMTs are certified. In addition to emergency service, the MEAS team offers Cardiopulmonary Resuscitation (CPR) and first-aid classes to community groups.

Special Services

Frequently, special facilities exist to serve specific groups such as the physically or mentally disabled. After surveying the immediate extracommunity area, no such facilities were located within a 10-mile radius of Rosemont.

Intracommunity Health Facilities

According to the Health Systems Agency (HSA) of Jefferson County, CT 4104 is a medically underserved area; CT 4107 is not.

The type and number of practitioners offering health services in Rosemont are listed in Table 11.15. A need for gynecologic and obstetric services was frequently expressed by female residents. Numerous people cited the need for family practitioners as well as bilingual health care providers. (One of the nurse practitioners speaks Spanish, but none speaks Vietnamese.) Rosemont residents with financial resources tend to select from extracommunity medical services, whereas indigent residents rely on medical services within the community. All private practitioners require payment when services are rendered or third-party reimbursement; the nurse practitioners use a sliding scale to calculate fees. In addition to private practitioners, two clinics—the Third Street Clinic and the Rosemont Health Center—are located in Rosemont.

Third Street Clinic

The Third Street Clinic was founded in 1968 by concerned citizens and church leaders in Rosemont. The clinic, located in the center of CT 4104, was initially financed by public donations and church-sponsored fundraisers. All professional time and supplies were donated. Today, the Third Street Clinic serves 30% to 40% of Rosemont residents and has an annual operating budget of $750,000, a reduction of $220,000 from 2 years ago. The majority of funds are from federal and state grants as well as from client fees and Medicare and Medicaid reimbursements. Although patients are charged according to a sliding scale, no one is denied care. Services provided at Third Street Clinic are summarized in Table 11.16. The clinic provides no acute or trauma care services. The staff includes one part-time physician, two part-time nurses, one social worker, one administrator, and a clerk. Both nurses speak Spanish, but none of the staff speaks Vietnamese. Optometry students and supervising faculty provide services 1 day a week, and one nurse-midwife provides antepartum care two mornings

TABLE 11.15 Practitioners in Rosemont

Type	Number
Dentist	6
General medical	1
Optometrist	2
Orthodontist	1
Osteopath	2
Podiatrist	1
Chiropractor	3
Nurse practitioner	2

Data from windshield survey, Chamber of Commerce, and phone directory.

TABLE 11.16 Services and Number of People Served at Third Street Clinic

Service	Description	Patient Visits (Weekly Average)
Family planning	Physical examinations, education, and prescriptions filled	24
Well-child examinations	Physical assessment, referral for illness, immunizations, and screening	19
Antepartum and postpartum	Physical assessment and monitoring	42
Optometry	Eye examinations and prescriptions filled	9
Podiatry	Assessment and treatment	6
Chronic disease counseling and treatment	Treatment and care instructions for hypertension, diabetes, and cardiovascular conditions	31

a week. The clinic is open Monday through Friday, 8 AM to 5 PM. On average, 125 people are seen weekly. Medical professionals and citizens form the board of directors. According to the clinic's director, immediate medical needs for the residents of CT 4104 include the following:

- Ill infant, child, adolescent, and adult assessment, treatment, and follow-up
- Dental assessment and restoration
- Counseling, referral, and, when possible, treatment for drug abuse and alcoholism
- Group health teaching, especially for pregnant women, parents of young children, and adolescents
- Wellness and self-care classes for all age groups
- Support groups for single parents and senior citizens

There are no consistent health education or counseling services. Transportation services from area neighborhoods to the clinic, as well as dental and home nursing care, were discontinued 2 years ago after grant reductions. The major problem confronting the clinic is the recruitment of health care providers, especially nurses and physicians. Clinic services cannot be expanded (or maintained at the present level) unless additional health care providers are recruited and retained.

Most Rosemont residents are aware of the Third Street Clinic, and many use the clinic's services routinely. The major impediment to clinic use is the 1- to 2-mile walk to the clinic for many residents (there is no direct bus connection for most people). Rosemont residents feel welcome at the clinic, and low staff turnover has fostered positive relationships between the staff and the community. Residents did, however, express a need for additional services at the clinic.

Rosemont Health Center

The Rosemont Health Center, centrally located in CT 4107, is a nonprofit clinic devoted to the diagnosis and treatment of STDs (including HIV infection). The clinic is open Monday through Saturday, 6 PM to 10 PM, and Sunday, 2 PM to 10 PM. The center reports 20% of the syphilis cases and 60% of the gonorrhea cases in Jefferson County. Approximately 600 patient visits occur monthly (200 new cases, 200 repeat cases, and 200 follow-ups). All 75 professional staff members are volunteers and donate 4 to 10 hours of service a month. The director of the clinic is employed part-time. The state donates penicillin, tetanus cultures, and Venereal Disease Research Laboratory (VDRL) tests. Initially, there were no fees for services. Now, a sliding scale fee is assessed to defray costs of equipment, rent, and utilities. No person is denied care. Ninety percent of the patients were gay men when the clinic opened. However, in recent years the demographic makeup of the clientele has shifted to more closely resemble the entire population of the area. Each patient is issued an identification number and card that is used with each visit. People in psychological crisis are referred to the city health department for counseling. Most patients drive or walk to the clinic.

The director of the health center discussed the immediate need for expanded counseling and support groups, especially for people who are HIV positive. A second need is for an orientation program and information update sessions for staff members, most of whom are former patients. The majority of patients are from the Rosemont area, although an increasing number of patients are commuting to the clinic from Hampton and surrounding Jefferson County. Patients surveyed in the waiting room rated the care as excellent; appointments are rarely canceled by patients.

Observations at the clinic revealed a warm, caring atmosphere where people were treated with respect and were provided privacy when needed. However, there was no visible emergency cart. There were no standard policy and procedure manuals and no posted protocol for an adverse treatment response (such as penicillin reaction) for the many volunteers who worked there.

Extracommunity Social Service Facilities

Because social service agencies are frequently located in office buildings, their location in the community may be difficult to determine during a windshield survey. It is preferable to use a directory such as the type compiled by the Chamber of Commerce or local planning board to begin identifying social service organizations relatively close to the community being assessed. If the community does not have a Chamber of Commerce, use the telephone directory.

Counseling and Support Services

The Hampton Comprehensive Counseling Center was founded in 1971 by concerned citizens of Hampton and Jefferson County for the purpose of providing counseling to adolescent drug users. Today, the center offers a comprehensive mental health program for all residents of Hampton. The center is located 2 miles south of Rosemont. Although people can self-refer to the center, most patients are referred from schools, clinics, and private practitioners. Fees are based on a sliding scale; third-party reimbursements are not accepted. Last year's operating budget was $1,800,000. The majority of revenue comes from clients, although numerous churches and social service agencies sponsor individuals and families. The staff consists of six professionals and two clerks. Services are outlined in Table 11.17. On average, 300 patients are

TABLE 11.17 Services Offered at the Hampton Comprehensive Counseling Center

Service	Description
Diagnosis	Screening procedure for the mentally handicapped; recommends services required for clients' needs
Information and referral	Liaison teams coordinate services with state schools for the mentally retarded and state hospitals for the mentally ill
Counseling and therapy	Group and play therapy provided
Alcohol and drug abuse services	Counseling services
Psychiatric evaluation and medical services	Psychiatric department provides evaluations and medications for clients
Emergency service	Handles crisis calls 24 hours/day, 7 days/week
Education and consultation	Center staff works with other community groups, including schools, police, and social service agencies, to solve local problems

Data from Hampton Comprehensive Counseling Center.

seen each month. The director describes the patient population as white and middle- to upper income, with more men than women. Most patients use private transportation to arrive at the clinic. No additional services are planned because the center staff believes they are adequately meeting the needs of the population. Rosemont residents queried were unaware of the existence of the counseling center, and no one knew of anyone having used the center, although all residents interviewed knew of several adolescent drug users.

The YMCA Youth Development Center borders Rosemont and offers a variety of educational and recreational programs. Adjacent to the "Y" is the YMCA Indo-Chinese Refugee Program, an agency that seeks to facilitate the resettlement of Asian immigrants. Major services include cultural orientation, job counseling and placement, and courses in English as a second language. The agency services have experienced a 200% increase in usage during the past 3 years. Presently, more than 100 people use the facility daily. Although all four staff members are bilingual, the staff is too small to meet the needs of the Vietnamese community—a large proportion of which lives in Rosemont. The staff believes the immediate need is for counseling and therapy programs for alcohol and drug abuse as well as teaching basic survival skills (e.g., finding a job, housing, and medical care). The staff estimates that 40% to 50% of the Asians using their services are from Rosemont. Asian residents in Rosemont agree that the "Y" is responsive to their needs, but, when asked, they do acknowledge long waiting periods (sometimes weeks) for classes and counseling.

Clothing, Food, Shelter, and Basic Welfare Services

Most churches and synagogues in the area have a food pantry, and many can arrange emergency shelter and provide clothing and essential transportation services. People are usually helped on a walk-in basis, but sometimes the church is referred to a family or individual in need. In Hampton, a special organization, The Metropolitan Ministries, serves as an interfaith link between the religious communities of Hampton and community residents in need of social services. The Metropolitan Ministries coordinates services, thereby avoiding duplication, and refers people to the program that can best meet their immediate needs.

Take Note

In most communities, churches must be contacted individually for a listing of services.

In addition to the churches, synagogues, and mosques, numerous clothing resale shops are located in shopping areas close to Rosemont. Residents are very knowledgeable about available retail stores and actively promote preferred merchants.

The Jefferson County Welfare Department and the Hampton Welfare Department screen and process applicants for food stamps, housing subsidies, and financial aid. Each welfare department has a division of child protection that investigates reports of child abuse and neglect. The division provides casework services, foster home placement, and emergency shelter for women and children, as well as parenting classes and child-therapy groups. Welfare departments are funded by federal, state, and local tax revenues.

Special Services

The United Way lists 42 private- and public-supported social service agencies located in Hampton or Jefferson County. The United Way directory includes identifying information for each agency, as well as services and fees. Agencies on the roster include the Society to Prevent Blindness, American Lung Association, March of Dimes, Hampton Area Woman's Center, Paralyzed Veterans Association, and the International Rescue Committee.

Take Note

In your community assessment material, this would be an ideal location to append a list of social service agencies, along with identifying information (such as address, phone number, major services, and contact person). Brochures describing services, eligibility, and so on are useful to include as well.

Intracommunity Social Service Facilities

Two churches in Rosemont, South Main Methodist and St. Martin Episcopal, have extensive social outreach programs, including preschool and day care services; benevolence funds for food, clothing, and shelter; and numerous support groups (e.g., Parents Without Partners, Singles, and Solitaires). St. Martin has a seniors' center open 8 AM to 6 PM daily. The seniors enjoy a variety of recreational and educational programs and a hot noon meal. In addition, volunteers assist with shopping and errands, minor home repairs, light housekeeping, and meals for seniors who are permanently or temporarily incapacitated. Noticeably absent from St. Martin were any support groups or programs directed at the large gay male population. When asked about this, staff members responded, "That problem does not exist in this community." South Main does offer a coffee klatch on Friday night and plans to offer additional services to the gay male population, although there is strong resistance from the older parishioners.

On the north side of CT 4107 is Lambda Alcoholics Anonymous (AA), a program specifically for gay men and women, a group originally not allowed to join Alcoholics Anonymous. Lambda AA in CT 4107 is an active group, with the present participation exceeding 200 people. All socioeconomic groups are represented in the meetings, and members take turns leading the support groups.

Economics

The economic subsystem includes the "wealth" of Rosemont (i.e., the goods and services available to the community) as well as the costs and benefits of improving patterns of resource allocation. It should be evident that extracommunity factors, such as the state of the United States and world economies, affect in great measure the local economy. Nevertheless, intracommunity economic factors impinge on all other subsystems, so they must be included in the assessment. Table 11.18 lists the suggested areas for studying a community's economy, along with sources of the data. The census data can be used to summarize most of these economic indicators. Two key indicators of a community's economic health are the percentage of households below the poverty level and the unemployment rate.

Financial Characteristics of Households

The two census tracts that comprise the Rosemont community vary greatly in income characteristics. The census data show the median income for households in CT 4104 to be $34, 878, whereas in CT 4107 it is $48,238. Table 11.19 lists the household income for the community and Hampton, comparing 2000 and 2010 figures. Sometimes midyear data may be used to continue looking at trends until the completion of the next census.

Businesses

Several high-rise office buildings are located on the northern boundary of the area along the Audubon Parkway, including the National General Life Insurance complex of three towers, the new National Tower, the National Service Corporation, and the Second Mortgage

TABLE 11.18 Economic Indicators and Sources of Information

Indicators	Source
Financial Characteristics	

Households
    Median household income
        % households below poverty level
        % households receiving public assistance
        % households headed by females
    Monthly costs for owner-occupied households and
    renter-occupied households
	Census records

Individuals
    Per capita income
        % of persons who live in poverty
	Census records

Labor Force Characteristics	

Employment Status
    General population (age 18 +)
        % employed
        % unemployed
        % not participating in employment (retired)
    Special groups
        % women working with children under age 6
	Chamber of Commerce
	Department of Labor
	Census records

Occupational Categories and Number (%) of Persons
    Employed
        Managerial
        Technical
        Service
        Farming
        Production
        Operator/laborer
	Census records

Union Activity and Membership	Local union(s) office

Corporation's building. Way-on-the-Bayou, a new office complex, is also being constructed at the corner of Way Drive and Buff's Bayou. These buildings all feature spacious land-scaped grounds, modern architecture, and covered parking. Some of the residents of the area are employed in these offices; however, most employees, according to local residents, live outside of Rosemont.

TABLE 11.19 Income Indices for the Years 2000 and 2010 for CT 4104, CT 4107, and City of Hampton

Income Indices	CT 4104		CT 4107		Hampton	
	2000	2010	2000	2010	2000	2010
Median household income ($)	28,247	31,878	34,798	48,238	42,598	42,598
% of families with incomes below poverty level	13.3	20.6	18.3	12.1	14.2	12.1
% of female-headed households	NA	29.6	NA	19.8	12.7	27.1

NA, data not available.
Data from Census of Population and Housing, selected characteristics.

The major area businesses include the Rose Milk Company factory at the northern edge of the area on Way Drive, the Sheet Metal Workers Union Local No. 54 at the corner of Way Drive and Jackson, and American Life Insurance Company on Green.

All of the main thoroughfares in the area are lined with locally owned businesses such as grocery stores, craft stores, antique shops, cleaners, and small restaurants (see the Physical Description section). In addition, these kinds of businesses are also dispersed throughout the area within the residential districts. The Hampton Lighting and Power Service Center is located near the northern edge of the area. Hampton's vehicle maintenance department and its street repair department are also located on West Pleasant in the northern part of the Rosemont area. There are also a considerable number of publishing houses (probably the largest concentration in Hampton) on the northern edge of the area, as well as the broadcast studios of the local CBS station (KHAM-TV).

According to local residents, the economic impact of these businesses on the Rosemont area is minimal because most residents are employed outside of Rosemont, and, although they do patronize neighborhood convenience stores, they tend to shop for major purchases in other areas of the city. The residents also indicated that the vast majority of the businesses do not directly participate in the life of the community. Selected industries of the area are listed in Table 11.20.

When there are major businesses within a community that employ a substantial number of community residents, a thorough assessment is required. See Chapter 19 for further information about workplace assessment.

Labor Force

Employment Status

As mentioned earlier, the unemployment rate is a key indicator of the economic health of the community. The labor force of a community is composed of people aged 16 years and above. Table 11.21 summarizes key data relating to the workforce of the Rosemont community as well as the city of Hampton and Jefferson County. The majority of workers are categorized under "private wage and salary," as shown in Table 11.22.

TABLE 11.20 Selected Industries in Rosemont

| | CT 4104 | | CT 4107 | |
	Number	Total %	Number	Total %
Manufacturing	92	10	430	15
Wholesale and retail trade	450	48	1,084	37
Professional and related services	387	42	1,423	48
TOTAL	929	100	2,937	100

Data from Census, selected characteristics.

TABLE 11.21 Rosemont Labor Force for CT 4104, CT 4107, City of Hampton and Jefferson County

	CT 4104	CT 4107	Hampton	Jefferson County
People age 16 and over	4,580	6,470	1,189,136	2,519,937
Labor force	1,825	5,472	850,389	1,653,892
Percentage of people age 16 and over	39.8	85.4	71.5	65.6

Data from Census of Population and Housing, selected characteristics.

TABLE 11.22 Class of Workers for CT 4104, CT 4107, and Jefferson County by Percentage of Work Force

	CT 4104	CT 4107	Jefferson County
Private wage and salary	67	76	82.6
Government	18	12	11.2
Local government	13	12	6.0
Self-employed	2	6	0.2
TOTAL	100	100	100

Data from Census of Population and Housing, selected characteristics.

TABLE 11.23 Occupations for Rosemont (CT 4104 and CT 4107)

	CT 4104		CT 4107	
	Number	%	Number	%
Managerial, professional, and related	117	7.1	2,238	42.1
Technical, sales, administrative support	198	12.1	1,813	34.1
Service	724	44.2	560	10.5
Farming	28	1.7	11	0.02
Precision production	186	11.3	463	8.7
Operators, fabricators, laborers	387	23.6	230	4.3
TOTAL	1,640	100	5,315	100

Data from Census of Population and Housing, selected economic characteristics.

Occupation

General occupational categories are included in the census. Table 11.23 lists the occupations of the citizens of Rosemont.

Take Note

Census occupational categories are quite general. To determine more precisely what sort of work is incorporated in a category, it is necessary to ask those who do the job or to look up the category in the Department of Labor publications.

Differences between the two census tracts that constitute Rosemont are clearly seen in the occupational makeup of the community. Whereas almost half of the workers in CT 4104 are categorized under "service," a similar percentage of workers in CT 4107 are classified under "managerial and professional specialty."

Safety and Transportation

Table 11.24 lists the major components of safety and transportation that affect the community.

TABLE 11.24 Safety and Transportation

Indicators	Sources of Information
Safety	
Protection services	Planning office (city, county, and state)
Fire	Fire department (local)
Police	Police department (city and county)

Sanitation
    Waste sources and treatment
    Solid waste
	Waste and water treatment plants

Air quality	Air control board (state, regional, and local offices)
Transportation	

Private
    Transportation sources
    Number of persons with a transportation disability
	Census data: Population and housing characteristics

Public
    Bus service (routes, schedules, and fares)
    Roads (number and condition; primary, secondary,
      and farm-to-market roads)
    Interstate highways
    Freeway system
    Air service (private and publicly owned)
	Local and city transportation authorities
	State highway department
	
	Local airports (Note: Local airports are frequently
	  owned and operated by city government.)

Rail service	In the United States, Amtrak is the primary source of intercity rail transportation

Protection Services

Fire, police, and sanitation services are provided by the city of Hampton. Rosemont residents pay for these services through their city taxes. Therefore, these services are extracommunity, located outside the community of Rosemont.

Fire Protection

The fire department and MEAS are combined in Hampton. (For a description of the MEAS, see the Health and Social Services section.) The fire station serving Rosemont maintains two fire trucks, one air boat (for evacuations during flooding), and 20 personnel. Firemen must complete 335 hours of basic certification courses. The fire captain reports a response time of less than 10 minutes. During the 90 days before the assessment, the station responded to 45 fires. This compares with 39 responses during the same period of the previous year. Forty responses were to homes—the major culprit being grease fires that started in the kitchen. Other leading causes of fires include lighted cigarettes and children playing with matches. In addition to responding to fires, personnel perform safety checks of homes; teach fire-prevention to school and community groups; and distribute window stickers that specify the location of children, elderly citizens, and pets for emergency alert during a fire.

Police Protection

The police substation serving Rosemont has a staff of 27 full-time employees, including 21 police officers and 6 civilians (4 dispatchers and 2 record clerks). Equipment includes five marked and four unmarked patrol cars, two motorcycles, and a complete computerized data storage and retrieval system. This station has one holding cell where people are detained until they can be transported to the Hampton Jail. According to the dispatcher, response time to Rosemont is 4 to 6 minutes. Crime statistics for CT 4104 and CT 4107 are presented in Table 11.25.

TABLE 11.25 Crime Statistics for CT 4104 and CT 4107

	2009		2010		2011	
	CT 4104	CT 4107	CT 4104	CT 4107	CT 4104	CT 4107
Murder	10	3	5	3	7	2
Rape	34	17	17	5	12	4
Robbery	328	186	345	157	320	146
Aggravated assault	94	29	76	25	57	20
Burglary	345	339	329	337	320	325
Theft	384	363	370	359	328	322
Vehicle theft	109	327	112	378	101	315
TOTAL	1,304	1,264	1,254	1,264	1,145	1,134

Data from City of Hampton police department.

The most frequent crimes are burglaries and thefts, which the police captain believes are committed mainly by nonresidents of Rosemont. Speeding and driving while intoxicated (DWI) are also frequent crimes in Rosemont; although, after the addition of two motorcycle police officers two years ago, the number of traffic accidents has decreased by 38%. The police department offers the following services to Rosemont residents:

- Housewatch—When residents are out of town, the police will check their house three times a day for up to 30 days.
- Identification—The police department loans an engraver to citizens who wish to engrave personal belongings. The department also provides household possessions registration and pamphlets on how to protect one's home from burglary.
- Fingerprinting—Fingerprinting is done and a record of the prints is provided to the person for personal identification as well as for immigration requirements. The police department is presently pursuing a special project, a citywide campaign to fingerprint all children and adolescents. A copy of the fingerprint record is given to parents, and the original remains with the police. After several weeks of radio and TV announcements, police personnel are now present at local shopping centers every weekend to explain and complete the fingerprinting process. This special project is in response to citizen concern and requests for police assistance in locating an increasing number of missing children.
- Animal Protection Officer—The city of Hampton has a leash and fence law for dogs. The animal protection officer picks up stray animals and detains them in the city kennel until the owner or an adopter can be found.
- Public Education—Crime prevention programs are offered to community and school groups.

Residents of Rosemont repeatedly voiced concern about their personal safety. Elderly citizens expressed fear of being mugged and related stories of friends who have been harassed and robbed during the day as they walked to and from local stores. (One grocery store owner reported that he has stopped cashing Social Security checks because so many patrons had been mugged after leaving his store.) The feeling of being a prisoner in one's own home was repeatedly expressed, as were questions regarding what people could do to protect themselves.

Gay men described experiences of perceived harassment by police as well as incidents of marked delay (up to 30 minutes) in police response time to requests for help. Residents reported that brawls, quarrels, and physical violence are becoming commonplace in Rosemont. The citizens are concerned for themselves and others; they want a safe place to live.

Sanitation

Water Sources and Treatment. The terrain of Rosemont is flat with minimal changes in elevation. Stagnant pools of water are common—a situation that promotes mosquito populations during the warm months. Drainage is toward the northeast and into Buff's Bayou, the only open stream in Rosemont. All storm water and sewage are gathered into Hampton's sewage system. There is no separate system for storm water disposal. As a result, raw sewage backs up during heavy rains, and residents complain about the smell and problems associated with toilets that cannot be flushed.

Sewage from Rosemont is treated at the 5th Street Plant. A sewage moratorium exists for Rosemont owing to overcapacity at the 5th Street Plant. Consequently, only single-family dwellings can be built on plotted lots. Builders requesting permits for multifamily dwellings are given the option of delaying building indefinitely or being assessed a fee based on projected occupancy of their building and the associated gallons of sewage that will be produced. The assessed fee is used to increase the capacity of the treatment plant. However, even if the assessed fee option is chosen, it may be 3 to 4 years before the permit is issued.

Potable (drinkable) water for Rosemont comes from Lake Hampton, located 20 miles north of the city. Residents are concerned about possible contamination of the drinking water with lead and other heavy metals. There is no routine testing of the drinking water except to meet state health department requirements for chlorine content. Fluoride is not added to Rosemont's drinking water, and it is not present naturally.

Solid Waste. Garbage is collected weekly from city of Hampton–provided individual household plastic cans at curbside; residents state that the service and frequency are adequate. The major complaint is that illegal dumping of large items, such as refrigerators, stoves, and so forth, has increased, and, despite numerous calls to proper authorities, the trash is not cleaned up with any regularity. Parents are concerned that children attracted by abandoned machinery and appliances may be hurt as they explore. In addition, inoperable automobiles are abandoned in parking spaces on the streets, and months can pass before the cars are removed by the city.

Air Quality

The Federal Air Quality Act of 1967 provided for the establishment of air-quality control regions. Regional offices maintain an inventory of air-pollution sources and monitor air status. In a similar fashion, individual states formed advisory boards that developed air-quality standards and long-range air-quality programs. Local air-monitoring stations sample and record information levels on such pollutants as ozone, carbon monoxide, sulfur dioxide, and nitrogen dioxide. In addition, some 30 to 40 suspended particles in the air (solids) are measured and recorded, as are certain gaseous substances (e.g., ammonia).

To assess the air quality of Rosemont, the Air Control Board was contacted; its recent reports document a rise in air pollution, which is attributed to an increase in industrial growth and a high population density. Some 25 miles east of Rosemont is a large industrial complex, and, although the daily emissions from the industries are within acceptable limits, certain wind and temperature patterns act to compound emissions. This causes a visible yellow haze to form that shrouds Rosemont and surrounding communities many days of the year. Area residents complain of eye irritation and increased frequency of respiratory conditions. The chemical reactions that lead to the haze and the contribution of automotive and industrial emissions, as well as potential health effects associated with the haze, are unknown and are presently being researched.

Take Note

Air pollution is a frequently used term; it is defined as the presence of one or more contaminants in such concentration and of such duration that they may adversely affect human health, animal life, vegetation, or property.

Despite the pollution increase and industrial growth, there has been no significant increase in the amount of pollutants introduced into the atmosphere surrounding Rosemont. This is attributed to compliance of industries with the Air Control Board regulations and the permit system for new industries. Citizens can contest industry construction permits and, through this process, provide a forum for public opinion and objections that regulation boards take into consideration during the permit decision-making process. Citizens are also entitled to complain to the board regarding a specific industry's emissions; the board will then investigate and file a report.

During the past year, Rosemont has experienced three air stagnation advisories. Because the pollution concentration is greater than usual, people with respiratory conditions such as bronchitis and emphysema are advised to remain indoors and limit outside activities until the air stagnation clears.

 Take Note

Air stagnation occurs when a layer of cool air is trapped by a layer of warmer air above it; the bottom air cannot rise and pollutants cannot be dispersed.

The board believes citizens are ill-informed regarding the meaning of and the appropriate actions that should be taken during air stagnation advisories as well as each citizen's responsibility in minimizing pollution. For example, citizens seem unaware that transportation sources (such as automobiles and buses), not industry, are the major contributors of air pollution problems and that a citizen who burns leaves or trash is releasing tiny particles of matter into the air that can irritate the eyes, nose, and lungs. To promote public awareness and understanding, the local office makes presentations to organizations, schools, and citizen groups. Numerous public television and radio programs were planned for the year after the assessment.

Transportation

The primary means of transportation in Rosemont include walking, bicycle riding, automobiles, Hampton city buses, Hampton city vans (special transportation for the elderly and handicapped), and school buses.

Private

The major source of private transportation is the automobile. Table 11.26 presents the types of transportation used to commute to work, and Table 11.27 indicates the number of people

TABLE 11.26 Transportation Sources to Work Used by Residents of CT 4104, CT 4107, and City of Hampton

	CT 4104		CT 4107		Hampton	
	Number	**%**	**Number**	**%**	**Number**	**%**
Drive alone	1,351	42.8	3,279	63.8	NA	75.7
Car pool	749	23.7	808	15.7		14.6
Public transportation	721	22.8	567	11		4.1
Walk	231	7.3	300	5.8		1.8
Other means	79	2.5	130	2.5		1.4
Work at home	27	0.9	58	1.2		2.4
Total	3,158	100	5,142	100		100

NA, data not available.
Data from Census of Population and Housing, selected characteristics.

TABLE 11.27 Noninstitutionalized People 16 Years of Age or Older by Transportation Disability Status for CT 4104 and CT 4107

	With Disability		Without Disability		Total	
	Number	%	Number	%	Number	%
Age 16–64						
CT 4104	221	5.9	3,495	94.1	3,716	100
CT 4107	15	0.3	5,908	99.7	5,923	100
Age 65 and over						
CT 4104	197	21.3	728	78.7	925	100
CT 4107	55	10.5	469	89.5	524	100

Data from Census of Population and Housing.

aged 16 years or older who have a transportation disability. According to the census data, mean travel time to work for Rosemont residents is 17.7 minutes as compared with 26.6 minutes for Hampton residents.

Public

The major source of public transportation within Rosemont and surrounding communities is the Hampton bus system. The city provides east–west bus service at half-hour intervals during the day on Pecan Drive and Live Oak Boulevard. The same service is provided on north–south routes for Way Drive, Rosemont Boulevard, and Hampton Street. For people who qualify (such as the elderly or handicapped), the bus company provides door-to-door service from the person's home to essential services such as food shopping or medical care visits. The cost of this service varies from $1.00 to $2.00 per trip, according to geographic area. Although all users agree the service is reliable, it is only available Monday through Friday, 8:30 AM to 5:00 PM, and reservations are required several days in advance—a requirement that is impossible to meet in some situations such as during acute illnesses.

Roads

Jefferson County (of which Rosemont is a part) has adequate primary, secondary, and farm-to-market roads. In addition, several miles of a freeway system circle Hampton. Two major interstate highways transect Hampton, and the state highway department has budgeted $2 billion for highway construction and maintenance for Jefferson County over the next 20 years. Recently, the residents of Jefferson County voted for an additional tax devoted entirely to improving intracounty transportation. Rosemont residents complain of congested freeways and damaged roads that go without repair for months. The need was expressed for a road system that efficiently handles local traffic.

Air Service

Jefferson County has four small, privately owned airports. The city of Hampton owns and operates two airports that provide national and international service.

Rail Service

Amtrak connects Hampton to other major cities in the state as well as to other states. METRO light rail began operation in Hampton on January 1, 2004. It was the first phase of a projected 73 miles of service by 2025. The rail runs near, but not through, Rosemont, serving downtown Hampton, a major sports stadium, two universities, the museum district, a city park, and the medical center. Fare is $1.00 one way, and for $2.00 the rider can purchase a 24-hour pass for unlimited rides.

Politics and Government

Rosemont falls within the city limits of Hampton, which has a mayor-council form of government. There are 14 council members (5 at-large), one of whom represents Rosemont and nearby communities. Each serves a 2-year term. The city council meets at City Hall on the first Tuesday of each month. The meetings are open to the public, and Rosemont residents often attend.

The city council and mayor comprise the policy-making body as well as the administrative head of Hampton. Their duties include the following: maintaining competent staff to operate all city services (the health department and police, for instance), passing ordinances, and appropriating funds to carry out policies.

The councilman for District Three, which includes Rosemont, is James Browning. Councilman Browning was elected by a wide margin of votes and has been popular with the Rosemont community because he spearheaded the fight against sexually oriented businesses (the "SOB Fight," as it is popularly called). This issue has not been settled, and the citizens are supporting Councilman Browning's reelection, so he may continue the fight.

The active participation in the Hampton council of Councilman Browning is only one indicator of Rosemont's politics. There are several politically oriented organizations and civic clubs in the area, all of which seek to improve the quality of life in Rosemont and help to support intercommunity activities.

A brief synopsis of several organizations that are politically active in Rosemont is presented in Table 11.28. (Contact person, address, and phone number should be included in such lists but have been omitted from this description.)

TABLE 11.28 Organizations Politically Active in Rosemont

Organization	Description
Neartown Business Alliance (Founded 1949)	Owners of businesses in the area meet monthly and work to promote the area and its businesses. The alliance contributes to campaigns of supporters of Rosemont.
Gay Political Caucus (Founded 1964)	This is a very active and visible group. It works to influence elections through voter registration, campaign work, and education. It has been credited with the election or defeat of certain candidates. Membership is open to all interested in community improvement. It meets on third Tuesday, 7:00 PM.
Rosemont Firehouse (Founded 1973)	This is a coordination and referral group; it operates a 24-hour crisis hotline. It is sponsored by donations from most of the area's churches as well as the civic groups, and most of the workers are community volunteers.
Rosemont Watch (Founded 1978)	The Watch works to prevent crime in the area through education and visible activities such as "Block Awareness Week." It coordinates activities with the Hampton City Police. All citizens are encouraged to become involved. It meets monthly.
Seniors for a Safe Community (Founded 1980)	Composed primarily of retired people (but open to all interested residents), this group was formed to address the problem of the mugging or robbing of senior citizens, especially on the days when Social Security checks arrived. The original small group has expanded, as have their goals, so now they are actively involved in promoting a better quality of life for all in the community (with a special emphasis on the elderly). This group is active in the "SOB Fight" and also works closely with Rosemont Watch.

Several other groups in the community are less visible and active unless an issue of particular interest becomes "hot." For instance, many voluntary agencies, such as the American Lung Association—Hampton Chapter, are located in the community and can be called on to assist specific campaigns (e.g., smoking-prevention programs in the schools or antipollution campaigns aimed toward extracommunity sources). The Community Services Directory lists all such organizations both by interest (heart, lung, crime, and so on) and general area (Rosemont groups can usually be found under "Southwest, near downtown").

Political activism is evident throughout Rosemont. During election years, there are campaign posters everywhere; talk at gathering places (barbershops, grocery stores, bars) inevitably turns to politics; and numerous rallies are held in support of candidates or issues. In Rosemont, there appear to be two major political factions. Voting records show CT 4107 residents to be more liberal than residents in CT 4104. This may reflect the fact that CT 4107 has more affluent, younger, and more professional residents than CT 4104.

Communication

Communication may be formal or informal. Formal communication usually originates outside the community (extracommunity) as opposed to informal communication, which almost always originates and is disseminated within the community. Salient components of formal and informal communication, as well as sources of data, are presented in Table 11.29.

Formal Communication

Hampton has one major newspaper, *The Hampton Herald*. Additional daily newspapers include a business journal, *Current Issues*; an African American-oriented paper; *Progress*; one Spanish-language paper, *La Prensa*; and a Vietnamese tabloid. Hampton has 12 AM radio stations and 10 FM stations, 6 commercial TV stations, and 1 educational network. Cable television is available to Rosemont residents on a monthly subscription basis. Residents receive home mail delivery.

TABLE 11.29 Communication

Components	Sources of Information
Formal	
Newspaper (number, circulation, frequency, and scope of news)	Chamber of Commerce
	Newspaper office
Radio and television (number of stations, commercial versus educational, and audience)	Telephone company
	Yellow Pages
Postal service	Telephone book
Telephone status (number of residents with service)	Census data on phone use
Informal	
Sources: bulletin boards; posters; hand-delivered flyers; and church, civic, and school newsletters	Windshield Survey
	Talking to residents
Dissemination (How do people receive information?)	Survey
Word of mouth	
Mail	
Radio, television	
Internet may be considered both formal and informal	Personal computer, workplace, public library, "Cyber" cafes

Informal Communication

Bulletin boards and posters dot community and municipal buildings in Rosemont. Posters are placed on trees and tacked to buildings throughout the community, and a rainbow of flyers can be seen tucked into fences and doors. Radio and television announcements herald forthcoming events and offer open forums on community issues. The Rosemont Civic Association publishes a bimonthly, four-page newsletter to notify residents of upcoming meetings and social activities. Polls and surveys are a regular feature of the newsletter, which is distributed free to all residents.

Key informants within Rosemont include the Civic Association secretary, local ministers, and fire and police personnel as well as community civic board members. People can be seen chatting throughout Rosemont, and, when asked how information is received, they mention all of the above formal and informal sources.

Education

The general educational status of a community can be summarized using census data. Census information lists the number of residents attending schools, years of schooling completed, and percentage of residents who speak English. To supplement this broad assessment, information is needed about major educational sources (e.g., schools, colleges, and libraries) located inside the community. Table 11.30 is a guide for assessing a community's educational sources.

 Take Note

It is sometimes difficult to decide which educational sources to include in the assessment. Community usage is probably the single most important indicator. Primary and secondary schools attended by the majority of children in a community, regardless of intra- or extracommunity location, are major educational sources and require a thorough assessment, whereas schools composed primarily of students from outside the community do not require such extensive appraisal.

TABLE 11.30 Education

Components	Sources of Information
Educational Status	
Years of school completed	Census data—Social characteristics section
School enrollment by type of school	Census data—Social characteristics section
Language spoken	Census data—Social characteristics section
Educational Sources	
Intracommunity or extracommunity (collect data for each facility)	Local board of education
Services (educational, recreational, communication, and health)	School administrator (such as the principal or director) and school nurse
Resources (personnel, space, budget, and record system)	School administrator
Characteristics of users (geographic distribution and demographic profile)	Teachers and staff
Adequacy, accessibility, and acceptability of education to students and staff	Students and staff

TABLE 11.31 Years of School Completed for CT 4104, CT 4107, and City of Hampton

	CT 4104	CT 4107	Hampton
Persons 25 years and over	3,459	4,948	888,269
Elementary			
0–4 years	611	26	41,695
5–7 years	665	164	66,775
8 years	409	101	37,373
High School			
1–3 years	800	278	136,179
4 years	661	914	240,320
% High school graduates	28.2	88.5	68.3
College			
1– 3 years	181	1,173	160,999
4 or more years	132	2,292	204,928

Data from Census of Population and Housing, social characteristics.

Educational Status

Table 11.31 presents the years of schooling completed by adults in CT 4104 and CT 4107. In a similar format, Table 11.32 lists school enrollment by type of school, and Table 11.33 presents the number and percentage of community residents who speak English poorly.

Intracommunity Educational Sources

Temple Elementary School

Temple Elementary School is located on the corner of Pecan and Magnolia Drives, close to the center of CT 4104. Asphalt lots bound three sides of Temple; two are used for vehicle parking, and one is for play. A small patch of grass persists on the remaining side, a fenced-in area that

TABLE 11.32 School Enrollment and Type of School for CT 4104, CT 4107, and City of Hampton

	CT 4104	CT 4107	Hampton
Type of School			
Public nursery school	94	44	20,735
Private nursery school	77	44	15,427
Public kindergarten	194	14	21,863
Private kindergarten	25	14	4,833
Public elementary (1–8 years)	1,258	186	198,367
Private elementary (1–8 years)	10	136	18,440
Public high school (1–4 years)	482	92	94,099
Private high school (1–4 years)	12	25	7,154
College	92	922	78,472
Total enrolled in schools (age 3 years and over)	2,120	1,258	413,536

Data from Census of Population and Housing.

TABLE 11.33 Ability to Speak English for CT 4104, CT 4107, and City of Hampton

| | Percentage Who Speak English Poorly or Not at All | |
	Age 5–17	Age 18 Years and Over
CT 4104	75.9	73.8
CT 4107	11	19.3
Hampton	21.4	26.2

Data from Census of Population and Housing.

contains several large trees, a swing set, and three teeter-totters. Several broken windows were seen, and no graffiti was noted. Temple is in its 74th year of continuous operation teaching grades kindergarten to eighth. Present enrollment is 924; 42% of the students are black, 33% are Asian, 18% are Hispanic, and 5% are white. Most of the children live in Rosemont and either walk to school or ride the school bus (provided for children living farther than 2 miles from Temple).

As part of the Hampton School District (HSD), Temple receives funding from the district revenues obtained from local property taxes, state coffers, and the federal budget. State monies to HSD are based on average daily attendance of students at each school. Most policies affecting Temple are formed and enforced by the HSD board. The board is composed of eight nonsalaried people, each elected from one of eight regions in the school district. Each term of office is 4 years. Board member Jane Roberts represents Rosemont; at the time of assessment, she was in the second year of her 4-year term. Responsibilities of the HSD board include prescribing qualifications of employees, establishing salary schedules, setting goals and objectives for the district, establishing the policies to implement the goals and objectives, and evaluating the performance of the district in relation to adopted goals and objectives. The general superintendent is the administrative head of the board and is salaried and recruited by the board.

Principal. Temple's principal cited truancy and the related problem of academic failure as the school's major problems. According to office records, some 6% to 8% of the student body is absent each day, and most of those absent are not ill. The principal reported that truancy is most common among seventh and eighth graders, especially among Hispanic boys.

Regarding bilingual education for non-English-speaking students, the principal believes that all classes should be in English and that the presence of bilingual education at Temple only slows the progress of the children who are learning English. There are two bilingual teachers at Temple; they reported that they have a list of over 100 students who have requested and have been assessed as needing the bilingual program.

Teachers. Teachers repeatedly stated the need for improved communication with parents. They believe that parents need to have current information about their child's learning needs and school performance as well as knowledge of specific techniques for fostering academic achievement. (School policy allows for two 20-minute parent–teacher conferences yearly—a time allotment that was rated as extremely inadequate by the teachers.) The teachers reported that 22% of the student body at Temple failed last year. Major impediments to learning were listed as poor English-speaking skills and understanding of English, stressful home environments, and inadequate adult supervision at home. Teachers felt overwhelmed and frustrated; the average employment stay at Temple is 2 years.

School Nurse. The school nurse at Temple is present 2 days a week; she is at West Hampton High the remaining 3 days. A review of the daily clinic register for the preceding 6 weeks noted a clinic attendance of 141; the majority (72%) of those visiting suffered from stomachache or headache. Although none of the stomach ailments required early dismissal, 60% of the headaches were associated with fever and necessitated early dismissal from school. Remaining complaints were sore throats and minor cuts or falls. All children were screened biannually for vision and hearing problems. The nurse recognized the need for yearly screening, but said she lacked the necessary time. She stated that if school policy would permit the recruitment and training of parent volunteers, then yearly screening would be feasible. In addition to vision and hearing testing, all children are screened for head lice twice a year; children found to be infected are dismissed from school and are not readmitted until they have been successfully treated.

Some 62% of the students participate in the free lunch program. The nurse expressed concern that several children who appear undernourished (displaying, e.g., low weight for height and small arm circumference for age) do not qualify for the lunch program, whereas others who appear to be well nourished do qualify. Eligibility is based on family size and income.

Major health problems as described by the nurse include lack of hygiene (children frequently come to school dirty and inadequately clothed for cold weather); dental caries; high (30% to 40%) annual incidence of head lice, especially in primary grades (kindergarten, first grade, and second grade); incomplete immunization status (92% of the children have up-to-date immunizations); and lack of parent follow-through for needed medical care and treatment during illnesses.

To assess dental status, the nurse performed oral assessment of children who came to the clinic during one 4-week period. She found that 62% of the children had discolored areas or cavities in the pits of their teeth or between teeth. Most of the children stated they had never been to a dentist, and many reported frequent tooth pain and difficulty chewing.

The nurse does not do any health teaching in the classroom because school policy mandates that the nurse be present in the clinic at all times. The ruling causes considerable frustration because the nurse's participation in the teaching and promotion of health habits is restricted to one-to-one clinic encounters (a time when the child is ill and not receptive to learning). When asked about staff and teacher usage of the clinic, the nurse discussed at length the need for health information expressed by both teachers and staff. Questions regarding exercise, stress, and diet modifications are common. The nurse would like to assess and identify specific health needs of staff and teachers.

Community Service. As a community service, Temple sponsors scout troops and basketball and softball teams, and provides a meeting place for several newly formed church and community action groups. In addition, Monday through Thursday nights, Temple houses extension courses from Hampton Community College. A full range of subjects is offered, including academic, vocational, and enrichment courses. Present enrollment exceeds 1,200, an increase of 22% from the previous year.

All Rosemont residents were familiar with Temple Elementary; most had children who attended Temple, or they themselves had attended Temple as children. Residents felt that Temple was a community landmark and a symbol of unity that links one generation to the next. The primary complaint, repeated by several families, was a perceived insensitivity of Temple's staff and teachers to ethnic and racial differences and needs. For example, all school notices are written in English, and all programs offered by the Parent Teachers Organization (PTO) are presented in English. Both Asian and Hispanic parents have brought specific concerns and needs to the staff and teachers at Temple, but have repeatedly been told that all parental requests must come from appropriate PTO committees—an organization that seems alien to many Asian and Hispanic parents.

Day Care

One day care center is located in CT 4104—the Busybee Nursery. There are no day care facilities in CT 4107. Housed in a renovated building, Busybee accepts children aged 2 to 5 years. Some 60 children are cared for by five staff members, and 43 children (primarily toddlers) are on the waiting list. The center is licensed by the state. Rosemont residents repeatedly lamented the lack of day care facilities. Many parents felt forced to leave their young children with other mothers or teenagers who have dropped out of school. Several mothers reported leaving their children daily with a babysitter who cares for 8 to 10 children.

Library

The Rosemont library is conveniently located adjacent to the main shopping district and offers a variety of adult, teen, and youth book programs, films, and special educational activities. Notices of all programs are published in the Rosemont Civic Association newsletter and posted on local bulletin boards.

Extracommunity Educational Sources

High school students from Rosemont attend Central Hampton High, a complex that houses 4,800 students and is located 8 miles from Rosemont. Concerned about truancy and grade failure, Central Hampton began a "Failproof" program 2 years ago. Some 82% of students and their parents have participated. As a result, school scores on state and national proficiency tests have improved, and truancy has decreased. The principal described numerous community outreach services offered by the school, including recreational programs in the evening and on the weekends, as well as a full complement of adult education courses.

The nurse at Central Hampton is present 5 days a week. The majority of visits to the clinic (an average of 30 daily) involve allergy-related complaints, gastrointestinal upsets, and minor sprains or strains that occur during physical exercise class. Because of HSD policies, the school nurse is prohibited from offering health education in the classroom.

The nurse's major concern is the increased number of teenage pregnancies and the HSD board's decision of 2 years ago not to permit sex education information in the classroom. Classes in sexuality, sexually transmitted disease, contraception, and decision making in the area of sexual activity had been offered at all high schools in Hampton before the new ruling. The nurse does not know the sequence of events that resulted in the sex education decision. A second major concern is the increased use of alcohol among students. A drug awareness curriculum was prepared by the state board of education and will be implemented during the next semester as part of the biology course.

Numerous private preschool and grade schools are available in Hampton, and some are used by the residents of Rosemont, especially by people in CT 4107. Some 20 colleges and universities are located in Hampton and Jefferson County; most offer a variety of general education and specialty training programs. One unique aspect of the area's educational resources is Hampton Community College, a junior college that provides classes in 21 public schools in Hampton and Jefferson County. Numerous residents state that they prefer Hampton Community College to other area resources because of its convenient locations, low tuition, and employment-oriented approach to education.

Recreation

The recreation facilities within and adjacent to Rosemont are listed in Table 11.34 and pictured in Figure 11.5. With the exception of the schoolyards, there is very little recreational area for children and almost none for adults and teenagers. Although there are funds in the budget of the Hampton Parks and Recreation Department for the acquisition of property, there are no plans for any development in the Rosemont area. However, the city has recently begun an improvement program along the banks of Buff's Bayou to create a "River Walk" similar to those in other cities with rivers. It will be several years before the project is completed.

The Rosemont Sports Association provides quality organized recreation opportunities for the local community. Programs consist of teams for bowling, softball, flag football, tennis, and so forth. The Rosemont Sports Association, however, is open only to members who pay a fee of $20 per year.

TABLE 11.34 Recreational Facilities in Rosemont and Adjacent Areas

	Acreage	Location	Facilities
San Juan	2.6	1650 Pleasant	Shelter building, playground equipment, softball field, and baseball field
Richards	1	1414 Redbud	Shelter building, playground equipment, picnic area, and basketball court (swimming pool recently filled in)
Applehurst	1.9	600 Water Oak	Recreation center, rest room, playground equipment, picnic area, tennis, basketball, and volleyball courts
Jeckle Park	0.08	1500 Maple	None
Buff's Bayou	?	"Greens" along the bayou	Park benches and jogging/bicycle trail

Data from City of Hampton, Parks and Recreation Department, interview with JB (Director), May 1994.

Churches of Rosemont (two were visited—see the Social Services section) offer a wide variety of activities for all ages. Exercise classes, craft classes, Mother's Day Out, preschool classes, senior citizens' groups, and many other programs are available to members. Although other community residents are welcome to take advantage of these activities, the people interviewed at the churches reported that their participants are almost all church members.

Several residents spoke of an area along the northern bank of Buff's Bayou (just east of Way Drive) that is used as a gathering place by residents who live nearby. Families take their children there on summer evenings, so parents can visit while the children play. The only facilities at this area are benches that have been placed along the grassy area.

A bicycle/jogging trail follows the bayou for several miles and is popular with the health-conscious residents who use it frequently, especially in the early morning and late evening hours. Some people have expressed fear of being mugged while using this trail, but there have been no official reports of crime in this area over the past year. The trail and all the land along the bayou are maintained by the city of Hampton.

The area residents of the east side tend to congregate for recreation on sidewalks and in neighborhood bars. The one playground in the area, other than the one at Temple Elementary, is located adjacent to the Audubon Parkway Village (the low-rent housing complex), and it is used exclusively by the residents of that complex. The playground equipment is in very poor repair, and there is virtually no grass left in the area. The Parks and Recreation Department has no plans to upgrade or replace the equipment or to replant the grass.

There is one movie theater and one theater for stage production in Rosemont, but movie theaters are accessible and near almost all areas surrounding the community. Other forms of evening entertainment are reflected in the numerous bars and restaurants that feature live music (as was mentioned in the physical examination of the community).

Extracommunity recreational facilities abound. A large city park that includes museums, a zoo, a band shell, and picnic areas is less than a mile to the south of Rosemont. Another city park in downtown Hampton, called Serenity Park, is less than a mile to the northeast.

Virtually every major league sport has a team in Hampton. The sports arenas are some distance from the area, but there is adequate bus service to them.

An abundance of music and theater is available to those who can afford it. Hampton has a symphony orchestra, a ballet, both grand and light opera, and a legitimate stage company, to name a few options. In addition, water activities, such as boating and fishing, are as close as 30 miles away. According to several residents of Audubon Parkway Village, a special day out includes crabbing along the bay—which is often a successful endeavor to fill the dinner pot as well as provide fun for the whole family.

Summary

The community assessment is never complete; however, we must pause at some point. Because we have addressed all parts of the model, this is where we will stop. A description of each community subsystem has been recorded. Note that at every step of the assessment, people in the community were included. Not only did we interview the professionals (e.g., school nurses, principal, police chief, and so on), but clients of the subsystems were also included (parents, shoppers, patients, and people on the street). The assessment, like all steps in the process, is carried out in partnership with the community. The next step is analysis, a process that synthesizes the assessment information and derives from it diagnoses specific to the community.

Crucial to community assessment is a model, or map, to direct and guide that process. The model (community assessment wheel) provided a framework, and the windshield survey tool guided the assessment of Rosemont. In the Further Readings list, several other approaches to community assessment are presented. As you are aware, there are other models you may wish to consider as you continue your practice of community health assessment.

Critical Thinking Questions

1. You are a member of many communities. Describe at least three communities of which you are a part. What makes each a community?

2. Describe one community you have identified above using the community assessment wheel. Find some basic demographic information about the community on the internet. Does it differ with your own view of that community?

3. What are some characteristics of your community that illustrate its *normal line of defense*? Give an example of your community's *flexible line of defense*.

4. What opportunities exist for you to become involved in your community? Are these related to your role as a community health nurse?

REFERENCES

Hancock, T., & Minkler, M. (2005). Community health assessment or healthy community assessment. In M. Minkler (Ed.), *Community organizing and community building for health* (pp. 138–159). New Brunswick, NJ: Rutgers University Press.

Neuman, B. N. (1972). A model for teaching total person approach to patient problems. *Nursing Research, 21*(3), 264–269.

World Health Organization. (1986). *Ottawa charter for health promotion.* WHO Regional Office for Europe. Copenhagen, Denmark: Author.

FURTHER READINGS

Beverly, C. J., McAtee, R., Costello, J., Chernoff, R., & Casteel, J. (2005). Needs assessment of rural communities: A focus on older adults. *Journal of Community Health, 30*(3), 197–208.

Clark, N., & Buell, A. (2004). Community assessment: An innovative approach. *Nurse Educator, 29*(5), 203–207.

Corso, L., Wiesner, P. J., & Lenihan, P. (2005). Developing the MAPP community health improvement tool. *Journal of Public Health Management and Practice, 11*(5), 387–392.

Escoffery, C., Trowbridge, J., & Miner, K. R. (2004). Conducting small-scale community assessments. *American Journal of Health Education, 35*(4), 237–241.

Green, L. W., & Kreuter, M. W. (2005). *Health promotion planning: An educational and ecological approach* (4th ed.). New York, NY: McGraw-Hill Higher Education.

Kretzman, J. P., & McKnight, J. L. (1993). *Building communities from the inside out: A path toward finding and mobilizing a community's assets.* Chicago, IL: ACTA Publications.

Kulbok, P. A., Meszaros, P., Bond, D. C., Botchwey, N. D., & Hinton, I. (2009). Partnering with rural youth and parents to design and test a tobacco, alcohol, and drug use prevention program model (Abstract). *Virginia Foundation for Healthy Youth.* Retrieved from http://healthyyouthva.org/vtsf/research/projects.asp

Pender, N. J., Murdaugh, C. L., & Parsons, M. A. (2011). *Health promotion in nursing practice* (6th ed.). Upper Saddle River, NJ: Prentice Hall.

Serafini, P. (1976). Nursing assessment in industry: A model. *American Journal of Public Health, 66*(8), 755–760.

CHAPTER 12

Community Analysis and Nursing Diagnosis

Elizabeth T. Anderson and Judith McFarlane

LEARNING OBJECTIVES

This chapter focuses on the second phase of the nursing process, analysis, and the associated task of forming community nursing diagnoses.

After studying this chapter, you should be able to:

1. Critically analyze community assessment data.
2. Formulate community nursing diagnoses.

Introduction

Analysis is the study and examination of data. These data may be quantitative (numerical) as well as qualitative. All aspects need to be considered. Analysis is necessary to determine community health needs and community strengths, as well as to identify patterns of health responses and trends in health care use. During analysis, any need for further data collection is revealed as gaps and incongruities in the community assessment data. The end point of analysis is the community nursing diagnosis.

COMMUNITY ANALYSIS

Analysis, like so many procedures we carry out, may be viewed as a process with multiple steps. The phases we use to help in the analysis are categorization, summarization, comparison, and inference elaboration. Each is described below.

Categorize

To analyze community assessment data, it is helpful to first categorize the data. Data can be categorized in a variety of ways. Traditional categories of community assessment data include the following:

- Demographic characteristics (family size, age, sex, and ethnic and racial groupings)
- Geographic characteristics (area boundaries; number and size of neighborhoods, public spaces, and roads)

- Socioeconomic characteristics (occupation and income categories, educational attainment, and rental or home ownership patterns)
- Health resources and services (hospitals, clinics, mental health centers, and so forth)

However, models are being used increasingly in the organization and analysis of community health data because they provide a framework for data collection and a map to guide analysis. Because the community assessment wheel (see Fig. 11.2) was used to direct the community assessment process in the Rosemont example, that same model can be used as a framework for analysis. Consider the core as the major focus for analysis, with the subsystems representing the context. Stressors and strengths (lines of resistance) may be contributed by either the core, the subsystems, or both.

Summarize

Once a categorization method has been selected, the next task is to summarize the data within each category. Both summary statements and summary measures, such as rates, charts, and graphs, are required.

Take Note

Most health care agencies and educational institutions have access to computerized information systems—systems through which formatted data can be retrieved in a variety of forms—including summary health statistics. For example, data entered into a computer system as census figures can be configured into population pyramids, and census and vital statistics information can be programmed to calculate birth, death, and fertility rates. Calculations that previously required hours to complete are now computed in seconds. In addition, your local health department will be able to furnish the rates for you (for instance, the infant mortality rate [IMR]). Note, however, that the denominator used may not be the community as you have defined it.

Compare

Additional tasks of data analysis include the identification of data gaps, incongruencies, and omissions. Frequently, comparative data are needed to determine if a pattern or trend exists or if data do not seem correct and if revalidation of original information is required. Data gaps are inevitable, as are mistakes in recording data; the important task is to analyze data critically and be aware of the potential for gaps and omissions. It is helpful to have professional colleagues as well as community residents review the analysis. Every person has a unique perspective; it is only through the sharing of views that a whole and comprehensive picture of community assessment data can evolve.

Take Note

The word *data* is plural for datum (a real or assumed thing used as a basis for calculations). So, when referring to data, use the appropriate (plural) verb form. For example, the data *were* collected by all members of our group; or, these data *reflect* a downward trend in the IMR.

Using the data from your community, compare them with other similar data. For instance, you calculate (or discover) an IMR of 12 per 1,000 live births. How does this compare with the city? The state? The nation? Is it for the entire infant population of your community? Is the IMR different based on race? (Note: This is a good time to review Chapter 2 to assist you with epidemiologic reasoning as you try to make sense of your data.)

Another important comparison—across time—is helpful to detect trends. If data are available for several years, you can compare those different times to discover whether the problem is improving. An example would be IMRs.

Other resources for comparison are the documents dealing with objectives—for the nation and for individual states. Healthy People 2020 presents national figures, such as incidence and prevalence when available, for our major health problems and proposes goals and objectives for each (see www.healthypeople.gov). Healthy People 2010—along with state and, if available, local health planning documents—can be invaluable to you both as you analyze your data and as you develop a plan based on those data.

Draw Inferences

Having categorized, summarized, and compared the data you have collected, the next phase is to draw logical conclusions from the evidence (i.e., to draw inferences that will lead to the statement of a community nursing diagnosis). It is in this phase that you synthesize what you know about the community (i.e., what do these data *mean*?). These conclusions or inferences will identify the community's stressors and strengths in succinct phrases. These phrases, then, form the basis for a community nursing diagnosis.

The next section of this chapter walks you through analysis of the data we collected in the community assessment of Rosemont. Following these analysis examples, information on how to form community nursing diagnoses is presented (see the Community Nursing Diagnosis section later in this chapter).

ROSEMONT SAMPLE COMMUNITY ANALYSIS

The analysis of the Rosemont assessment data, as in the assessment process, begins with the community core, because it is the core (the people and their health) that is of interest to the community health nurse. Recall that the core is affected by (and affects) all of the subsystems depicted in the model surrounding it. Some subsystems will influence certain problems more than others, but it is important to assess the subsystems because of their contribution to the causes and alleviation of problems in the core.

Community Core

An analysis of Rosemont's core is presented in Table 12.1. Community core data include many demographic measures, a type of data especially amenable to graphs and charts. The adage "one picture is worth a thousand words" is particularly meaningful for demographic characteristics.

Perhaps, the most graphic illustration of the age and sex composition of a population is the population pyramid. Population pyramids for census tracts (CTs) 4104 and 4107 appear in Figure 12.1. A population pyramid for Rosemont is shown in Figure 12.2. Several other graphic display methods (pie chart, frequency graph, bar chart, and map) may be used. An example of each is included in Figure 12.3.

TABLE 12.1 Analysis of Rosemont's Core

Categories of Data	Summary Statements/Measures	Inferences
History		
	Cultural and ethnic diversity	Community revitalization
	Renovation of businesses and homes	Community pride
	Pride and concern evident	
Demographics		
Age	42.5% of population <19 years	Large % of children and adolescents
CT 4104	53% of population >19 years or <65 years	High dependency ratio*
	10% of population >65 years	Large % of elderly compared with Hampton and Jefferson County
Data gap: Need prior census data to determine if demographics are consistent or changing		
CT 4107	7.5% of population <19 years	Small % of children and adolescents
	15.2% of population <19 years or >65 years	Low dependency ratio
	7.7% of population >65 years	
Data gap: Need census data on 5-year increments to construct population pyramids		
Sex		
CT 4104	48% of population is male	Equal % of males and females
	45% of population aged 20–64 is male	
CT 4107	65% of population is male	High % of males
	69% of population aged 20–64 is male	
Data gap: Need prior census data to determine if demographics are consistent or changing		
Race/ethnicity		
CT 4104	Diversity: black 54%; Asian 19%; white 12%; Hispanic 9%	Racial and ethnic diversity
CT 4107	Homogeneity: white 89%	Racial and ethnic homogeneity
Data gap: Need census data from 1990 to determine if demographics are consistent or changing		
Household types		
CT 4104	83% of households are families	Family households dominate
CT 4107	36% of households are families	Nonfamily households dominate
Marital status		
CT 4104	15% single, 60% married, 14% divorced	Small % of single adults
		Majority of adults married
CT 4107	53% single, 24% married, 15% divorced	Large % of single adults
		Small % married
Data gap: Need prior census data to determine if demographics are consistent		
Vital Statistics (Refer to Chapter 3 for rate calculation)		
Births	Rate per 1,000	(When compared with Hampton and Jefferson County data)
CT 4104	30.5	A higher birth rate
CT 4107	17.3	A lower birth rate
Hampton	19.4	
Jefferson County	25.2	
Data gap: Need general fertility rate and age-specific birth rate		
Deaths	Rate per 1,000	(When compared with Hampton and Jefferson County Data)
CT 4104		
Infant	33.3	A higher death rate for all ages
Neonatal	23.8	
Fetal	76.2	
CT 4107		
Infant	17.1	A higher infant and neonatal rate
Neonatal	17.1	
Fetal	8.5	
Crude	6.2	

TABLE 12.1 Analysis of Rosemont's Core (continued)

Categories of Data	Summary Statements/Measures	Inferences
Data gap: Need vital statistics from previous 3–5 years to determine if rates are consistent or changing		
Hampton		
Infant	12.1	
Neonatal	7.9	
Fetal	12.6	
Crude	6.0	
Jefferson County		
Infant	12.3	
Neonatal	8.3	
Fetal	15.3	
Crude	7.3	
Causes of Death	See Table 11.8	(When compared with Hampton and Jefferson County data)
CT 4104		A much higher % of deaths due to diseases of infancy, homicides, suicides
CT 4107	See Table 11.8	A higher % of deaths due to cerebrovascular disease
		A lower % of deaths due to heart disease

*Dependency ratio describes the potentially self-supporting portion of the population and the dependent portions at the extremes of age. The dependency ratio is usually computed as follows:

$$\frac{\text{population under age 20} + \text{population age 65 and over}}{\text{population age 20 to 64 years of age}} \times 100$$

The dependency ratio for CT 4104 is 91, meaning for every 100 persons aged 20 to 65 (supposedly self-supporting because of age), there are 91 persons under age 20 or over age 65 needing support (because of age). In contrast, the dependency ratio for CT 4107 is 19.

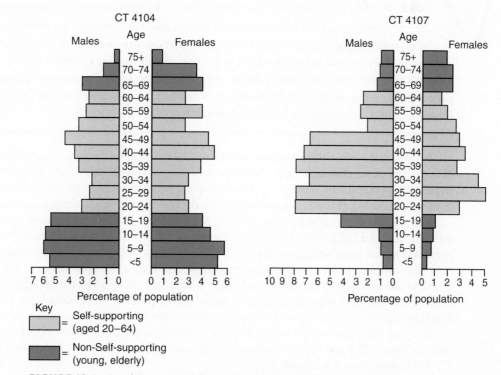

FIGURE 12.1   Population pyramid: Age and sex structure of CT 4104 and CT 4107.

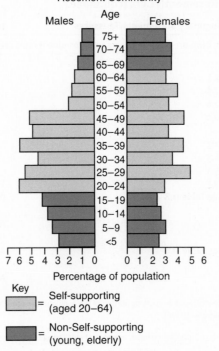

FIGURE 12.2   Population pyramid of Rosemont: Age and sex structure.

    Take Note

The population pyramid is formed of bars; each bar represents an age group. Usually, 5- or 10-year age groups are used, although adaptations can be made for smaller or larger age ranges. Bars are stacked horizontally, one on another, with bars for males on the left of a central axis and those for females on the right. The percentage of males and females in a particular age group is indicated by the length of the bars, as measured from the central axis. All age groups in a pyramid should use the same interval.

To construct a population pyramid, use Table 12.2 to calculate the percentage contribution of each age and sex class and Table 12.3 for actual pyramid construction. Note that parts of the population pyramids in Figure 12.1, those depicting people younger than 20 years and older than 65, are shaded; this was done to denote the dependent portions of the population.

Studying the population pyramids for CT 4104 and CT 4107 reveals striking age and sex differences, and this illustrates an important lesson. If the demographics of Rosemont had been presented as one population pyramid (see Fig. 12.2), important age and sex differences might have been minimized or have gone unrecognized, and their associated age- and sex-related health needs would be left unmet. This hazard in data analysis is referred to as aggregating or pooling the data. It is important to divide data along all possibly meaningful lines, so important information is not overlooked. Be alert to this problem as you proceed with your analysis.

Studying the inferences presented in Table 12.1, in conjunction with the population pyramids in Figures 12.1 and 12.2, the following statements can be made about Rosemont's core. In CT 4104, there exists the following:

- A large percentage (42.5%) of children and adolescents
- A high dependency ratio
- An equal percentage of adult men and women aged 20 to 64 years

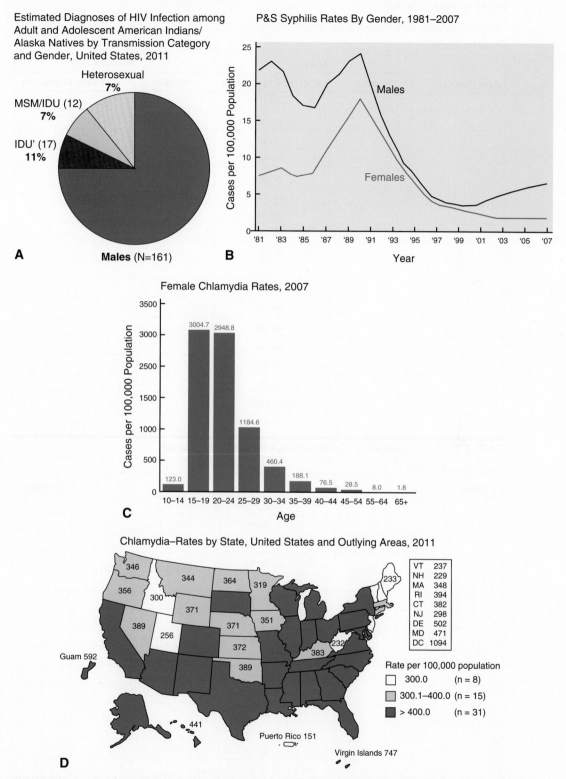

FIGURE 12.3   Graphic models to display assessment data (Adapted from http://www.cdc.gov/hiv/risk/racialEthnic/aian/, www.cdc.gov/std/stats07/trends.htm [top right and bottom left], and http://www.cdc.gov/std/stats11/figures/3.htm).

TABLE 12.2 Calculating the Percentage Contribution of Each Age and Sex for a Population Pyramid

Community Name, Census Tract, or Geographic Boundaries: _____

Total Population: _____

Ages (Years)	Males		Females	
	Number	% of Total Population	Number	% of Total Population
		Total		
		Younger than 5		
		5–9		
		10–14		
		15–19		
		20–24		
		25–29		
		30–34		
		35–39		
		40–44		
		45–49		
		50–54		
		55–59		
		60–64		
		65–69		
		70–74		
		75 and over		

TABLE 12.3 Calculations for Constructing a Population Pyramid

Population Pyramid For: _____

Males							Females
					75 and Over		
					70–74		
					65–69		
					60–64		
					55–59		
					50–54		
					45–49		
					40–44		
					35–39		
					30–34		
					25–29		
					20–24		
					15–19		
					10–14		
					5–9		
					Younger than 5		
8	9	4	2	0	2	4	6	8

Percentage of population

- A larger percentage (10%) of elderly than Hampton or Jefferson County
- A small percentage (15.2%) of single adults
- A moderate percentage (60.7%) of married adults
- A predominance (83%) of family households
- A mixed racial/ethnic composition with 54% black, 19% Asian, 12% white, and 9% Hispanic
- A high infant and neonatal death rate:
  - IMR (33 per 1,000 live births)
  - Neonatal mortality rate (24 per 1,000 live births)
- A higher birth rate (31 per 1,000 population) than Hampton (19 per 1,000 population) or Jefferson County (25 per 1,000 population)
- A higher crude death rate (10 per 1,000 population) than Hampton (6 per 1,000 population) or Jefferson County (7 per 1,000 population)
- A much higher percentage of deaths caused by diseases of early infancy, homicide, suicide, and tuberculosis than Hampton or Jefferson County
- A slightly higher percentage of deaths caused by cerebrovascular disorders than Hampton or Jefferson County
- In contrast, it can be seen that CT 4107 has the following factors:
- A small percentage (7.5%) of children and adolescents
- A low dependency ratio
- A larger percentage (7.7%) of elderly than Hampton or Jefferson County
- A high percentage (69%) of adult males aged 20 to 64 years
- Racial and ethnic homogeneity, with 89% of the population white
- A predominance (64%) of nonfamily households
- A large percentage (53%) of single adults
- A small percentage (24%) of married adults
- A lower birth rate (17 per 1,000 population) than Hampton, Jefferson County, or the state
- A higher infant mortality (17 per 1,000 live births) and a higher neonatal mortality (17 per 1,000 live births) than Hampton, Jefferson County, or the state
- A lower crude death rate (6.2 per 1,000 population) than Hampton or Jefferson County
- A higher percentage of deaths from accidents, diabetes mellitus, and congenital anomalies than Hampton, Jefferson County, or the state
- A lower percentage of deaths due to heart disease than Hampton or Jefferson County

Having analyzed the core characteristics of Rosemont, it is evident that major differences exist between CT 4104 and CT 4107, although both are part of Rosemont. In the following sections, this finding will be explained in more detail as each subsystem in our community assessment wheel model is analyzed.

Physical Environment

To study the physical components of Rosemont, data were collected that began with community inspection in the windshield survey and concluded with a systems review and laboratory studies (in other words, census and chamber of commerce data). Table 12.4 presents an analysis of the physical examination data.

Studying the inferences in Table 12.4, the following statements about Rosemont's physical components can be made:

- Rosemont is a community of contrasts and diversity.
- Densely populated residential areas, composed mainly of older homes, abut businesses of various types.
- Industry is minimal and is concentrated entirely in CT 4104.
- Housing values increased greatly in CT 4107; in both CT 4104 and CT 4107, only rents rose greatly.

TABLE 12.4 Analysis of Rosemont's Physical Examination Data

Categories of Data	Summary Statements/ Measures	Inferences
Inspection		
Windshield survey (Learning about the community on foot)	A community of contrast: bustling business areas and quiet neighborhoods Ethnic diversity evident in foods	Ethnic and business diversity Congested streets lined with homes or businesses Minimal industry Little "open" space
Vital Signs	Flat terrain and mild climate Densely populated (14 persons per acre) Posters abound, sharing information and heralding forthcoming events	Mild climate, abundant flora Densely populated (14 persons per acre) Note: In CT 4104, there are 221 persons per acre at one housing development
Systems Review Land usage		
CT 4104	37% of land in commercial usage, 28% single family, 8% multifamily, and 9% open	CT 4104 has almost twice the commercial usage of land (37%) compared with CT 4107 (20%)
CT 4107	20% of land in commercial usage, 32% single family, 15% multifamily, and 18% open	CT 4107 has twice the percentage of open space (18%) compared with CT 4104 (9%)
Housing Values		
CT 4104	From 2000 to 2010, average home values increased 17%, and average rents increased 19%	Sharp contrast between average home values; in CT 4104, average home value is $55,720, compared with $92,400 in CT 4107
CT 4107	From 2000 to 2010, average home values increased 29%, and average rents increased 46%	Average rent is higher in CT 4107, a reflection of "gentrification" in the area

Note: No data gaps identified; data for this area are complete.

Health and Social Services

An analysis of the health and social services in Rosemont is presented in Table 12.5. Because the data were categorized initially as extra- and intracommunity health and social services, the same format has been used in the analysis. Notice that statements from health care providers have been reported separately from those of health care recipients. This distinction has been made because health care providers frequently have a different concept of the adequacy, accessibility, and acceptability of health services than health care recipients. Be sure to collect and analyze data from both perspectives.

After reviewing Table 12.5, the following statements can be made about Rosemont's health services:

- The Sunvalley Clinic, operated by the city health department, has inadequate antepartum services for Rosemont women; this results in
  - Many women delivering at Jefferson Memorial with no antepartum care
  - Women forced to deliver at home because they do not meet eligibility requirements at Jefferson Memorial
- There are no practicing private obstetric, gynecologic, or family practitioners, nor are there any nurse-midwives in Rosemont.

TABLE 12.5 Analysis of Health and Social Services in Rosemont

Categories of Data	Summary Statements/Measures	Inferences
Health Facilities		
Extracommunity		
Hospitals	Most are referral or private. One public hospital, Jefferson Memorial, has problems of • Long waits (≥8 h) • Fragmented care • Inaccessibility	Only one public hospital; users complain of lengthy waits and fragmented care
Private care	Numerous options, including HMOs	Variety of private care options
Health department (Sunvalley Clinic)	Health providers feel Sunvalley Clinic has • Inadequate antepartal services; women wait 8–10 weeks for an initial appointment that is often after their expected date of confinement • Inadequate nursing services to meet elderly's needs Rosemont residents feel the clinic is Inaccessible (no direct bus connection) Impersonal (no primary care providers)	Inadequate antepartal services Many women deliver at Jefferson Memorial with no antepartal care Many women are forced to self-deliver at home because they do not meet eligibility requirements at Jefferson Memorial Inaccessibility and unacceptability of Sunvalley services

Data gap: Number of Rosemont residents using
  Well and ill infant, child, adolescent, adult services
  Mental health counseling and referral services
  User's perception of adequacy, accessibility, and acceptability of the above services

Home health	One large Visiting Nurse Association (VNA) Numerous home health agencies; most require fee-for-service or third-party reimbursement	Numerous options for home health care

Data gap: Frequency and type of VNA services used by Rosemont residents

Continuing care	Two long-term licensed facilities close (8 miles) from Rosemont	Two long-term licensed facilities

Data gap: Adequacy of facilities as perceived by health administrators, staff, and patients

Emergency services: Medical emergency ambulance service (MEAS)	Cardiac and cerebrovascular accident (CVA) are major reasons for MEAS visits to Rosemont	Cardiac and CVA are major reasons for MEAS visits, followed by accidents and home falls

Data gap: Number of persons using MEAS and their age, sex, race, and ethnic characteristics

Intracommunity Health Services		
Health care practitioners	Rosemont has no • Obstetric, gynecologic, or family practitioners • Bilingual health practitioners	Lack of OB/GYN and family practitioners No bilingual health practitioners
Clinics		
Third Street Clinic	Health care providers feel immediate health needs include • Ill infant, child, adolescent, and adult assessment, treatment, and follow-up • Dental assessment and restoration • Counseling, referral, and treatment for substance abuse	Inadequate health services for ill persons (all ages) Dental assessment and restoration Counseling and treatment for substance abuse

(continued)

TABLE 12.5 Analysis of Health and Social Services in Rosemont (continued)

Categories of Data	Summary Statements/Measures	Inferences
	• Group health teaching	Health education
	• Support groups for single parents and senior citizens	Self-help/support groups
	Additional needs of the clinic include recruitment and retainment of health care providers	
	Many Rosemont residents use the clinic routinely; people feel welcomed and comply with medical care	Rosemont residents state that care at Third Street Clinic is acceptable and accessible
	Residents agree that additional services are needed	

Data gap: Number of persons requesting services that health care providers believe are needed
Characteristics of people requesting medical care services

Rosemont Health Center	Director of clinic feels immediate needs are	Highly acceptable, accessible, and affordable care for STDs
	• Formation of counseling and support groups	Inadequate counseling and support groups
	• Orientation program and inservice for staff (all are volunteers)	Lack of orientation and inservice for the staff
		Lack of procedure manuals and posted protocols for emergency care
		Lack of safety procedures including visible emergency cart and proper syringe disposal

Data gap: What do staff perceive as needs? What do residents perceive as needs?

Social Facilities
Extracommunity

Hampton Community Counseling Center (HCCC)	HCCC offers counseling to adolescent drug users	HCCC is close to Rosemont and offers needed counseling for substance abuse, yet HCCC is not used by Rosemont residents
	Most patients are middle- or upper-class males; all are white	
	Staff believe they are meeting community needs	
	Rosemont residents are not aware that the center exists	
YMCA Indo-Chinese Refugee Program	Cultural-orientation programs for Asian immigrants; staff perceive immediate needs are for programs on the following:	Insufficient number of cultural programs, resulting in long waiting periods and frustration
	Substance abuse	
	Basic life survival skills (e.g., employment, self-health care)	
	Many Rosemont residents use the YMCA services; all agree the programs are excellent, but state the waiting period for classes is long and frustrating	

Intracommunity
Churches

South Main	Extensive social service programs	Social outreach programs offered by both churches
Westpark	Extensive social service program	
Lambda Alcoholic Anonymous (AA)	Active AA program for gay men: membership exceeds 120	Active chapter of Lambda AA

- The Third Street Clinic has inadequate health services, specifically a lack of
  - Assessment and treatment of people who are ill
  - Dental assessment and restoration
  - Counseling and treatment programs for substance abuse
  - Health-education programs responsive to residents' needs
  - Support and self-help groups as needed and requested by residents
- The Rosemont Health Center offers acceptable, accessible, and affordable services for sexually transmitted diseases (STDs); however, there is a lack of
  - Orientation and education for the staff
  - Procedure manuals and posted protocols for emergency care
  - A visible emergency cart

The following deductions can be made about Rosemont's social services:

- Hampton Community Counseling Center (HCCC) is located close to Rosemont, but is not used by Rosemont residents, although residents repeatedly expressed a wish for substance-abuse counseling programs.
- The YMCA Indo-Chinese Refugee Program is heavily used by Asians in Rosemont; however, present programs of cultural orientation are inadequate to meet the demand. Both the YMCA staff and Rosemont residents see a need for additional programs.
- South Main and Westpark churches offer numerous social service programs; however, only South Main offers a social program, especially for the gay male population—a program that is resisted by older parishioners.
- An active chapter of Lambda Alcoholic Anonymous (AA) is located in Rosemont.

Economics

An analysis of the economic and financial characteristics of Rosemont is presented in Table 12.6. The analysis begins with individual wealth indices (such as income), proceeds to indicators of business and industrial wealth, and concludes with employment status of community residents. As with other subsystems, the categories for data assessment have become categories for data analysis.

After studying Table 12.6, the following statements can be made about the economic status of Rosemont. Striking differences exist in the financial characteristics between households in CT 4104 and CT 4107.

In CT 4104, it was found that:

- The median household income of $31,878 is less than 40% of the median income in CT 4107 and Hampton.
- One fifth of families (20.6%) have incomes below the poverty level.
- Thirty percent of all households are headed by females.
- One third of all families receive public assistance/welfare.

In CT 4107, the following factors exist:

- The median household income of $48,238 is much greater than that of CT 4104, but less than that of Hampton.
- Twelve percent of families have incomes below the poverty level.
- Twenty percent of all households are headed by females.
- Only 4.3% of families receive public assistance/welfare.

Striking differences also exist between the labor force characteristics of CT 4104 and CT 4107.

In CT 4104, it was found that:

- Only 39.8% of the population is of employable age (16 years or older).
- Most people (67.8%) work in service or operator/labor occupations.

TABLE 12.6 Economic Indicators of Rosemont

Categories of Data	Summary Statements/ Measures	Inferences
Financial Characteristics of Households Median household income (2010)		
CT 4104	$31,878	Median household income in CT 4107
CT 4107	$48,238	is considerably higher than in
Hampton	$52,598	CT 4104
% of families with incomes below poverty level (2000)		
CT 4104	20.6%	In CT 4104, one fifth of all families have
CT 4107	12.1%	incomes below the poverty level
Hampton	12.1%	
% of families on public assistance/welfare		
CT 4104	36.4%	In CT 4104, 36.4% of all families are
CT 4107	4.3%	on public assistance/welfare compared
Hampton	3.4%	with 4.3% in CT 4107 and 3.4% in Hampton
Business/industry characteristics (2000)		
CT 4104	Nearly equal percentage of wholesale/retail (48%) and professional (42%)	In CT 4104, equal percentage of wholesale and professional businesses
CT 4107	Predominance of professional (48%) over wholesale/retail (37%)	In CT 4107, professionals predominate
Labor force characteristics (2000):		
Age (% of persons >16 years of age)		
CT 4104	39.8%	Only 40% of persons in CT 4104 are of
CT 4107	85.4%	employable age (>16) compared with
Hampton	71.5%	85% in CT 4107 and 71% in Hampton
Occupational groups		
Managerial/professional		Striking differences between CTs by
CT 4104	7.1%	managerial occupational categories
CT 4107	42.1%	
Technical/sales		In CT 4104, 67% of workers are in
CT 4104	12.1%	service or operator occupations
CT 4107	34.1%	compared with 14.8% in CT 4107
Service		In CT 4107, 76% of workers are in
CT 4104	44.2%	managerial or technical occupations
CT 4107	10.5%	compared with 19% in CT 4104
Operators/laborers		Almost a quarter of workers in CT are
CT 4104	26.3%	operators/laborers
CT 4107	4.3%	

Note: No data gaps identified; data in this area are complete.

CT 4107 presented a contrasting picture:

- Of the population, 85.4% is of employable age (16 years or older).
- Most people (76.2%) work in managerial or professional positions.

Safety and Transportation

An analysis of the safety and transportation services in Rosemont is set forth in Table 12.7. Reviewing the data, the following statements can be made about Rosemont's safety (protection) services and associated concerns:

- Grease fires are the major cause of house fires.
- Thefts and burglaries are the major reported crimes, followed by robbery and vehicle theft; elderly people and gay men feel especially victimized. Both groups related numerous stories of harassment and violence.

TABLE 12.7 Analysis of Safety and Transportation Services in Rosemont

Categories of Data	Summary Statements/Measures	Inferences
Safety *Protection Services* Fire	45 fires during past 90 days; of these, 40 occurred in homes (usually a grease fire)	Major cause of fires within last 90 days was grease

Data gap: Obtain additional data (12 months) and determine if grease fires are major cause
Document age, sex, and racial characteristics, as well as time of day and associated circumstances

Police	Crime statistics for past 4 years show thefts as the leading crime, followed by burglary. Frequency of occurrence is high for both CTs. Robbery is twice as prevalent in CT 4104 compared with CT 4107, and vehicle theft is three times more common in CT 4107. Residents expressed fear and related stories of muggings and violence directed especially toward the elderly and gay male populations	Thefts and burglaries are the major crimes; the elderly and gay men feel especially victimized

Data gap: Assess residents' knowledge about self-protection measures against crime
Assess residents' interest and past participation in crime prevention programs
Assess available crime prevention programs

Sanitation Sewage	Sewage moratorium exists owing to overcapacity of present facility	Inadequate sewage treatment facilities, resulting in building restrictions
Potable water	No fluoride in drinking water No routine testing of drinking water for arsenic or heavy metals (elements that residents believe may be contaminating the water)	Lack of fluoride in drinking water No routine tests of drinking water for arsenic or heavy metals

Data gap: Assess history of fluoride issue. Has fluoride been proposed, voted on? What is the present position of the health department, city council, civic associations, and the general public?
Regarding arsenic and heavy metals: Is Lake Hampton tested for arsenic or heavy metals? What is the position and plan of the health department, city council, and civic associations?

Solid waste	Increased illegal dumping of machinery and appliances; inoperable autos are parked on the streets for months before removal by the City of Hampton	Potential for accidents (with consequences such as trauma and suffocation) as people explore abandoned objects and automobiles

Data gap: Document laws and fees for illegal dumping. Are signs posted to notify persons of law and associated fines?
What actions have been taken by residents, civic associations, and businesses?

Air	Rise in air pollution attributed to increase in industrial growth and population density. Residents complain of eye irritation and increased number of respiratory conditions	Increased air pollution
	Air Board feels citizens are inadequately informed regarding actions needed during an air stagnation advisory and individual responsibility to decrease pollution	Citizens may be inadequately informed regarding personal actions needed during an air stagnation advisory to decrease air pollution

Data gap: Assess if public awareness programs have occurred. If so, when, and what was the response? What do residents understand about air pollution, air advisories, and their role in decreasing air pollution? Do residents desire more information about air pollution?

Transportation *Private (to work)* CT 4104	43% of people drive alone, 24% carpool, and 23% use public transportation	Almost half (43%) drive alone to work, with equal percentages (24%) carpooling or using public transportation
CT 4107	64% of people drive alone, 16% carpool, and 11% use public transportation	Most people (64%) drive alone to work, some carpool (16%), and only a few use public transportation (11%)

(continued)

TABLE 12.7 Analysis of Safety and Transportation Services in Rosemont (continued)

Categories of Data	Summary Statements/Measures	Inferences
Transportation Disability		
CT 4104	6% of persons aged 16–64 and 21% of over age 65 have a disability	When compared with CT 4107, a large percentage of residents in CT 4104
CT 4107	0.3% of persons aged 16–64 and 11% of those over age 65 have a disability	have a transportation disability, especially those over age 65

- There is no fluoride in Rosemont's drinking water, neither is there routine testing for arsenic or heavy metals, substances that residents fear are contaminating the water.
- Abandoned vehicles and dumping of machinery and appliances places residents, especially children, at increased risk of accidental injury.
- Air pollution has increased; the Air Control Board believes that citizens are inadequately informed about air pollution advisories as well as personal actions that can be taken to decrease pollution.

Regarding Rosemont's transportation services, the following deductions are made:

- A large percentage of residents in CT 4107 drive to work alone (64%) compared with those in CT 4104 (43%); however, 47% of the residents in CT 4104 use car pools or public transportation to get to work, compared with 27% in CT 4107.
- Compared with CT 4107, a substantially larger percentage of the population in CT 4104 has a transportation disability, especially among those over age 65.

Politics and Government

A rich diversity of political organizations exists in Rosemont. However, at this point in the nursing process—analysis—it is sufficient to describe the organizations and identify key persons. Consider your information about the political system and form of government to be reference material that will be useful at the next stage of the nursing process—program planning with the community.

Communication

Ample formal and informal communication sources exist in Rosemont. No analysis is required of the data. Consider the communication data to be reference material that will be useful at the next stage of the nursing process—program planning with the community.

 Take Note

If sufficient information is collected regarding a community's communication system (refer to Table 11.29 in Chapter 11 for components to assess), then there is no need to further analyze the data.

Education

An analysis of Rosemont's general educational status (characteristics of school enrollment, years of schooling completed, and language spoken) and specific educational sources (e.g., public and private schools, both intra- and extracommunity) is presented in Table 12.8.

TABLE 12.8 Analysis of Educational Sources in Rosemont

Categories of Data	Summary Statements/ Measures	Inferences
Educational Status		
Years of schooling completed: % high school graduates		
CT 4104	28%	In CT 4104, only 28% of persons
CT 4107	89%	over age 25 are high school
Hampton	68%	graduates, compared with 89% in CT 4107 and 68% in Hampton

	School enrollment: % elementary, % high school, % college	
CT 4104	59%, 23%, 4%	The majority of persons attending
CT 4107	15%, 7%, 73%	school in CT 4104 are elementary
Hampton	48%, 23%, 19%	grade students; in CT 4107, the majority of those attending school are in college

Language spoken: % of population with poor English proficiency			
Age 5–17	Age	18+	In CT 4104, some 75% of the
CT 4104	76%	74%	population has poor English
CT 4107	11%	19%	proficiency, compared with small
Hampton	21%	26%	percentages in CT 4107

Educational Sources
Intracommunity

Temple Elementary	Grades K to eighth
	Enrollment 924
	Ethnicity
	  42% black
	  33% Asian
	  18% Hispanic
	  5% white
		Mixed ethnicity, predominance of black children

	Principal feels major problems are • Truancy • Academic failure • Principal wants to stop bilingual classes	According to staff, major problems are • Truancy • Academic failure (22%) • Inadequate parent–teacher relationships • English insufficiencies • Stressed home environments, with inadequate adult supervision

Data gap: Explore the principal's statement about bilingual education. Why the opposition? What is the position and policy on bilingual education in Hampton Independent School District (HISD)?
What is the principal's perception of parental concerns?

	Teachers believe major impediments to student learning are • Inadequate parent–teacher communication • Poor English proficiency • Stressed home environment • Inadequate adult supervision	Same as above

Data gap: Explore teachers' perceptions of bilingual education. What are teachers' perceptions of parental concerns?

Temple Elementary	*Nurse believes* major health problems of youngsters are • Poor hygiene Dental caries • Prevalence of head lice Incomplete immunizations • Lack of parent follow-through for needed medical care	Major student health problems are • Inadequate hygiene • Control of dental caries • Control of head lice • Parent follow-through with needed medical care • Health education

(continued)

TABLE 12.8 Analysis of Educational Sources in Rosemont (continued)

Categories of Data	Summary Statements/ Measures	Inferences
Data gap: Document age, sex, ethnicity, and racial characteristics of children with specific health problems		
	Nurse believes more health teaching and screening would be possible with parent volunteers Present policy restricts nurse to clinic, permitting no classroom teaching	Same as above
Data gap: Document school policy regarding Recruitment and training of parent volunteers The nurse's presence and role in the clinic Explore nurse's attitude toward health education Discuss options for health programs for students, staff, and parents		
Temple Elementary	Parents believe Temple is a community strength, but the present staff members are insensitive to ethnic and racial needs; attempts to discuss these concerns with Temple's staff have been frustrating	Parental concern and involvement are evident; however, attempts to discuss concerns with staff have been frustrating
Data gap: Identify officers and key people (committee chairs) of Temple's PTO. Are these officers/key people aware of ethnic and racial needs? Identify students' perceptions of their school. What activities do they enjoy? Are there afterschool activities? Who participates? What activities are needed?		
Busybee Day Care Extracommunity Central Hampton High	One day care center in CT 4104; no facility in CT 4107 Truancy and grade failure reversed with "Failproof" program Increased number of teenage pregnancies Decision by school board not to permit sex education classes Increased use of alcohol	Inadequate day care facilities Parents leave children in crowded homes Increased number of teenage pregnancies Increased use of alcohol among high school students Sex education classes not permitted in high school
Data gap: Number of pregnancies during last 3–5 years (for comparison) and age, grade level, racial, and ethnic characteristics of girls		
History and reason for HISD Board decision to stop sex education Document scope of alcohol use and characteristics of users		

Major differences exist between the general educational status of CT 4104 and CT 4107. The status in CT 4104 is as follows:

- A small percentage of residents are high school graduates (28%), with the majority of persons enrolled in school attending elementary grades.
- Some 75% of the population has limited English proficiency.

In contrast, the CT 4107 data show that:

- A large percentage of residents are high school graduates (89%), and the majority of the persons who attend school are in college.
- Only 19% of the residents have limited English proficiency.

With regard to specific educational sources, Temple Elementary is the primary educational resource in Rosemont. Temple has an enrollment of 924 students. The principal, teachers, nurse, and parents were interviewed during the assessment process. To summarize the situation at Temple, it has been concluded that:

- Problems of truancy exist, especially among Hispanic boys. There are large numbers of academic failures (22% of students last year).
- Large numbers of students have English-skills insufficiencies, further documented by general educational data.
- Inadequate working relationships exist between parents and teachers, compounded by the language barrier.
- Student health problems consist of:
  - Dental caries (62% of students)
  - Head lice, especially in grades kindergarten to second
  - Incomplete immunizations
  - Poor hygiene
  - Inadequate parental follow-through of needed medical care
  - Inadequate health-education program
- There is parental concern and involvement and a desire to communicate needs to staff.

One day care facility exists in Rosemont—the Busybee. This facility is extremely inadequate. As a result, parents are forced to leave children in conditions that may be crowded and undersupervised.

The major extracommunity educational facility is Central Hampton High. The major problems of Central Hampton High, according to the school nurse, include:

- Increased number of teenage pregnancies
- Lack of sex education classes
- Increased use of alcohol

Central Hampton has succeeded in reducing truancy and grade failure through a program called "Failproof."

Recreation

Recreational space and facilities are minimal. A sum of 5.6 acres of public recreational space is available for a population of 13,631 (combined populations of CT 4104 and CT 4107). The organized sports and recreational programs that are available through churches and associations require membership and usually charge a fee. There are no public recreational programs, and the few pieces of public recreational equipment that exist are in need of repair.

COMMUNITY NURSING DIAGNOSIS

The community's core and subsystems, its lines of defense and resistance, its stressors, and its degree of reaction comprise assessment parameters for the community nurse who views the community as partner. Analyzing data on these parameters with the community leads to the *community nursing diagnosis*. Note the similarities and differences between a nursing diagnosis of an individual and a community nursing diagnosis depicted in Table 12.9.

In the preceding pages, each subsystem of the Rosemont example has been analyzed in relation to its effect on the core (the people), and inferences have been drawn. The final task of analysis is the synthesis of the inference statements that include stressors and strengths into community nursing diagnoses. A diagnosis is a statement that synthesizes assessment data. A diagnosis is a label that both *describes a situation* (or state) and *implies an etiology* (reason).

A *nursing diagnosis* limits the diagnostic process to those diagnoses that represent *human responses to actual or potential health problems that nurses are licensed to treat*. This stipulation

TABLE 12.9 Community Nursing Diagnoses

Community Response/ Concern/Problem (Actual or Potential)	Etiology Related to . . .	Documentation Signs and Symptoms as Manifested by . . .
Stress and anxiety of being criminally victimized	Increased episodes of thefts and burglaries Inadequate knowledge on the part of residents regarding self-protection measures	Police crime statistics of past 4 years Personal testimony of residents, especially the elderly
Potential for accidents (such as trauma and suffocation) as children and adults explore abandoned goods	Illegal dumping of machinery and appliances Abandonment of automobiles Nonenforcement of city ordinances	Parental concern for safety Observation of persons exploring abandoned goods
Potential for health problems associated with air pollution (such as initiation and exacerbation of respiratory conditions)	Increased air pollution Lack of knowledge regarding personal action required during an air stagnation advisory to decrease air pollution	Air Board reports of current air pollution levels Residents' complaints of eye irritation and increased number of respiratory conditions
Truancy and academic failure at Temple Elementary	Large number of students with poor English proficiency Stressed home environment in CT 4104, where 30% of homes are headed by females and 21% of families are below poverty level Inadequate communication links between parents and school personnel	Records at Temple Elementary
Stress within Rosemont between the homosexual and heterosexual populations	Differing lifestyles of gay men Lack of acceptance of gay male lifestyle	Lack of social programs for gay men in Westpark Church Resistance of older church members in South Main to existing program for gay men Large percentage of single males in CT 4107
Potential for inadequate coping of single parents, the elderly, and persons with STDs	Lack of support groups and programs for single parents, the elderly, and persons with STDs Inadequate resources at Third Street Clinic to offer programs, although the need is recognized Inadequate resources at Hampton Health Center to offer programs, although the need is recognized	Health providers' perceptions of the Third Street Clinic Health providers' perceptions of the Rosemont Health Center High percentage of deaths owing to homicides and suicides in CT 4104
Unsafe working environment at Rosemont Health Center	Lack of orientation and inservice programs for staff Lack of procedure manuals and posted protocols for emergency care Lack of safety procedures	Visual assessment Perceptions of administration Perception of volunteer nurse
Potential for inadequate cultural assimilation of Asian immigrants	Lack of programs to meet present needs Lack of staff at Indo-Chinese Refugee Program Increased need for programsLarge Asian population in CT 4104 (19%) Large percentage of population in CT 4104 (75%) with poor English proficiency	Perceived needs of Asians in Rosemont

TABLE 12.9   Community Nursing Diagnoses (continued)

Community Response/ Concern/Problem (Actual or Potential)	Etiology Related to . . .	Documentation Signs and Symptoms as Manifested by . . .
Incomplete immunization status of children at Temple Elementary	Inadequate communication between parents and school's staff Inaccessibility and unacceptability of Health Department's Sunvalley Clinic Inadequate income in CT 4104 to purchase immunizations	School health records at Temple Elementary
High infant, neonatal, and fetal mortality rate	Inadequate antepartum care at Sunvalley Clinic Lack of obstetric and family practitioners in Rosemont Lack of bilingual practitioners in Rosemont Inadequate income in CT 4104 to purchase essential medical care	Vital statistics
Potential for boredom and associated consequences (violence, vandalism)	Lack of public, no-fee recreational programs Minimal public recreational areas and equipment	A total of 5.6 acres of public recreational space in Rosemont Visual inspection of available land and equipment
High prevalence of pediculosis capitis among children at Temple Elementary	Crowded living conditions Knowledge deficit regarding transmission and treatment	Cases reported by school nurse at Temple Elementary

is based on the American Nurses Association (ANA) Social Policy Statement (see Further Readings section at the end of the chapter). Although no standard format exists, most nursing diagnoses have three parts:

1. A description of the problem, response, or state
2. Identification of factors etiologically related to the problem
3. Signs and symptoms that are characteristic of the problem

A *community nursing diagnosis* focuses the diagnosis on a community—usually defined as a *group, population, or cluster of people with at least one common characteristic* (such as geographic location, occupation, ethnicity, or housing condition). To derive a community nursing diagnosis, community assessment data are analyzed and inferences are presented. Inference statements shape nursing diagnoses. Some inference statements form the descriptive part of the nursing diagnosis (i.e., they testify to a potential or actual community health problem or concern); for example:

- High IMR in Rosemont
- High prevalence of dental caries among children at Temple Elementary School in Rosemont

Other inference statements are *etiologic* and document the possible reasons for the health problem or concern. Etiologic statements are linked to the descriptive statements with a "*related to*" clause, for example:

- High infant mortality in Rosemont is related to
  - Inadequate resources at the health department's Sunvalley Clinic to meet antepartum care needs
  - Inaccessibility and unacceptability of present antepartum services at the Sunvalley Clinic
  - Lack of obstetric and family practitioners in Rosemont
  - Absence of nurse-midwives in the community

- High prevalence of dental caries among children at Temple Elementary School in Rosemont is related to
  - Lack of dental assessment and treatment at the Third Street Clinic
  - Lack of fluoride in Rosemont's drinking water
  - Low median household income in CT 4104 and associated limited economic resources for purchasing dental care
  - No dental hygiene education offered at Temple Elementary

Finally, the *signs and symptoms* of the community nursing diagnosis are the inference statements that document the duration or magnitude of the problem. Examples of documentation include record accounts, census reports, and vital statistics. This final piece of the community nursing diagnosis is linked to the first two parts with an *"as manifested by"* clause, for example:

- High IMR in Rosemont is related to
  - Inadequate resources at the health department's Sunvalley Clinic to meet antepartum care needs
  - Inaccessibility and unacceptability of present antepartum services at the Sunvalley Clinic
  - Lack of obstetric and family practitioners in Rosemont
- As manifested by
  - IMR in CT 4104 = 30.5; in CT 4107 = 17.3 (per 1,000 live births)
  - Specific data from clinic about lack of appropriate personnel
  - No city bus to Sunvalley Clinic
  - Clinic hours are 8 am to 5 pm, Monday to Friday, not accessible to working people
  - Shortage of needed practitioners (include numbers if available)
  - No certified nurse-midwives live or work in the community
- High prevalence of dental caries among children at Temple Elementary School in Rosemont is related to
  - Lack of dental assessment and treatment at the Third Street Clinic
  - Lack of fluoride in Rosemont's drinking water
  - Low median household income in CT 4104 and associated limited economic resources for purchasing dental care
  - No dental hygiene education offered at Temple Elementary
- As manifested by
  - No dental program at the Third Street Clinic
  - City of Hampton does not have naturally occurring fluoride in the water and does not add fluoride to the water supply
  - Median income is $28,247
  - No health-education programs are offered at Temple

Although a single problem is stated, the etiology and signs and symptoms may be multiple. Also notice that, although the health problem inference is drawn from the analysis of one subsystem (such as the health and social services subsystem or the educational subsystem), the etiologies may be, and usually are, drawn from several subsystems. For example, regarding the health problem of dental caries among children at Temple Elementary, etiologic inferences were derived from four subsystems: educational, health and social services, safety and transportation, and economic. This example sums up a most important lesson of community health nursing: *All community factors (subsystems) join to determine the health status of a community. No one subsystem is more important or crucial than any other in determining a community's health.*

The process of deriving community nursing diagnoses always remains the same. First, assessment data are categorized and studied for inferences that are descriptive of potential or actual health problems amenable to nursing interventions; next, associated inferences are identified that explain the derivation or continuation of the problem; and last, documentation is presented. Additional community nursing diagnoses for Rosemont are presented in Table 12.9. There is no particular order to the list, neither is the list conclusive. Determining the order of priority among community nursing diagnoses is part of program planning and depends on existing community goals and resources as well as the community's priorities. This important skill is discussed in Chapter 13.

There has been criticism that the diagnoses do not include the positive aspects of the community; however, as depicted in the model, the positives (lines of resistance or strengths) are part of the assessment and are considered in the statement of the degree of reaction (diagnosis). It is in the planning and intervention phases that you will want to build on the community's strengths, and you will have already identified what they are.

Deriving community nursing diagnoses requires critical decision making and astute study; it is a challenging and vital task. The completeness and validity of the diagnoses that have been derived will be tested during the next stage of the nursing process and will form the foundation of that stage—the planning of a health program.

Take Note

This is an excellent time to share your assessment data with colleagues and people in the community to solicit their own analysis. Because we all have opinions and values that color our perceptions, group critiquing and analysis of assessment data are ways to foster objectivity.

Summary

Critical analysis of the Rosemont community has been completed using the community assessment wheel as a guide. Subsequently, community nursing diagnoses were formulated, based on the inferences of the analyses. Although the use of community nursing diagnoses is relatively new to practice, community health nurses have, since the profession's inception, derived inferences from assessment data and acted on those data. However, the terminology and format that have surrounded these informally produced inferences (diagnoses) have been inconsistent. There is considerable discussion, and some controversy, regarding the structure and terminology that would be optimal for community-focused nursing diagnoses. In your practice, you will be exposed to various formats for making community nursing diagnoses; evaluate and test the usefulness of each. It is only through collaboration and vigorous testing that a standard format will evolve. In the Further Readings list, there are additional sources to help you as you develop community nursing diagnoses.

Critical Thinking Questions

1. Using data from your community, develop a diagnosis that begins with "At risk for . . ."
   a. Include a clearly stated potential problem.
   b. List the possible etiologies (the "related to" statements).
   c. Include the data (and sources) that point to these "related to" statements.

2. Develop hypothetical information (etiologies and data) for the following community problem: "Potential for high-risk sexual behavior in high school teens."

3. Where would you obtain the necessary data for the problem in #2?

FURTHER READINGS

American Nurses Association. (2010). *Nursing's social policy statement*. Washington, DC: Author.

Best, A., Stokols, D., Green, L. W., Leischow, S., Holmes, B., & Buchholz, K. (2003). An integrative framework for community partnering to translate theory into effective health promotion strategy. *American Journal of Health Promotion, 18*(2), 168–176.

del Rio, A. (2005). Community health diagnosis as a curriculum component: Experiences of the faculty of health sciences, Walter Sisulu University, Eastern Cape, South Africa. *MEDICC Review, 8*(8), 22–25.

Jha, N. (2011). Community diagnosis program – A multi-professional education and team approach for medical, dental and nursing students. *Health Renaissance, 9*(1), 41–44.

Muecke, M. (1984). Community health diagnosis in nursing. *Public Health Nursing, 1*(1), 23–35.

Racher, F. E., & Annis, R. C. (2005). Community partnerships: Translating research for community development. *The Canadian Journal of Nursing Research, 37*(1), 169–175.

Racher, F. E., & Annis, R. C. (2008). Community health action model: Health promotion by the community. *Research and Theory for Nursing Practice, 22*(3), 182–191.

CHAPTER 13

Planning a Community Health Program

Elizabeth T. Anderson and Judith McFarlane

LEARNING OBJECTIVES

This chapter covers the planning of nursing actions to promote community health.

After studying this chapter, you should be able to:

1. Validate community nursing diagnoses with your community.

2. Use principles of change theory to direct the planning process.

3. In partnership with the community, plan a community-based health program that includes:

   - Measurable goals and behavioral objectives

   - A sequence of actions and a time schedule for achieving goals

   - Resources needed to accomplish the plan

   - Potential obstacles to planned actions and revised actions

   - Revisions to the plan, as goals and objectives are achieved or changed

   - A recording of the plan in a concise, standardized, and retrievable form

Introduction

Once a community's health has been assessed, the data have been analyzed, and community nursing diagnoses have been derived, it is time to consider nursing interventions that will promote the community's health by formulating a community-based plan. Each of the three parts of the diagnosis statement—the descriptions of the actual or potential problem, its causes, and its signs and symptoms—directs planning efforts for the nurse. All three provide equally important information from which to plan. Figure 13.1 displays the process for deriving a community nursing diagnosis and summarizes how the parts of the diagnosis both describe the community assessment and give direction for program planning, intervention, and evaluation. Community-based plans are based on the nursing diagnoses and contain

Assessment

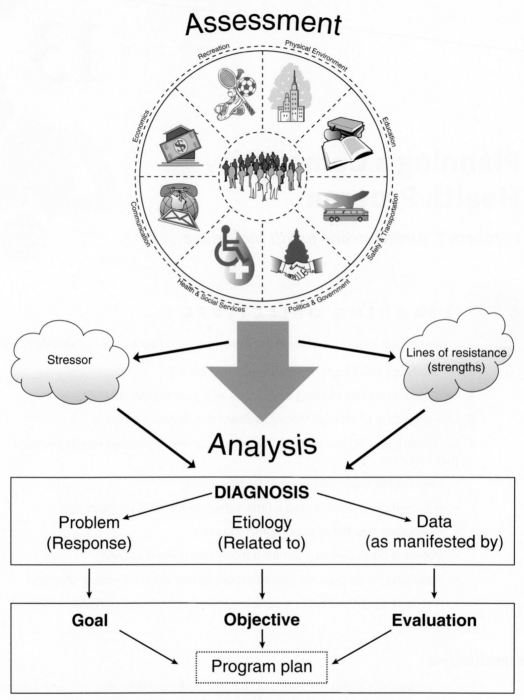

FIGURE 13.1   The process of program planning from the community nursing diagnosis.

specific goals and interventions for achieving desired outcomes. Planning, like assessment and analysis, is a systematic process completed in partnership with the community.

In addition to forming a partnership with the community, the community health nurse must consider the influences of social, economic, environmental, and political issues. Many (if not all) community health issues are directly and profoundly affected by larger policy issues. For example, the high prevalence of dental caries among students at Temple Elementary is related as much to the lack of fluoride in Rosemont's drinking water as it is to the lack of dental hygiene education at the school. In turn, each etiologic antecedent is influenced by city, county, state, and national legislative actions and policies. None of the nursing diagnoses for Rosemont can be considered to be separate from the remaining diagnoses; all diagnoses document the health status of Rosemont and must be considered as a whole during the community-based planning.

 Take Note

Before proceeding, let's stop and consider the word *partnership* and its implications for community health nursing. Recall that a community is a social group determined by geographic boundaries and common values and interests. Community members function and interact within a particular social structure that both creates and exhibits behaviors and values. The normative behaviors and value systems of individuals, families, and the community that you have assessed may be very different from your own individual and family behaviors and values as well as the shared values of the community in which you reside. This difference creates a potential conflict. What may appear to you as a primary health problem of the community (e.g., the incomplete immunization status at Temple Elementary in Rosemont) may not hold the same importance for the community's residents. They may be far more concerned about the possibility of being criminally victimized. Hence, there is a real need to validate community nursing diagnoses with the community. There is one question to ask: Are the community nursing diagnoses of importance to community residents? Methods of validating community nursing diagnoses are presented in this chapter.

Additional considerations of the nurse who is involved in community-based health planning are the health needs of populations at risk. Special at-risk groups reside in all communities: the homeless, the poor, people infected with HIV, pregnant women, infants, children, and the elderly are groups at increased risk for decreased health status. The health needs of at-risk groups must be considered as part of all community health plans.

Last, community-based planning involves an awareness and application of planned change—a process of well-thought-out actions to make something happen. Planned change is discussed in detail later in this chapter.

VALIDATING COMMUNITY NURSING DIAGNOSES

In reviewing the community nursing diagnoses for Rosemont (see Table 12.9), it can be seen that several diagnoses focus on population. Many diagnoses seem to affect all residents, such as the stress and anxiety of being criminally victimized. It may be helpful to stop and review your community nursing diagnoses and categorize them according to the population most affected. A categorization of Rosemont's diagnoses appears in Box 13.1.

Because several diagnoses focus on children and the age and dependency status of children place them at increased risk of decreased health status, a decision was made to begin the planning process by validating the diagnoses that focused on children.

Validating your community nursing diagnoses with the community residents is an important step for establishing and maintaining the partnership. Equally important is the right of community leaders, organizations, and residents to confidentiality of privileged information and the right to choose not to participate in health planning. Communities have the right to

---

Box 13.1 Community Nursing Diagnosis for Rosemont by Population Group

Children
- Potential for accidents (e.g., trauma or suffocation as children explore abandoned machinery)
- Specific to Children at Temple Elementary
- Truancy and academic failure
- Incomplete immunization status
- High prevalence of pediculosis capitis
- High prevalence of dental caries
- Lack of health promotion information including nutrition, exercise, and safety

Infants
- High infant, neonatal, and fetal mortality rate

All Rosemont Residents
- Stress and anxiety of being criminally victimized
- Potential for health problems associated with air pollution
- At Rosemont Health Center, unsafe working environment

---

identify their own health needs and to negotiate with the community health nurse with regard to interventions and specific programs. In turn, the community health nurse has the responsibility to provide or assist with the development of information needed for this process. The American Nurses Association's *Code of Ethics for Nurses With Interpretive Standards* (http://www.nursingworld.org/MainMenuCategories/EthicsStandards/CodeofEthicsforNurses/Code-of-Ethics.pdf) provides a guide for the many human rights issues that the community health nurse encounters.

PLANNED CHANGE

We all experience change. As you read these words, your knowledge level is changing. Yet planned change differs from change that is not planned in that actions occur in a definite sequence, with each one serving as preparation for the next. Planned change is a well-thought-out effort designed to make something happen; all efforts are directed and targeted to produce change. (Many theorists have written about planned change; several works are listed at the end of this chapter.) An adaptation of Reinkemeyer's stages of planned change is presented in Box 13.2. The stages are like a recipe; it is helpful to follow them to produce the intended outcomes.

Box 13.2 An Adaptation of Reinkemeyer's Stages of Planned Change

Stage 1   Identification and development of a felt need and desire for change
Stage 2   Development of a change relationship between the community health nurse and the community
Stage 3   Clarification or diagnosis of the community's problem, need, or objective
Stage 4   Examination of alternative routes and tentative goals and intentions of actions (planning)
Stage 5   Transformation of intentions into actual change (intervention)
Stage 6   Stabilization and evaluation
Stage 7   Termination of the relationship between the community health nurse and the community

Source: Reinkemeyer, A. (1970). Nursing's need: Commitment to an ideology & change. *Nursing Forum, 9*(4), 340–355.

Box 13.3 Lewin's Stages of Planned Change and Their Application to the Planning Process

Lewin's Stages of Planned Change	Application to the Planning Process
• Unfreezing	• Identification of a need for change
	• Moving process
	• Presence of a change agent
	• Identification of problems
	• Consideration of alternatives
	• Adaptation of plan to circumstances
• Refreezing	• Implementation of the plan
	• Stabilization of the situation

Source: Lewin, K. (1958). *Group decision and social change*. In E. Maccoby (Ed.), *Readings in social psychology* (3rd ed.). New York, NY: Holt, Rinehart and Winston.

One early change theorist, Kurt Lewin (1958), described three stages of planned change: unfreezing, moving, and refreezing, as shown in Box 13.3. During the unfreezing stage, the client system (in other words, the organization, community, or at-risk population) becomes aware of a problem and the need for change. Then the problem is diagnosed, and solutions to the problem are identified. From these alternative solutions, one is chosen that seems most appropriate for the situation. In the moving stage, the change actually occurs. The problem is clarified, and the program for solving the problem is planned in detail and begun. Finally, the refreezing stage consists of the accomplished changes becoming integrated into the values of the client system. In this stage, the idea is established and continues to be influential. Lewin also addressed forces that help or hinder change, labeling them the driving forces and the restraining forces, respectively. Using our own model, these may be the lines of resistance and the stressors.

Theories of planned change are important because they can be used to guide and direct the planning process.

APPLYING CHANGE THEORY TO COMMUNITY HEALTH PLANNING

To validate our nursing diagnoses and initiate the planning process, Reinkemeyer's stages of planned change have been chosen as a guide.

Stage 1: Identification and Development of a Felt Need and Desire for the Change

To initiate a felt need and desire for change within the Rosemont community, those organizations that reported actual or potential health concerns of children were contacted, and a meeting was suggested to report the findings of the Rosemont community assessment. Meetings were arranged with the staffs of Temple Elementary, the Third Street Clinic, and the YMCA Indo-Chinese Refugee Program. During the meetings, input from all staff members was sought regarding their observations and perceptions of child health needs as well as their desire to become involved in a planned program of health promotion.

Temple Elementary requested that the assessment data be shared with representatives of the Parent Teacher Organization (PTO) as well as with the school's newly formed parent–teacher liaison group. Both the Third Street Clinic and the YMCA Indo-Chinese Refugee Program requested a presentation to their community advisory boards.

Stage 2: Development of a Change Relationship Between the Community Health Nurse and the Community

Both stages 1 and 2 were completed during the assessment presentations. All staff members were keenly aware of child health needs, and each organization desired to become involved in the planning process. To expedite planning, the Rosemont Health Promotion Council was formed. Each of the three organizations, Temple Elementary, the Third Street Clinic, and the YMCA Indo-Chinese Refugee Program, decided to send one staff member and one interested parent to the planning meetings. At this point, the community health nurse functioned as a change agent to guide and facilitate, but not to direct the planning process. The council elected a chairperson and agreed on meeting dates. The purpose of the council was to coordinate interagency planning for a community-based health promotion program.

Stage 3: Clarification or Diagnosis of the Community's Problem, Need, or Objective

The third stage is the time to validate the community nursing diagnoses. At the conclusion of each presentation, the community health nurse proposed a survey questionnaire to assess the target population's perception of their health concerns. Revisions were solicited from staff and community groups, and the final, agreed-on questionnaire is presented in Box 13.4. Notice that the questionnaire is directed to parents, yet the nursing diagnoses are focused on children. Some council participants believed two questionnaires were necessary—one for the parents and one for the children. What do you think? Because of the age of the children (some had not learned how to read) and the associated time and costs of two questionnaires, it was decided to use one questionnaire directed at the parents.

Although the Rosemont questionnaire focuses on child health, the same format could be used to validate assessed health concerns of the elderly, well adults, teenagers, or pregnant women. The process of checking your assessed community data against the perceptions of the target population can be completed by a survey questionnaire (such as the one in Box 13.4) that can be mailed or conducted as an interview. Or you may choose to validate assessed data by interviewing community leaders and civic groups that are representative of the target population. The word *representative* is very important. For example, the Temple Elementary PTO would not be representative of parents in Rosemont because, as was noted during the assessment, most parents are not active in the organization.

Before we continue, a few words are needed about composing questionnaires. Everyone is confronted daily with people asking questions. Questionnaires arrive in the mail, and people call on the phone. Frequently, the interviewees learn neither the purpose of the questionnaire nor how the information will be used. When you draft a questionnaire, begin with introductory information that states who you are and what the purpose of the questionnaire is. Emphasize that participation is voluntary and that the information will be kept confidential. Sign your name and, if the questionnaire is to be mailed, include a phone number where you can be contacted. Write questions that can be answered quickly (the whole questionnaire should not take longer than 10 minutes to complete). Ideally, place all questions on one side of a standard 8½-inch by 11-inch piece of paper that, if it is to be mailed, can be refolded so that

Box 13.4 Questionnaire to Validate Community Nursing Diagnosis

Dear Parent:

We are nursing students who are interested in learning more about what you think are the most important health needs of your family. Answering a few short questions will help us plan some information sessions for you about how to keep your family healthy. Please either place a √ in the appropriate box or fill in the line. Your participation is voluntary. All information is confidential, and you will not be identified in any way. If you have questions, please feel free to call us at 713-480-0000. Thank you.

Virginia Brown
Ricardo Guerrero
Ann Nguyen
Alice Washington

1. How many children do you have? _____
2. What are their ages? _____
3. If you have a baby, do you breast-feed? Yes [ ] No [ ]
4. If you have a baby, do you bottle-feed? Yes [ ] No [ ]
5. What other foods do you feed your baby? _____
6. What foods do you usually feed your children? _____
7. Would you like to know more about what to feed your baby and children to keep them healthy?
   Yes [ ] No [ ]
8. Would you like to know where you can take your children for health care, both when they are well and sick? Yes [ ] No [ ]
9. Check (√) the following common problems you would like to know more about.

   [ ] Vomiting   [ ] Worms
   [ ] Diarrhea   [ ] Fever
   [ ] Colds and allergies   [ ] Temper tantrums and angry behaviors
   [ ] Skin rashes   [ ] Refusal to do homework or go to school
   [ ] Cuts and falls   [ ] Poor school grades
   [ ] Head lice

10. Other concerns that you would like information about (this can include information for yourself, a friend, or a child):

   _____

   _____

11. Have you ever felt that you, a sibling, or another adult hurt your child when the child was punished?
    Yes [ ] No [ ]
12. Would you like to learn about ways to keep from hurting children when adults are angry?
    Yes [ ] No [ ]
13. Circle the best days and times for you to attend information sessions.

Monday	AM	PM	Friday	AM	PM
Tuesday	AM	PM	Saturday	AM	PM
Wednesday	AM	PM	Sunday	AM	PM
Thursday	AM	PM			

14. Circle the best place for you to attend information sessions.
    Temple Elementary
    Third Street Clinic
    YMCA
    Other (specify where)

a return address shows. Before sharing the questionnaire with agencies or community residents, administer it informally to friends and family; any comments made (such as "What do you mean by _____?" or "I don't understand _____.") signal the need for rewriting and clarification.

Because Rosemont has large populations of Spanish- and Vietnamese-speaking residents, staff at Temple Elementary and the YMCA Indo-Chinese Refugee Program volunteered to translate the questionnaire into these languages. The questionnaire was then ready for distribution.

After several discussions by the Rosemont Health Promotion Council, it was decided to distribute the questionnaire from Temple Elementary by sending one form home with each child. The questionnaires were color-coded by language, and each child was given a questionnaire in the language that was spoken commonly at home.

Take Note

How should the questionnaire be administered? Should the questionnaire be mailed to all households of children at Temple Elementary? Should the questionnaire be given to all adults who bring their children to the Third Street Clinic? Or should the questionnaire be used as an interview and given to a selected number of parents at Temple Elementary, or to clients at the Third Street Clinic, or to adults attending the YMCA Indo-Chinese Refugee Program? (Recall from research that people who have been randomly selected can be considered representative of the total population.) What would you recommend? Before making a decision, list each option and consider the benefits and drawbacks of each. Here is some information for your decision making: Mailed questionnaires have about a 50% return rate that can be increased somewhat with a reminder postcard or telephone call, whereas questionnaires administered as an interview potentially have a 100% return rate. However, interviews require interviewers and about 5 minutes per person per page of questionnaire, whereas mailed questionnaires require less labor but have the financial consideration of postage.

Within 2 weeks, 410 of the 736 questionnaires had been returned. The results were tabulated and summarized by the community health nurse and the student nurses from the local university who were helping her. The summaries were then presented to the Rosemont Health Promotion Council. Examples of the summarized data are presented in Tables 13.1 through 13.4. Why do you think the information was presented by ethnicity? What differences do you notice between family composition and ethnicity, health information desired and ethnicity, and further concerns and ethnicity? Of what importance are these ethnic differences for community health planning?

TABLE 13.1 Family Composition by Ethnicity

Number of Children	Hispanic		Vietnamese		Other*	
	N	%	N	%	N	%
One	82	57	44	61	31	16
Two	12	8	3	4	112	58
Three	24	17	10	14	34	18
Four or more	26	18	15	21	17	8
Total	144	100	72	100	194	100

*Primarily white and black.

TABLE 13.2 Health Information Desired by Ethnicity

	Hispanic		Vietnamese		Other*	
	N	%	N	%	N	%
Vomiting	124	86	65	90	22	11
Diarrhea	134	93	71	98	34	18
Skin rashes	114	79	11	15	52	29
Cuts/falls	45	31	60	83	5	3
Colds/allergies	46	32	5	7	62	32
Head lice	24	17	10	14	74	38
Worms	85	59	70	97	10	5
Fever	132	92	69	96	93	48
Tantrums/angry behavior	10	7	4	5	175	90
School refusal	5	3	6	8	165	85
Poor grades	4	3	2	3	132	68
Total respondents	723		373		824	

*Primarily white and black.

TABLE 13.3 Percentage of Respondents Noting Other Concerns by Ethnicity

	Hispanic (%)	Vietnamese (%)	Other* (%)
Legal issues (child support, custody rights)	32	15	64
Finances/budgeting	23	26	51
Child-care programs	82	12	75
Adult health (weight reduction, birth control)	75	11	68
Employment	82	95	75
Crime prevention, especially prevention of rape and child molestation	88	84	89

*Primarily white and black.

TABLE 13.4 Percentage of Respondents Answering Yes to Questions 11 and 12 by Ethnicity

	Answered Yes		
	Hispanic (%)	Vietnamese (%)	Other (%)*
Question 11: Have you ever felt that you, a sibling, or another adult hurt your child when the child was punished?	89	92	94
Question 12: Would you like to learn about ways to keep from hurting children when adults are angry?	94	95	98

*Primarily white and black.

Take Note

The Rosemont questionnaires were categorized by ethnicity (surmised from the language commonly spoken in the home). However, depending on the community, responses may be categorized by urban versus rural residence, age of respondents, or other meaningful variables. Once summarized, no preferred day and time emerged for the classes. However, a definite preference was shown for location, with all Vietnamese-speaking families preferring the YMCA location and Spanish-speaking clients preferring the Third Street Clinic.

Stage 4: Examination of Alternative Routes and Tentative Goals and Intention of Actions (Planning)

Having validated the community nursing diagnoses, the Rosemont Health Promotion Council was anxious to establish a plan. Much discussion followed the presentation of the questionnaire results. Representatives from Temple Elementary focused on questions 9 and 10 and were eager to present a series of effective parenting seminars on discipline. Temple also felt the high percentage of white and black families who requested information about school phobias and poor grades merited sessions on that topic. Temple's staff discussed how programs to meet the questionnaire needs were consistent with the school's goal of improved communication between teachers and parents as well as with the goals of their failproof program. In addition, recent state programs developed to prevent child abuse were proposed for presentation.

The staff of the Third Street Clinic focused on the families with infants and the associated desire for information on nutrition and the care of common health conditions. The Third Street Clinic had recently initiated a Healthy Baby Program, consisting of evening and Saturday well-child and prenatal clinics, as well as a total service day on Friday when clients could drop in without appointments for immunizations and screening tests for blood pressure, vision, and hearing. Informal counseling was also offered on Friday. The goal for the next 6 months was to invite various service providers, such as optometry and dental hygiene students as well as Medicare and State Employment Commission representatives, to use the clinic space for information sessions and services. After considering the results of the questionnaire, the staff began to discuss the possibility of offering health promotion classes on Fridays that would focus on weight reduction, exercise and fitness, and information about common health conditions. The idea of inviting the police department to make presentations on crime prevention and legal rights was proposed and agreed on by everyone.

Representatives from the YMCA Indo-Chinese Refugee Program believed that, because of cultural taboos against discussing topics such as birth control in public, the information would be best accepted if offered at the YMCA by a respected member of the Vietnamese community. The YMCA was beginning a day care service for mothers of preschoolers, and staff members believed that some of the information on child care could become part of the new program as well as basic child health screening services of development, vision, and hearing. The YMCA representatives were equally concerned that Vietnamese refugees be culturally assimilated into the Rosemont community, and they wanted to plan interagency programs about crime prevention and legal rights that would bring the Vietnamese into more contact with other Rosemont residents. The suggestion was made that a program on crime prevention would bring not only residents of different cultures together, but also residents of different lifestyles. Keenly aware of the tension and stress between the homosexual and heterosexual populations, a community awareness program on crime prevention that would involve all three agencies and all residents of Rosemont was suggested and approved.

Take Note

Notice that each agency is considering how information learned from the questionnaire can be assimilated into existing or planned programs. All agencies have budgets and a set number of staff members to deliver services. Agencies must be as cost-efficient as possible and will want to consider how to include new services (such as information desired by parents) into an existing program. Community health nurses can facilitate this process by becoming familiar with the organizational structure and purpose of each agency. When you establish a planned-change relationship with an agency, ask about their organizational structure (most agencies have an organizational chart with positions arranged according to authority). Decision making usually follows the organizational chart, with consent from all levels being required before major changes can be made or a new program can be begun. Learn the names of the staff members and their position on the organizational chart. (An organizational chart for the Third Street Clinic appears in Figure 13.2.) Ask for a statement of the agency's mission and goals. Ask if you can attend a board meeting and pertinent committee meetings. Your purpose is to learn as much as possible about the services and decision-making process of the agency to facilitate the planned-change nursing interventions.

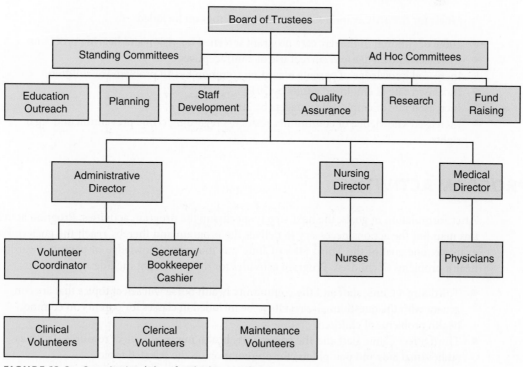

FIGURE 13.2   Organizational chart for Third Street Clinic.

COMMUNITY HEALTH GOAL

Now is the time to transform the ideas and proposals of each agency into a community-based goal and concrete intentions of action. After validating the nursing diagnoses with the community, the community-based goal was to provide health promotion programs on issues desired by the community residents, using methods acceptable to cultural norms and offered in an accessible location at an affordable cost to the community.

This statement is very comprehensive and can be considered an umbrella goal for the Rosemont community under which each agency will have goals. Goals specific to Temple Elementary included:

● Reduce truancy 20% by the end of one school year
● Reduce grade failures 20% by the end of one school year
● Increase immunization levels to 95% within 1 year
● Improve communication between parents and teachers
● Increase parental knowledge on how to protect children from molestation

Goals for the Third Street Clinic that were congruent with the community goal included:

● Increased knowledge of community residents regarding crime prevention and legal rights
● Increased knowledge of parents regarding common health problems of children
● Increased knowledge and practice of effective parenting skills
● Increased percentage of adults who practice healthy lifestyle practices, including:
  ● Exercise fitness
  ● Weight control
  ● Stress management

Goals for the YMCA Indo-Chinese Refugee Program included:

● 100% of children in the day care program screened for vision and hearing problems
● Increased knowledge and correct use of contraceptives
● Increased knowledge of parents regarding common health problems of children
● Increased rate of employed adults by 50%
● Increased rate of employed teenagers by 20%
● Increased knowledge of community residents regarding crime prevention and legal rights

PROGRAM ACTIVITIES

After formulation of goals, the next step is specifying the program activities. Program activities map out the actions necessary to deliver the program and thereby reach the goal(s). For example, one goal of the Third Street Clinic was increased knowledge of parents regarding health problems of children. Program activities for the goal might include:

● Third Street Clinic staff and the community health nurse will select topics that are congruent with the questionnaire results to be included in classes for parents on common health problems of children.
● Third Street Clinic staff and the community health nurse will select resources (such as audiovisual aids and pamphlets) for presentation on the selected topics.
● Third Street Clinic staff and the community health nurse will decide on a day, time, and presentation schedule that are congruent with the questionnaire results.

Each program activity deals with planning the program and is written as sequential steps, each step being required to reach the goal. In addition, each program activity needs a date of accomplishment (e.g., "By June 15, the Third Street Clinic staff and the community health nurse will . . .").

LEARNING OBJECTIVES

Once program activities have been established, learning objectives are written. Learning objectives are derived from a goal and describe the precise behavior or changes that will be required to achieve the goal. Whereas program activities map out the actions necessary to deliver the program, learning objectives specify what changes in knowledge, behaviors, or attitudes are expected as a result of program activities.

Learning objectives focus on the learner and state what changes the learner can expect as a result of participating in the program. For example, one topic selected for presentation during the classes on common health problems of children was fever assessment and home management. The learning objectives were as follows: After the class and practice session on fever assessment and management of the fever at home, each participant will be able to:

- Demonstrate how to take a rectal and axillary temperature
- Discuss common causes and dangers of fever during childhood
- State what constitutes a fever
- Explain at least three methods to reduce a fever
- Describe danger signs that require a medical assessment

Both program and learning objectives can be written in sequential steps that are required to reach the goal, or each objective may have different aspects that, when combined, achieve the goal. Goals and objectives need to be measurable. To make statements measurable, use precise words. Examples of precise terms and less precise terms appear in Box 13.5.

In addition, strive for each goal and objective to include:

- A time frame for attaining the change (e.g., "By June 15 . . .")
- The direction and magnitude of the change (e.g., "Increase immunization levels to 95%")
- The method of measuring the change (e.g., "After the session, each participant will demonstrate _____ ")

Goals and subparts of the goals (objectives) help to clarify a program and establish the expected changes that will result from the program. Although much has been written on the mechanics of writing goals and objectives, little information exists on the collaborative relationship that must exist between the community health nurse and community agency(ies) before meaningful goals and objectives can result.

Box 13.5   Examples of Less Precise and More Precise Terms

Less Precise Terms (Many Interpretations)

To know	To appreciate
To understand	To be aware
To realize	To lower

More Precise Terms (Fewer Interpretations)

To identify	To compare and contrast
To discuss	To state
To list	To decrease by 20%

COLLABORATION

What is meant by a collaborative relationship? Recall from the initial community assessment data that the staff of Temple Elementary had voiced concerns about truancy and grade failure; these same concerns are their first two goals. However, when the nursing diagnoses were validated with the community, parents were more concerned about ways in which they could protect their children from molestation. Could the concerns of the parents and those of the Temple Elementary staff be addressed in the same program? If they could, what would be the program goal? The objectives? This process is an example of collaborative planning and is the essence of community health nursing. You may wonder how to establish collaborative planning and inform agencies about the usefulness of goals and objectives. Although you may be convinced of the value of planned change, how do you convince others, especially because planned change is not commonly practiced in agencies? Role modeling is probably the best strategy. After reviewing the community nursing diagnoses and validating data with an agency, propose goals and objectives that are congruent with the agency's purpose and organizational structure. Solicit input from the group, and continue to revise the goals and objectives until a consensus is reached.

RESOURCES, CONSTRAINTS, AND REVISED PLANS

Once goals and objectives have been written, the next step is to identify available resources and any constraints to the plan. These are analogous to Lewin's driving and restraining forces. Last, revised plans are proposed to the planning group. Resources are all the available means for accomplishing a task, including staff and budget as well as physical space and equipment. Recall that part of your community assessment included the identification of strengths. As you consider resources, include those strengths that may facilitate meeting program goals and objectives. For program planning, it is important to identify the resources needed as well as the resources available. Constraints are obstacles that restrict or limit actions and can include a lack of staff, budget, physical space, and equipment. Constraints may be thought of as the difference between needs and resources. Revised plans are actions that are proposed based on the knowledge of resources and constraints.

Following much discussion and self-examination, each agency of the Rosemont Health Promotion Council formed program goals and objectives. Then, alongside each goal and objective, necessary resources were listed. For example, at the Third Street Clinic, the following resources and constraints were identified as crucial to the goal:

GOAL: *To increase the knowledge of parents regarding common health problems of children.*

Resources Needed

- Staff member to develop and assemble existing information on common health problems of children
- Staff member to present the information materials in English, Spanish, and Vietnamese
- Physical space and necessary equipment (e.g., thermometers and basins) to teach assessment and home care skills

Resources Available

- Staff members who speak English and Spanish
- Staff nurse knowledgeable about the care of children
- Physical space and some necessary equipment
- Staff interest and desire to offer information requested by parents

Constraints

It may be helpful to consider constraints as the mismatch between resources needed and resources available. Constraints at the Third Street Clinic include:

- No staff member who speaks Vietnamese
- Discomfort of staff because of inexperience in developing and adapting learning materials
- Time limitations
- Staff members' insecurity about their ability to perform group teaching (all previous teaching was performed on a one-on-one basis)
- Lack of resource material (e.g., audiovisual aids and brochures on care of common childhood problems)

 Take Note

Universal constraints are staff and money—agencies never have enough. An additional constraint is resistance to change. All people are reluctant to change existing routines and patterns of behavior. Initially, change is uncomfortable, and, until new roles are learned, anxiety exists. Making people aware of the natural discomfort associated with change can help build rapport and establish a collaborative relationship.

When each agency had listed its program goals, objectives, and activities, along with resources and constraints, several alternative actions became apparent. For example, a constraint of the Third Street Clinic was lack of staff members who spoke Vietnamese. A similar constraint of the YMCA Indo-Chinese Refugee Program was lack of staff with necessary knowledge to offer classes on contraception or the care of children with common health problems. Therefore, the following revised plan was proposed:

REVISED PLAN A bilingual (English–Vietnamese) staff member from the YMCA would attend the classes offered in English at the Third Street Clinic and then offer the classes in Vietnamese at the YMCA.

Both the Third Street Clinic and the YMCA noted a lack of resource materials as a constraint to program implementation. Further assessment of community health resources by the community health nurse revealed that the Sunvalley Clinic, as part of the Hampton Health Department, had access to various audiovisual aids and printed materials on the subjects; however, all materials were in English.

REVISED PLAN One Spanish- and English-speaking staff member from the Third Street Clinic and one Vietnamese- and English-speaking staff member from the YMCA would translate the materials into Spanish and Vietnamese free of charge with the provision that they be given copies of all the translated materials.

REVISED PLAN The community health nurse would provide instruction in basic principles of group teaching, including methods of presenting information. In addition, the community health nurse would participate in the development and adaptation of materials and the teaching of classes.

For each constraint, a revised plan was proposed, discussed, and adopted. This is a period of intense collaboration between the community health nurse and community agencies, and only at the completion of this stage is the community ready for stage 5 of planned change—transformation of intentions into actual behavior change. This transformation of intentions is the actual program implementation (which is covered in the next chapter). However, before the plan is implemented, it must be recorded.

RECORDING

Community plans must be recorded in a standardized, systematic, and concise form that clearly communicates to others the purpose and actions of the plan as well as the rationale for revisions and deletions of actions. Discuss with each agency its present recording system, and decide on a format and system for recording the plan. The format need not be elaborate, and a simple one such as that used at the Third Street Clinic would be adequate if agreed on by the agency.

Summary

Before concluding, let's review the learning objectives for this chapter and their application to community health nursing. The planning process begins with validation of the community nursing diagnoses—a process that establishes the community's perception and value of community health needs. Next, using theories of planned change, the community health nurse and the community form a collaborative partnership to establish program goals and objectives. Last, based on resources and constraints, plans are proposed, recorded, and adopted. Although only one example is offered here, the process of community health planning was the same for all eight programs that were developed by the Rosemont Health Promotion Council.

The next two chapters address stages 5 through 7 of planned change (transformation of intention into actual change [intervention]; stabilization and evaluation; and termination of the relationship between the community health nurse and the community). Stage 5 is implementation and stage 6 is related to evaluation. You will recognize that stage 7 may lead to further assessment, thereby bringing the process full circle.

Critical Thinking Questions

Using the data you generated for Critical Thinking question #2 in Chapter 12, develop a plan for the community diagnosis, "Potential for high-risk sexual behavior in high school teens."

1. What is the goal?
2. Name two objectives to reach the goal.
3. What actions do they require?
4. How will you evaluate the actions?

REFERENCES

Lewin, K. (1958). Group decision and social change. In E. Maccoby (Ed.), *Readings in social psychology* (3rd ed.). New York, NY: Holt, Rinehart and Winston.
Reinkemeyer, A. (1970). Nursing's need: Commitment to an ideology & change. *Nursing Forum*, *9*(4), 340–355.

FURTHER READINGS

Campbell, M. K., Hudson, M. A., Resnicow, K., Blakeney, N., Paxton, A., & Baskin, M. (2007). Church-based health promotion interventions: Evidence and lessons learned. *Annual Review of Public Health, 28*, 213–234.

Green, L. W., & Kreuter, M. W. (2005). *Health program planning: An educational and ecological approach.* Mountain View, CA: Mayfield/McGraw-Hill.

Issel, L. M. (2009). *Health program planning and evaluation: A practical and systematic approach for community health.* Sudbury, MA: Jones and Bartlett.

Keller, H. H., Hedley, M. R., Wong, S. S., Vanderkooy, P., Tindale, J., & Norris, J. (2006). Community organized food and nutrition education: Participation, attitudes and nutritional risk in seniors. *The Journal of Nutrition, Health & Aging, 10*(1), 15–20.

Li, Y., Cao, J., Lin, H., Li, D., & He, J. (2009). Community health needs assessment with precede-proceed model: A mixed methods study. *BMC Health Services Research, 9*(10), 181.

Li, L.-C., Chen, Y.-C., Hsu, L.-L., Lin, C.-H., & Chrisman, N. J. (2012). The effects of an educational training workshop for community leaders on self-efficacy of program planning skills and partnerships. *Journal of Advanced Nursing, 68*(3), 600–613.

Lippitt, G. (1973). *Visualizing change: Model building and the change process.* La Jolla, CA: University Associates.

Rew, L., Chambers, K. B., & Kulkarni, S. (2002). Planning a sexual health promotion intervention with homeless adolescents. *Nursing Research, 51*(3), 168–174.

Thackery, R., Neiger, B. L., & Hanson, C. L. (2007). Developing a promotional strategy: Important questions for social marketing. *Health Promotion Practice, 8*(4), 332–336.

Zoellner, J., Motley, M., Wilkinson, M., Jackman, B., Barlow, M. L., & Hill, J. L. (2012). Engaging the Dan River Region to reduce obesity: Application of the comprehensive participatory planning and evaluation process. *Family & Community Health, 35*(1), 44–56.

CHAPTER 14

Implementing a Community Health Program

Elizabeth T. Anderson and Judith McFarlane

LEARNING OBJECTIVES

Implementation is the action phase of the nursing process: it is the carrying out of the community-based plan. Implementation is necessary to achieve goals and objectives, but, more important, the implementation of nursing interventions acts to promote, maintain, or restore health; to prevent illness; and to effect rehabilitation.

This chapter discusses the process of implementing a community-based health program. Intervention strategies are presented, along with resources that are helpful in program implementation.

After studying this chapter, you should be able to:

1. Suggest strategies to the community for implementation of health programs.

2. List specific interventions for population-based nursing in partnership with the community:

   • Implement planned programs

   • Review and revise interventions based on community responses

   • Use interventions to formulate and influence health and social policies that have an impact on the health of the community

Introduction

Once goals and objectives have been agreed on and recorded during the planning stage, all that remains for implementation is to actually carry out the activities to meet those objectives. This probably seems straightforward and simple. Indeed, at this point, you will have spent considerable time assessing, analyzing, and planning a program. You will be ready and eager to begin. But this very eagerness (and the associated impatience of the intervention stage) is a danger. You must take time to consider how you can promote community ownership, a unified program, and a clear health focus.

Take Note

This chapter focuses on the *process* of intervention and provides you with some general resources that may prove helpful in your community work. Many excellent examples of interventions in which community health nurses work as partners with the community are included in Part 3 of this text.

PROMOTING COMMUNITY OWNERSHIP

Essential to achieving the desired outcomes of the interventions is the active participation of the community. The meaning of partnership and collaboration was discussed in the preceding chapter, but the present concern is ownership. The people of the community need to feel a sense of ownership of the program or event, which can only come with their full participation in the decisions regarding planning as well as their assuming some responsibility for implementation. Herein lies a potential conflict. The profession of nursing is one of nurturing, sustaining, and caring for others. It is part of our profession to do for others what they would do for themselves if they were able. Indeed, most nurses interact professionally with people during an altered health state that requires nurses to do for others; but this is not true in community health nursing. Stepping into the community requires an attitude of doing *with* the people, not doing things *to* them or *for* them. When things are done to us or for us, our emotional commitment remains limited.

How might you ensure community ownership for a proposed program and planned interventions? How can you facilitate involvement? In Rosemont, the Rosemont Health Promotion Council coordinated interagency planning for a community-based health promotion program. When the planning was completed, the council directed its attention to the coordination of activities for the program's implementation. The important point in this example is that a coordination group was already in place. Usually, the planning committee can coordinate implementation.

Take Note

When the Rosemont Health Promotion Council and designated staff in charge of program implementation reviewed the program objectives, it became evident that resources had to be selected before the program could proceed. (Resources refer to audiovisual aids, pamphlets, and other material for presentation of the program.) Council and staff members began to ask where such materials could be obtained. What was available in Rosemont? What could you have suggested at this point?

Examining the initial assessment of Rosemont, it was noted that the United Way listed 42 private and publicly supported social service agencies located in Hampton or Jefferson County. The United Way listing included identifying information for each agency along with services and fees. Reviewing the list with the council and participating staff, the community health nurse suggested that selected agency representatives be invited to discuss programs and resources that they could make available, such as films and speakers. It was found that several agencies could provide relevant material. The March of Dimes was sponsoring a campaign in Hampton to increase public awareness of the importance of a healthy pregnancy for the birth of a healthy child. The Mental Health Association had developed teaching modules on effective parenting, and the police department and the Woman's Center were offering programs on crime prevention. All of these programs had recently received a brief description, including the names of their contact persons, in the *Hampton Herald*. At this point, it was decided to complete program and learning objectives for each of the health promotion goals established by the Rosemont Council. Therefore, as various agency personnel discussed their program with the council, decisions could be made on the appropriateness of the material for the Rosemont community.

Take Note

Do not panic at this point and feel that you must be knowledgeable about all agencies and their programs in the community that you have assessed. At the implementation stage, do refer to your initial assessment and consider logically which service agencies may have resources helpful to the planned program(s). Then contact selected agencies, request information on their purpose and present programs, share with the agency your community-based program plans, and solicit recommendations with regard to materials and resources.

Box 14.1 lists voluntary organizations that have professional staff at the national and local levels and an affiliated or community linkage structure. These voluntary organizations have ongoing programs for a wide variety of health issues, and most acknowledge health promotion as a vital part of their mission. The list is not inclusive and is meant to serve only as a guide.

Box 14.1 Voluntary Organizations (A Partial Listing)

American Association of Retired Persons (http://www.aarp.org)
American Cancer Society (www.cancer.org)
American Heart Association (www.americanheart.org)
American Lung Association (www.lungusa.org)
American Red Cross (www.redcross.org)
Association of Junior Leagues, Inc. (www.ajli.org)
Boy Scouts of America (www.scouting.org)
Boys' Clubs of America, Inc. (www.bgca.org)
Cooperative Extension Service (www.csrees.usda.gov/extension)
Girl Scouts of America (www.girlscouts.org)
Girls' Clubs of America, Inc. (www.bgca.org)
March of Dimes (www.marchofdimes.com)
National Board of the YMCA of the USA (www.ymca.net)
National Board of the YWCA of the USA (www.ywca.org)
National Coalition of Hispanic Mental Health and Human Services Organizations (COSSHMO)
　　(www.hispanichealth.org)
National Council on Alcoholism and Drug Dependence (www.ncadd.org)
National Health Council (www.nationalhealthcouncil.org)
National Kidney Foundation (www.kidney.org)
National Recreation and Parks Association (www.nrpa.org)
National Safety Council (www.nsc.org)
National Urban League (www.nul.org)
United Way of America (www.liveunited.org)

TABLE 14.1 Office of Disease Prevention and Health Promotion: Selected Programs and Initiatives

Program	Description	Contact
Healthy People	Launched in 1979; guides efforts to identify objectives for nation	http://www. healthypeople.gov
Healthfinder	A gateway website to link consumers and professionals to health and human services information from the federal government. Reliable information via the internet	http://www.healthfinder.gov
National Health Information Center	Central health information referral service for consumers and professionals	http://www.health.gov/nhic
Dietary Guidelines for Americans	Published with the U.S. Department of Agriculture; federally mandated nutrition education activities	http://www.health.gov/dietaryguidelines
Healthy Communities, Worksites, and Schools	With National Coalition for Healthier Cities and Communities, focuses on ways that communities can adapt the national Healthy People objectives for local use	http://odphp.osophs.dhhs.gov/pubs

Source: http://odphp.osophs.dhhs.gov/odphpfact.htm

In addition, the Office of Disease Prevention and Health Promotion (ODPHP), located within the Public Health Service (PHS; which, in turn, is located within the U.S. Department of Health and Human Services [DHHS]), publishes a tremendous amount of information that is designed to promote health and prevent disease among Americans. Special attention is given to facilitating the prevention activities of the five PHS agencies: the Alcohol, Drug Abuse, and Mental Health Administration; the Centers for Disease Control and Prevention (CDC); the Food and Drug Administration (FDA); the Health Resources and Services Administration (HRSA); and the National Institutes of Health (NIH). Several special programs, termed initiatives, are sponsored by ODPHP. A partial listing of the initiatives, services, and information available, along with web sites, is included in Table 14.1.

Having discussed the importance of community participation and ownership of the program, the remaining issues to consider are a unified presentation of the program and an emphasis on health, not the program itself.

IMPLEMENTING A UNIFIED PROGRAM

Because of limited resources, staff constraints, and other situations beyond the control of the planners, many good programs are implemented in a piecemeal fashion that minimizes their impact. A unified program requires collaboration and coordination between the agency personnel who will implement the program and the program's recipients (the target population). Allowing plenty of time for publicizing the program (and how you perform the mechanics of publicity—the how, where, and to whom) can make a crucial difference in whether people attend and what the subsequent impact will be.

Coordinated Publicity

After a time and place have been selected (based on initial input from the survey questionnaires), how might you publicize a program? Public service announcements, notification in the newspapers, bulletin inserts for civic and religious associations, flyers sent home with school-age children, and posters and notices in community service buildings and local shopping centers are some of the methods to consider. The Rosemont Health Promotion Council decided to publicize the first program on child health by sending home a flyer with each child at Temple Elementary. The flyer thanked the parents for their participation during the survey and invited them to programs at the Third Street Clinic and the YMCA Indo-Chinese Refugee Center. Public service announcements were made on the radio, and feature articles about the Rosemont Health Promotion Council and upcoming programs appeared in the Vietnamese and Spanish newspapers as well as in the *Hampton Herald* and Rosemont Civic Association's newsletter. Posters were placed in local grocery stores, churches, and other gathering places (again, use your assessment to identify the best places). Because the parents on the Rosemont Health Promotion Council had expressed a concern that parents with young children might not be able to attend programs, arrangements were made for child care, and a separate health program for preschool and school-age children was planned during the adult programs. The program publicity was focused on health promotion for the whole family and not just on programs for selected family members.

Unified Goals: Healthy People

The idea of a health program based on unified goals and objectives is central to the Healthy People documents. The following subsections show how this idea has evolved through the years.

Health Goals for 1990

In 1979, the first "health" initiative for the United States (Healthy People: The Surgeon General's Report on Health Promotion and Disease Prevention) promoted five goals. These broad goals focused on reducing mortality among targeted age groups—infants, children, adolescents, young adults, and adults—and on increasing the independence of older adults. These were the first "health" goals for the nation, and their target date was 1990 (U.S. Office of the Assistant Secretary for Health and Surgeon General, 1979).

Health Goals for 2000

Healthy People 2000 (U.S. Department of Health and Human Services, Public Health Service, 1990) was developed through broad collaborative efforts among government, voluntary organizations, professional organizations, businesses, and individuals. Three goals provided the framework:

1. Increase the span of healthy life for Americans;
2. Reduce health disparities among Americans; and
3. Achieve access to preventive services for all Americans.

In addition, organized under the approaches of health promotion, health protection, and preventive services, over 300 objectives were included under 22 priority areas.

Health Goals for 2010

Healthy People 2010 was, according to its Introduction,

> . . . distinguished from Healthy People 2000 by the broadened prevention science base; improved surveillance and data systems; a heightened awareness and demand for preventive health services and quality health care; and changes in demographics, science, technology and disease spread that will affect the public's health in the 21st century (U.S. Department of Health and Human Services, 1998, Introduction 1).

Two broad goals (eliminate health disparities, and increase quality and years of healthy life) provided the framework and were incorporated into the model for Healthy People 2010.

Health Goals for 2020

Healthy People 2020, which was launched in December 2010, has four main goals:

1. Attain high-quality, longer lives free of preventable disease, disability, injury, and premature death;
2. Achieve health equity, eliminate disparities, and improve the health of all groups;
3. Create social and physical environments that promote good health for all; and
4. Promote quality of life, healthy development, and healthy behaviors across all life stages.

There are nearly 600 objectives in Healthy People 2020, with more than 1,300 measures organized into more than 40 topic areas. In that these objectives are based on national data, as well as rigorous criteria (Table 14.2), they can be used as standards against which we can compare local data. They also provide excellent examples of clearly written, measurable objectives. The topic areas, listed alphabetically (ranging from "Access to Health Services" to "Vision"), are easily retrieved online (http://www.healthypeople.gov/2020/topicsobjectives2020/default.aspx).

 Take Note

Are the goals and objectives for your community realistic in terms of the past and in relation to trends over time? Do the goals and objectives for your community-based program further the national goals and objectives? When the Rosemont Health Promotion Council reviewed its goals and objectives, each was found to be congruent with the national plan, as well as with Rosemont's state health department objectives for improved health.

TABLE 14.2 Criteria for Objectives Development

Objective Attribute	Notes
Important and understandable	Relate to framework and have broad audience
Prevention oriented	Should address health improvements that can be achieved through population-based and health-service intervention
Drive action	Including suggestion of steps that will achieve the proposed targets
Useful and relevant	Should be usable by states, localities, and private sector to target schools, communities, worksites, health practices, and other settings
Measurable	Should include a range of measures (health outcomes, behavioral and health-service interventions, and community capacity) directed toward improving health outcomes and quality of life
Build on prior Healthy People goals	To provide continuity and comparability
Scientifically supported	Based on scientific evidence
Address population disparities	To recognize that there are disparities that affect health
Valid, reliable, nationally representative data, and data systems	General criteria needed for any objectives that relate to the health of populations

Source: http://www.healthypeople.gov/2010/HP2020/Objectives/selectionCriteria.aspx

MAINTAINING A HEALTH FOCUS

There is one remaining question to ask before initiating the program: Does it focus on health? This may seem to be a strange question. You might wonder, don't all community health programs focus on maintaining, restoring, or promoting health? Sometimes, the answer is no.

In Rosemont, the council and designated staff had become very involved in planning specific activities and information modules associated with the community health program. Several programs had been enlarged to include screening and health fairs; additional activities were suggested at each council meeting. The initial goal of promoting the health of Rosemont residents had seemingly changed to providing Rosemont residents with lots of activities and information about health. What had happened? Remember, we discussed the impatience and eagerness that are often associated with new programs. This situation is normal. Committees tend to overemphasize activities and knowledge and forget the initial reason for the program—to improve health. But it should be remembered that it is the sustained, day-to-day use of knowledge and lifestyle practices that improves health. Frequently, a program begins with enthusiastic momentum; media publicity attracts people to screening and information sessions—and then the program is over. Objectives are evaluated as having been achieved successfully, and another program is planned and implemented. But was there any real improvement in health? Did the participants change lifestyle practices? Will the changes be maintained and continued for a week? a month? a year? Most important, are the changed lifestyle or health practices supported by the surrounding environment and culture?

Environmental and Cultural Support

Many parents in Rosemont responded affirmatively to the survey questions about discipline. These parents believed that they or another person had hurt a child when the child was punished; the parents wanted to learn ways to keep from hurting children when adults were angry. The Rosemont Health Promotion Council responded with a series of programs on effective parenting that included information on various nonphysical strategies for disciplining youngsters, as well as role-playing and open discussion periods. However, as part of the community assessment, the community health nurse had recorded that the Hampton Independent School District (HISD) used physical punishment as a primary discipline method. Students at Temple Elementary were hit on the buttocks with a wide board that frequently left large bruises. The conflict between the effective parenting programs and punishment methods at Temple Elementary was obvious. What could be done? What would you suggest?

In Rosemont, part of the planned effective-parenting classes included discussion sessions on the difference between discipline and punishment and the importance of inquiring as to disciplinary and punitive procedures when parents left their children for supervision (e.g., at child care facilities and schools or with babysitters). Parents were asked to voice their feelings about the school district's policy on physical punishment. Although some parents were unaware of the school district's policy, most were aware of the punishment but believed the procedure could not be changed. After a discussion of parental rights and responsibilities, a group of parents made an appointment with the principal of Temple Elementary to discuss the situation. (After additional meetings with school board members, an open public hearing on public school discipline, and letters to state school board officials, the HISD changed the discipline policy to exclude physical punishment. The process took 2 years.)

Countless such incongruities exist between healthy lifestyles and environmental and cultural practices and policies. Here is one additional example: Recall that one community nursing diagnosis for children at Temple Elementary was a high prevalence of dental caries. During the effective-parenting discussions, several parents commented that their children were given hard candy as a reward for good behavior. When the nurse at Temple Elementary was contacted, it was verified that children exhibiting good behavior were given hard candy. This occurred on a daily basis.

Take Note ──

Identify the environmental and cultural practices and policies that are in conflict with the proposed community-based health program that resulted from your community assessment. What can be done to increase community awareness of these conflicts, and how can change begin? To focus on health and the maintenance of healthy lifestyles, all of the community must be involved.

Levels of Prevention

The best way to maintain a focus on health and not on the activities of the program is to use your nursing practice model as a guide. The nursing practice model built and described in Chapter 11 (see Fig. 11.1) defines intervention as primary, secondary, and tertiary levels of prevention. Do the programs proposed for Rosemont address these three levels of prevention?

Recall that *primary prevention* improves the health and well-being of the community, making it less vulnerable to stressors. Health promotion programs are primary prevention, as are programs that focus on protection from specific diseases. Usually, health promotion is nonspecific and directed toward raising the general health of the total community (e.g., teaching youngsters about nutritious foods or conducting adult exercise/fitness and stress-reduction sessions). Primary prevention can also be very specific, such as providing immunization against certain diseases. Additional primary prevention measures include the wearing of seat belts and the purification of public water supplies.

Secondary prevention begins after a disease or condition is present (although there may be no symptoms). Emphasis is on screening, early diagnosis, and treatment of possible stressors that may adversely affect the community's health. The tine test for tuberculosis, the Denver Developmental Screening Test for developmental delays, blood pressure assessments, breast self-examinations, and mammograms are secondary prevention interventions.

Tertiary prevention focuses on restoration and rehabilitation. Tertiary prevention programs act to return the community to an optimum level of functioning. Adequate shelters for battered women and counseling and therapy programs for sexually abused children are examples of tertiary prevention.

The distinction between prevention levels is not always clear. Is a program on the assessment of fever in children (and the prevention of febrile convulsions and dehydration through use of tepid baths and extra fluids) secondary or tertiary prevention? How would you classify an effective-parenting program, support groups for single parents, a crime-prevention program, and sessions on stress reduction and physical fitness? Can some programs be primary, secondary, and tertiary depending on the needs of the people who attend? Certainly effective-parenting classes for the parent with a child who has a behavior problem will have a different purpose than classes designed for expectant parents of a first child. Likewise, the corporate executive who has been diagnosed with cardiovascular disease and placed on a low-cholesterol diet has very different nutritional learning needs from those of the senior citizen on a fixed income. Few programs pertain to only one level of prevention.

The important point is to evaluate your programs (the implementation phase of the nursing process) and ask if the nursing interventions are consistent with the nursing practice model. If the focus is prevention, are the programs directed toward prevention?

Levels of Practice

In addition to level of prevention, we need to consider the level of practice. This text promotes the community as partner; therefore, the level of practice is considered community- and systems-based. Individual-focused practice may also be incorporated into population-based nursing, but is primarily aimed at one-on-one activity.

Box 14.2 Interventions for Population-Based Nursing Practice

Community organizations
Coalition building
Collaboration
Counseling
Health teaching
Delegated functions
Case management
Advocacy
Referral and follow-up
Screening
Outreach
Disease and health event investigation
Surveillance
Policy development and enforcement
Social marketing

Source: Minnesota Department of Health, Division of Community Health Services, Public Health Nursing Section. (2001). *Public health interventions—Applications for public health nursing practice.* Retrieved December 31, 2013, from http://www. health.state.mn.us/divs/opi/cd/phn/docs/0301wheel_manual.pdf.

Specific interventions for population-based nursing practice have been identified by the Public Health Nursing Section of the Minnesota Department of Health (2001). The interventions are included in Box 14.2. Consider these interventions as you develop plans to address the problems identified in your community.

 Take Note

The model for population- and community-based practice is public health nursing. Now, many nurses consider their practice to be population- and community-based. We use the term *community health nurse* to incorporate these nurses. Criteria—cornerstones—for public health nursing are listed below to describe this specialty practice:

- Focuses on entire populations
- Reflects community priorities and needs
- Establishes caring relationships with the communities, families, individuals, and systems that comprise the population that community health nurses serve
- Is grounded in social justice, compassion, sensitivity to diversity, and respect for the worth of all people, especially the vulnerable
- Encompasses the mental, physical, emotional, social, spiritual, and environmental aspects of health
- Promotes health through strategies driven by epidemiologic evidence
- Collaborates with community resources to achieve those strategies, but can and will work alone if necessary
- Derives its authority from the Nurse Practice Act

Source: Minnesota Department of Health, Public Health Nursing Section (2004).

Summary

Having considered the importance of community ownership of the program, the need to offer a unified program, and maintain a focus on health, there remains one step in the process—evaluation. Before a program is implemented, the manner in which it is to be evaluated must be established. The following chapter explains why this final stage of the nursing process is essential before implementation.

Critical Thinking Questions

For the objectives you developed for the diagnosis, "Potential for high-risk sexual behavior in high school teens," in Chapter 13, identify one intervention.

1. What level of prevention does it represent? Give your rationale.
2. Is there an objective in Healthy People 2020 related to this intervention?
3. What is the health focus of this intervention?

REFERENCES

Minnesota Department of Health, Division of Community Health Services, Public Health Nursing Section. (2001). *Public health interventions—Applications for public health nursing practice.* Retrieved December 31, 2013, from http://www.health.state.mn.us/divs/opi/cd/phn/docs/0301wheel_manual.pdf

Minnesota Department of Health, Public Health Nursing Section. (2004). *Cornerstones of public health nursing.* Retrieved December 31, 2013, from http://www.health.state.mn.us/divs/opi/cd/phn/practicecouncil/docs/1102phncouncil_relevantchallenges.pdf

U.S. Department of Health and Human Services, Public Health Service. (1990). *Healthy People 2000: National health promotion and disease prevention objectives.* Washington, DC: U.S. Government Printing Office.

U.S. Office of the Assistant Secretary for Health and Surgeon General. (1979). *Healthy People: The surgeon general's report on health promotion and disease prevention.* Washington, DC: U.S. Government Printing Office.

FURTHER READINGS

Andrews, J. O., Bentley, G., Crawford, S., Pretlow, L., & Tingen, M. S. (2007). Using community-based participatory research to develop a culturally sensitive smoking cessation intervention with public housing neighborhoods. *Ethnicity and Disease, 17*(2), 331–337.

Asset-Based Community Development Institute. This site has numerous resources and "tool kits" to assist in community work. Retrieved from http://www.abcdinstitute.org/abcd09/

Brownstein, J. N., Chowdhury, F. M., Norris, S. L., Horsley, T., Jack, L., Jr., Zhang, X., & Satterfield, D. (2007). Effectiveness of community health workers in the care of people with hypertension. *American Journal of Preventive Medicine, 32*(5), 435–437.

Fisher, J. W., & Peek, K. E. (2009). Collaborating for change: Creating a women's health network. *Women's Health Issues, 19*(1), 3–7.

Fletcher, B. J., Himmelfarb, C. D., Lira, M. T., Meininger, J. C., Pradhan, S. R., & Sikkema, J. S. (2011). Global cardiovascular disease prevention: A call to action for nursing community-based and public health prevention initiatives. *European Journal of Cardiovascular Nursing, 10*(2), S32–S41.

Frieden, T. R. (2014). Six components necessary for effective public health program implementation. *American Journal of Public Health, 104,* 17–22.

Graves, B. A. (2008). Integrative literature review: A review of literature related to geographical information systems, healthcare access, and health outcomes. *Perspectives in Health Information Management, 5,* 5–11.

Kulbok, P. A., Meszaros, P., Bond, D. C., Botchwey, N. D., & Hinton, I. (2009). *Partnering with rural youth and parents to design and test a tobacco, alcohol, and drug use prevention program model (Abstract).* Virginia? Foundation for Healthy Youth. Retrieved from http://healthyyouthva.org/vtsf/research/projects.asp

Lucey, P., & Maurana, C. A. (2007). Partnerships to address social determinants of health. *Nursing Economics, 25*(3), 179–182.

Racher, F. E., & Annis, R. C. (2008). Community health action model: Health promotion by the community. *Research and Theory for Nursing Practice, 22*(3), 182–191.

Stephens, P. C., Sloboda, Z., Stephens, R. C., Teasdale, B., Grey, S. F., Hawthorne, R. D., & Williams, J. (2009). Universal school-based substance abuse prevention programs: Modeling targeted mediators and outcomes for adolescent cigarette, alcohol and marijuana use. *Drug and Alcohol Dependence, 102*(1–3), 19–29.

Vasquez, E. P., Pitts, K., & Mejia, N. E. (2008). A model program: Neonatal nurse practitioners providing community health care for high-risk infants. *Neonatal Network, 27*(3), 163–169.

Yoo, S., Butler, J., Elias, T. I., & Goodman, R. M. (2009). The 6-step model for community empowerment: Revisited in public housing communities for low-income senior citizens. *Health Promotion Practice, 10*(2), 262–275.

CHAPTER 15

Evaluating a Community Health Program

Elizabeth T. Anderson and Judith Mcfarlane

LEARNING OBJECTIVES

Evaluation is determining the worth (or value) of something. During the evaluation process, information is collected and analyzed to determine its significance and worth. Changes are appraised, and progress is documented. This chapter discusses evaluation and the nursing practices that are necessary to plan and implement it.

After studying this chapter, you should be able to:

1. Establish evaluation criteria that are timely and comprehensive.

2. Use baseline and current data to measure progress toward goals and objectives.

3. Validate observations, insights, and new data with colleagues and the community.

4. Revise priorities, goals, and interventions based on evaluation data.

5. Document and record evaluation results and revisions of the plan.

6. Participate in evaluation research with appropriate consultation.

7. Appreciate the complexity of program evaluation, as well as the multiple paradigms that affect its implementation.

Introduction

The nurse evaluates the responses of the community to a health program to measure progress that is being made toward the program's goals and objectives. Evaluation data are also crucial for revision of the database and the community nursing diagnoses that were developed from analysis of the community assessment data.

Do you feel as though we are talking in circles? Evaluation is the "final" step of the nursing process, but it is linked to assessment, which is the first step. Nursing practice is cyclic as well as dynamic, and, for community-based interventions to be timely and relevant, the community database, nursing diagnoses, and health program plans must be evaluated routinely. The effectiveness of community nursing interventions depends on continuous reassessment of the community's health and on appropriate revisions of planned interventions.

Evaluation is important to nursing practice, but of equal importance is its crucial role in the functioning of health agencies. Staffing and funding are frequently based on evaluation findings, and existing programs are subject to termination unless evaluation evidence can be produced that answers the question: *What has been the program's impact on the health status of the community?* There has been a growing focus on program evaluation; training programs on evaluation are commonplace; and evaluation has become big business. Even a cursory review of online resources about evaluation can be an overwhelming experience (see, for example, the CDC website, http://www.cdc.gov/evaL/resources/index.htm [retrieved 1/4/14]). Unfortunately, evaluation is sometimes practiced separately from program planning. It may even be tacked onto the end of a program just to satisfy funding sources or agency administration. The problems of such an approach are evident. Effective community health nursing requires an integrative approach to evaluation; it is a unique aspect of the field.

EVALUATION PRINCIPLES

Congruent with the theoretical foundations of working with the community as partner, we base our program evaluation on principles explicated by the W. K. Kellogg Foundation (1998). These principles are summarized below.

1. *Strengthen programs.* Our goal is health promotion and improving the self-reliance of the community. Evaluation assists in attaining this goal by providing an ongoing and systematic process for assessing the program, its impact, and its outcomes.
2. *Use multiple approaches.* In addition to multidisciplinary approaches, evaluation methods may be numerous and varied. No single approach is favored, but the method chosen must be congruent with the purposes of the program.
3. *Design evaluation to address real issues.* Community-based programs, rooted in the "real" community and based on an assessment of that community, must contain an evaluation to measure those criteria of importance to the community.
4. *Create a participatory process.* Just as the community members were part of assessment, analysis, planning, and implementation, so too they must be partners in evaluation.
5. *Allow for flexibility.* "Evaluation approaches must not be rigid and prescriptive, or it will be difficult to document the incremental, complex, and often subtle changes that occur" (W. K. Kellogg Foundation, 1998, p. 3).
6. *Build capacity.* The process of evaluation, in addition to measuring outcomes, should enhance the skills, knowledge, and attitudes of those engaged in it. This includes both professionals and nonprofessionals.

THE EVALUATION PROCESS

There is a burgeoning body of literature on evaluation (see Further Readings at the end of this chapter). Program or project evaluation has become a specialty, with entire departments and consulting firms focused on measurement and evaluation.

For our purposes (i.e., to provide an introduction to program evaluation), we will use a three-part model (Table 15.1). In this model, we look at the *process* of implementing the program, the program's *impact*, and the *outcome* of the program.

TABLE 15.1 A Model for Program Evaluation

	Process (Formative)	Impact (Summative; Short-Term Outcome)	Outcome (Long-Term Outcome)
Information to collect	Program implementation, including • Site response • Recipient response • Practitioner response • Competencies of personnel	Immediate effects of program on, for example: • Knowledge • Attitudes • Perceptions • Skills • Beliefs • Access to resources • Social support	Incidence and prevalence of risk factors, morbidity, and mortality
When to apply	Initial implementation of a program or when changes are made in a developed program (e.g., moved to a new site, provided to a different population)	To determine if factors that affect health—both within the individual and in the environment—have changed. For example, did the person's behavior change? Was the new policy implemented?	To measure if incidence and prevalence have been altered. For example, has the immunization rate of 2-year-olds increased? Did the rate of admissions for illnesses decrease? Did the industry filter its polluting smoke stack?

Source: Green, L. W., & Lewis, F. M. (1986). *Measurement and evaluation in health education and health promotion.* Palo Alto, CA: Mayfield.

Our focus in this text is on health promotion, and health promotion programs are designed "to enable people to increase control over their health and its determinants by developing personal skills, embracing community action, and fostering appropriate public policies, health services and supportive environments." (WHO, 2005, p. 1).

Process or formative evaluation answers the question: Are we doing what we said we would do? That is, did we deliver the program, provide a place to meet, include handouts at our meeting, and so forth? For example, when the first effective-parenting training program was offered in Rosemont from 8 PM to 9 PM, only five parents attended. They stated that the time was too late for them to return home and complete bedtime activities for their school-age children. As a result of this formative evaluation, the time was changed to 7 PM to 8 PM, and attendance increased to 20 parents. Some authors (Green & Lewis, 1986) make a distinction between formative and process evaluation by using processes to denote the evaluation conducted during the program, whereas formative may be applied (as the name implies) at formative or preprogram stages.

Impact (or summative) evaluation is concerned with the immediate impact of a program on a target group. If your program is aimed at changing a group's knowledge and behavior relating to sexually transmitted diseases (STDs), for instance, you might build in a test to find out what they learned and what their intent is about modifying behavior. In the case of effective-parenting classes, summative evaluation criteria might include parental self-reports of changes in their attitudes toward physical punishment and disciplinary practices before and following the program, any alteration in discipline policies at Temple Elementary, and change in the number of reported incidents of child abuse.

It is in the long-term outcome evaluation, however, that you find out if the changes had a lasting and real effect. That is, did the incidence of STDs drop in this group? Because we are getting closer to the cause–effect question, careful evaluative research is needed to determine the actual contribution of the program to the outcome being measured.

Take Note ——————————————————————————

An in-depth review of evaluation research is beyond the scope of this text. There are several excellent texts that focus on evaluation research, and two examples of evaluation research are included later in this chapter.

Before considering specific evaluation strategies, it is important to consider the "evaluability" of the program. To do this, review the program plan and ask yourself the following questions:

- Are program activities stated in precise words whose concepts can be measured?
- Has a time frame for attaining the change been included?
- Are the direction and magnitude of the change included?
- Has a method of measuring the change been included?
- Are the data that will be needed to measure the objectives available at a reasonable cost?
- Are the program activities that are designed to meet the objectives plausible?

If you find in your practice that any of these questions cannot be measured in one of your plans, review Chapter 13 and amend the plan to make it as concise and complete as possible.

Take Note ——————————————————————————

A positive response to each of the above questions would be an ideal state that few programs attain. Therefore, do not despair if your program is less than perfect, but rather strive to increase your sensitivity to the issues that need to be considered in program planning to achieve optimum program evaluation.

COMPONENTS OF EVALUATION

Why collect evaluation data? To whom will the evaluation data be given, and for what purpose will they be used? What programs or activities will result from or be discontinued as a result of the evaluation? Before a strategy or method of evaluation can be selected, the reasons for and uses of the evaluation data must be established. An evaluation strategy appropriate for answering one type of evaluative question may not be useful for another. For example, if the Rosemont Health Promotion Council wanted to know the relevancy to community needs of a program on crime prevention, then questions would be asked of the participants concerning the usefulness and adequacy of the information that was given. Possible questions would cover a range of topics: Did the information make a difference as to how residents protect themselves from crime? What protection behaviors do the residents practice now that were not practiced before the program? Did the program answer the residents' questions? Did the program meet perceived needs? However, if the council wanted to know the outcome of the crime-prevention program (such as if the program decreased the incidence of crime experienced by the participants), then self-reports and community crime statistics would be monitored. Usually, questions of evaluation focus on the areas of relevancy, progress, cost-efficiency, effectiveness, and outcome.

Relevancy

Is there a need for the program? Relevancy determines the reasons for having a program or set of activities. Questions of relevancy may be more important for existing programs than for new programs. Frequently, a program, such as a blood pressure screening, is planned to meet an expressed community need. Then, the program continues for years without an evaluation of relevancy. The question should be asked routinely: Is the program still needed? Clearly, evaluation is necessary not just for new programs, but for all programs. A common constraint to beginning a new program is inadequate staff or budget. A remedy to that constraint can be a relevancy evaluation of existing programs. Staff and budgets from a program that is no longer needed can be redirected to the new program.

Progress

Are program activities following the intended plan? Are appropriate staff and materials available in the right quantity and at the right time to implement the program activities? Are expected numbers of clients participating in the scheduled program activities? Do the inputs and outputs meet some predetermined plan? Answers to these questions measure the progress of the program and are part of process or formative evaluation.

Cost-Efficiency

What are the costs of a program? What are its benefits? Are program benefits sufficient for the costs incurred? Cost-efficiency evaluation measures the relationship between the results (benefits) of a program and the costs of presenting the program (such as staff salary and materials). Cost-efficiency evaluates whether the results of a program could have been obtained less expensively through another approach. Cost–benefit analysis requires skills beyond the scope of this text, but references abound, particularly in economics and management literature.

Effectiveness (Impact)

Were program objectives met? Were the clients satisfied with the program? Were program providers satisfied with the activities and client involvement? Effectiveness focuses on formative evaluation as well as the immediate, short-term results.

Outcome

What are the long-term implications of the program? As a result of the program, what changes in behavior can be expected in 6 weeks, 6 months, or 6 years? Effectiveness measures the immediate results, whereas outcome evaluation measures whether the program activities changed the initial reason for the program. The fundamental question is this: Did the program meet its goal? (Was health improved?)

EVALUATION STRATEGIES: DATA COLLECTION AND ANALYSIS

Program evaluation incorporates consistent and ongoing collection and analysis of information, which is then used for decision making (W. K. Kellogg Foundation, 1998). As such, the choice of approach or method to collect the information is an important decision in itself and needs to be agreed on by all involved from the beginning. Realize that there is no one best approach to evaluation, but whichever approach is chosen needs to fit the questions you wish to answer.

Four key points need to be considered as you decide which method of data collection to use:

1. What resources are available for the evaluation tasks?
2. Is the method sensitive to the respondents/participants of the program?
3. How credible will your evaluation be as a result of this method?
4. What is the importance of the data to be collected—to the overall program? To participants? (W. K. Kellogg Foundation, 1998).

Consider, too, that there are several frameworks or paradigms that may inform your choices. A summary of five such paradigms is included as Table 15.2.

Taking the key points and paradigms into consideration, let us review the various methods of data collection.

Case Study

A case study looks inside a program to determine its adequacy to meet stated needs. The case-study method provides insight into an entire program and, unlike many forms of evaluation, can be started at any time during the program. The data collected during a case study include observation of program activity, reports prepared by the program, unstructured conversations with program personnel, statistical summaries of program activities, structured or unstructured interview data, and information collected through questionnaires. Subjective data and objective data can both be collected. Subjective data include information collected primarily through observations of participants or program staff. Objective data are collected

TABLE 15.2 Paradigms for Evaluation

	Natural Science Research Model	Interpretivism/ Constructivism	Feminist Methods	Participatory Evaluation	Theory-Based
Roots	Western "science"; European, white, male	Anthropology	Feminist research, power analysis	Education, community organization, public health, anthropology	Application in comprehensive community programs
Key points	Control of variables	Study through ongoing and in-depth contact with those involved	Women, girls, and minorities historically left out; conventional methods are seriously flawed	Create a more egalitarian process, make process more relevant to all, democratizing	Every social program is based on a theory—the key to understanding what is important is through identifying the theory
Approach	Hypotheticodeductive methodology, statistics	In-depth observations, interviewing	Contextual, inclusive, experiential, involved, socially relevant	Practical, useful, empowering	Developing a program logic model—or picture—to describe what works
Purpose	To explain what happened and show causal relationships between outcomes and "treatments"	To understand the targets of the program and the program's meaning to them	To include the feminine voice in all aspects of evaluation, being open to all voices	Actively engage all in process, capacity building	Revealing what works in comprehensive, community-based programs

Source: Minkler, M. (Ed.). (1997). *Community organizing and community building for health*. New Brunswick, NJ: Rutgers University Press; W. K. Kellogg Foundation. (1998). *Evaluation handbook*. Battle Creek, MI: Author.

from the organization or program documents or structured questionnaires and interviews. The distinction between subjective and objective is not readily perceptible. All questionnaires, regardless of how carefully written, have a subjective component, and, likewise, "objective" records or documents are all written by people and, therefore, introduce a subjective factor. It is best to have a mix of both objective and subjective data.

Techniques of the case study method include observation and interviews, nominal group, and Delphi technique.

Observation and Interviews

Observation is one method of collecting data for a case study. Observation can be participatory or nonparticipatory. The participant observer assumes a working role in the agency or organization and collects data about the program while working within the group. The nonparticipant observer remains an "outsider," does not assume a working role within the agency, and reviews and examines the program for designated periods.

The types of observations that are made are determined by the questions that have been asked about the program. For example, if the question is one of relevancy, the observer would concentrate on who, what, why, and when of the program. Who is using the services? Record the demographics of age, ethnicity, geographic location, educational level, and employment status. What services are the participants receiving? (For example, what services are offered in the well-child clinic? Immunizations? Physicals? Health teaching? Screening? How often are the services offered, and what are the ages of the children who use the services?) Why is the population using the offered services? (Availability? Affordability? No other options?) Lastly, when are the services accessed? (Do people come at appointed times or only when they are ill? Or do people tend to cluster at opening and closing times?)

Some data can be collected from agency records; other information can be collected by informal conversations with the participants—both the professional health care providers and the clients. When interviewing, always have a checklist of topics you want to consider, arranged in a logical sequence, along with the who, what, why, and when questions. Informal conversations, sometimes referred to as "unstructured interviews," afford the opportunity to explore with the participants their perceptions of the program. The results of unstructured interviews provide specific areas from which a "structured" interview can be developed. Recall from Chapter 13 that an interview is administered by an interviewer, whereas a questionnaire is self-administered. Observations and interviews share the problem of selective perception.

Selective Perception

Selective perception is the natural tendency of everyone to consciously classify into categories the behaviors or statements of others. These categories have been established by our cultural values, learning, and life experiences. To a certain extent, this process is desirable because it limits the number of observations that need conscious consideration and permits the rapid and effective handling of information. For example, if it was observed that a client waited 1 hour for a scheduled appointment, most people, based on the common orientation to time, would classify that observation as a negative aspect of the clinic's functioning.

Herein lies the major problem of selective perception. Statements and behaviors are classified according to the selective perception of the observer, which may be completely different from the selective perception of the client or other health care providers. The most dangerous effect of selective perception in program evaluation is when the observer has a preconception that a program will be successful or unsuccessful. This can produce a self-fulfilling prophecy because the biased observer may unconsciously record only data that support the preconceived belief. Both selective perception and self-fulfilling prophecy are sources of subjective data. Perhaps the most important point is that you should be aware of the problem of selective perception and share your observation and interview data with a mixed group of clients and health care providers. Ask the group for categorization and summation implications.

Interactiveness

Interactiveness is an additional event to be aware of during all observations. When an observer, whether participant or nonparticipant, observes and records program activities, the person's presence affects and shapes the activities observed. Productivity may increase because staff members are aware of being observed or because they are concerned about client satisfaction or dissatisfaction. All evaluation strategies can have an interactive component, but perhaps the interactive consideration is strongest in case studies because of the presence of an observer.

Nominal Group

Both the nominal group and the Delphi technique are based on the belief that the people in a program are the most knowledgeable sources on its relevancy. The nominal group technique uses a structured group meeting, during which all individuals are given a judgmental task, such as to list the functions of the program, problems of the program, or needed changes in the program. Each member is asked to write a response on paper and to not discuss it with other people. At the end of 5 to 10 minutes, all members present their ideas, and each idea is recorded (without discussion), so everyone can see all the suggestions. Once all ideas have been presented, a discussion begins, during which ideas are clarified and evaluated. After the discussion, the group votes to determine the order in which to address different areas. The nominal group technique allows all individuals to present their ideas before the entire group. Involving the entire group both decreases selective perception and promotes individual cooperation with the group's decisions because people believe they have been involved in the decision-making process.

Delphi Technique

The Delphi technique tends to be used in large survey studies, but is also useful as a case-study method. It involves a series of questionnaires and feedback reports to a designated panel of respondents. An initial questionnaire is distributed by mail to a preselected group (this could be all nursing staff members, a group of clients, or program administrators). Independently, respondents express their thoughts through the questionnaire and return it. Based on the responses of the group, a feedback report and a revised version of the questionnaire are sent to the respondents. Using the feedback information, the respondents evaluate their first answers and complete the questionnaire again. The process continues for a predetermined number of feedback rounds.

Usefulness to Evaluation

The case-study method of program evaluation can help answer questions of *relevance*. Questioning clients and health care providers helps to explore perceptions of how well the program is meeting its defined goals and to ascertain problem areas and possible solutions. The case-study method would not point to any one solution, but rather would offer several possible choices.

Questions of *progress* can also be addressed through the case-study method. The extent to which a program is meeting predetermined standards of service indicates progress. Because the case study provides an examination of the program, much can be learned if program activities are already in place.

Cost-*efficiency* of the program is difficult to evaluate using a case-study method. First, to evaluate if the program could have been offered more economically, a comparable program must exist; and, second, the case-study method is designed to look at only one program.

The method is not formatted to look at two programs and compare them. However, judgments can be made as to the operating efficiency of the program. These judgments must be based on the experience and knowledge of the evaluator and cannot be based on comparisons with other operating programs.

Effectiveness determines if the program has produced what it intended to produce immediately after the program, as opposed to the outcome, which measures long-term consequences. Although the case-study method may determine aspects of effectiveness, such as whether the aims of the program have been met in the short run, it is very difficult to measure long-term consequences unless the case-study method is conducted over a long period that allows a retrospective view of the program.

Surveys

A survey is a method of collecting information and can be used to collect evaluation information. Surveys are usually completed by self-administered questionnaires (the process used in Rosemont to determine community perception of health information needs) or by personal interviews. Surveys are formulated to describe (*descriptive* surveys) or to analyze relationships (*analytic* surveys). (Actually, most surveys can be used both to describe and to analyze.)

Surveys can be used to describe the need for a program, the actual operations of a program, or a program's effects. Along with the descriptive information, questions of analysis can be answered through a survey. For example, a survey could be used to *describe* the composition of the groups that attend crime-prevention or weight-reduction classes, as well as to *analyze* the relationship between descriptive data of sex, for instance, and weight-reduction success.

Surveys are usually performed for summative (impact) evaluation. Did the program accomplish what it was proposed to do? Was the program perceived as successful by clients? By personnel? If the program was considered successful, what parts were most helpful? Least helpful? What should be changed? Left unchanged? The questions asked by the survey are determined by the initial list of questions about program evaluation.

Like the case-study method, the answers on surveys come from the perceptions, values, and belief systems of the respondents. The response given to questions of program usefulness by the nurse who planned and implemented the program may be very different from the answers of the participants. Awareness of perception bias can direct evaluation efforts to consider the perceptions of all persons (providers, clients, and management) involved in program implementation.

Reliability and Validity

Surveys that are used for program evaluation must be concerned with the *reliability* and *validity* of the information collected. Reliability deals with the repeatability, or reproducibility, of the data (i.e., if the same questions were asked of the same people 1 week later, would the same responses be recorded?). Validity is the correctness of the information. If questions are written to evaluate knowledge, and the answers of the respondents reflect behaviors, then the questions are not valid because they do not measure what they claim to measure.

Usefulness to Evaluation

Surveys can be very valuable to answer questions of *relevance*, or the need for proposed or existing programs, especially if the perceptions of clients, providers, and management are solicited. In a similar fashion, surveys can measure *progress*. People critiquing surveys as an evaluation strategy may be concerned with the subjectivity of the survey—indeed, individual perception affects every response to every question. However, most decisions are based on subjective judgments, not objective reality. It is important to understand whose subjective impression is being used as a basis for judgment; it is imperative for community health nurses to ensure that clients' perceptions are represented alongside those of health care providers and managers.

Cost-efficiency, effectiveness, and outcome are difficult to measure using a survey. Although a survey can measure the perceived efficiency of the program or ideas on alternative ways of operating to make the program more cost-efficient, these perceptions are formed only in the context of the existing program. There is no other comparison program against which recorded perceptions can be measured. A survey can provide information on the characteristics of program activities that are perceived by the respondents to have caused changes in their health status, but these impressions are reported in the absence of any comparison group. A comparison group is especially important with regard to effectiveness and impact because it is impossible to tell if an alternative program (or no program at all) might have been more or less effective in accomplishing the same objectives.

Take Note

You may be wondering if a comparison group is so important and if perceptions cloud the evaluation with subjective impressions, then why use surveys at all? Two pluses exist for surveys: a great deal of information for program evaluation can be obtained, especially about the activities of the program from the perception of several groups; and important evaluation data can be inferred if the instrument (questionnaire or interview schedule) is reliable and valid.

Experimental Design

Completed correctly, an experimental design study can provide an answer to the crucial questions: Did the program make a difference? Are health behaviors, knowledge, and attitudes changed as a result of the program activities? Is the community healthier because of the programs offered by the Rosemont Health Promotion Council? However, the problem with experimental studies in program evaluation is that they require selective implementation, meaning that people who participate are selected through a process such as random assignment to a control group and an experimental group. For many ethical, political, and community health reasons, selective implementation is difficult to complete and is sometimes impossible. Despite these problems, the experimental study remains the best method to evaluate summative effects (outcomes) of a program and the only way to produce quantified information on whether the program made a difference.

Take Note

Reviewing the steps of the research process at this point may be of help to you in understanding the examples to follow. Indeed, each issue—such as a theoretical framework, sampling, reliability, and validity—must be addressed if an experimental design is proposed for evaluation. Your basic research text may be of help to you at this point.

The following designs are the most feasible and appropriate to health care settings. Apply the research process to each design.

TABLE 15.3 Pretest–Posttest One-Group Design

	Time 1		Time 2
Experimental group	Observation 1	Experiment	Observation 2

Pretest–Posttest One-Group Design

The pretest–posttest design applied to one group is illustrated in Table 15.3. Two observations are made, the first at Time 1 and the second at Time 2. The observation can be the prevalence of a health state (e.g., the percentage of adults in Rosemont who exercise regularly, the teenage pregnancy rate, cases of child abuse, and so on), knowledge scores, or other important community health facts. Between Time 1 and Time 2, an experiment is introduced. The experiment may be a planned program aimed at a target group, such as teen sexuality classes, or with a community-wide focus, like a crime-prevention program. The evaluation of the program is measured by considering the difference between the health state at Time 1 and the health state after the program at Time 2.

If the experiment in Table 15.3 was teen sexuality classes for 10th-grade girls at Hampton High School, Time 1 was a teen pregnancy rate of 5 per 100, and Time 2 (1 year later) was a teen pregnancy rate of 3 per 100 among the girls taking the classes, then would you agree that the teen sexuality program was responsible for the decrease in teenage pregnancies? What other information do you need to know in order to decide? (Are there other factors that could account for the decrease in the teen pregnancy rate? Perhaps family-planning programs have been focused on teenagers, or maybe local churches and social service agencies have sponsored teen sexuality programs. Teen access to and the use of contraceptive methods may have increased, or laws regarding teen access to contraceptive methods may have changed.) None of these factors can be eliminated as unassociated with the decrease in the teen pregnancy rate. To eliminate other possible explanations for program effectiveness, a control group must be added.

Pretest–Posttest Two-Group Design

A pretest–posttest with a control group design is illustrated in Table 15.4. The design has both an experimental group and a control group. At Time 1, an observation is made of both the experimental and control groups. Between Time 1 and Time 2, an experiment is introduced with the experimental group. At Time 2, second observations are made on both the experimental and control groups. Program evaluation is the difference between Observations 1 and 2 for the experimental group when compared with the comparison group (which has been selected to be as similar as possible to the experimental group). Will the pretest–posttest with a control group design eliminate the effect of outside factors that occurred simultaneously with the experiment and that might account for the change between Observation 1 and Observation 2, the very problem that plagued the pretest–posttest one-group design? The answer is yes if the experimental and control groups are similar.

To explain, let us return to Rosemont and the idea of a teen sexuality class for 10th-grade students at Hampton High School. If 10th-grade students, similar in social, economic, and geographic characteristics, were randomly selected and then randomly assigned to the

TABLE 15.4 Pretest–Posttest Two-Group Design

	Time 1		Time 2
Experimental group	Observation 1	Experiment	Observation 2
Control group	Observation 1		Observation 2

experimental or control group, it could be assumed that any other factors that influenced the experimental group would also affect the control group. However, frequently the decision is made that all students must be given the same program, thereby eliminating a comparison group. This also becomes an ethical problem: If we think this is an effective program and the teens will benefit from it, is it ethical to withhold it from any of the teens?

At the Rosemont Health Promotion Council, when the information was received that all 10th graders must be given a teen sexuality program that had been proposed by the school nurse as a response to an increasing number of teen pregnancies, the suggestion was made that perhaps another high school could be used as a control group. How would you respond to that suggestion? Perhaps another high school class of 10th graders could be used, if the students were similar in social, economic, and geographic characteristics to the students at Hampton High (an unlikely situation).

Another possibility mentioned by the Rosemont Health Promotion Council was to offer the program in one school year to one half of the Hampton High 10th graders (using the other half as a control) and then in the following year to offer the program to the remaining students. This method would ensure that all students would be given the program, but would also allow for an experimental pretest–posttest design for evaluation.

A third method that was suggested to ensure an experimental design was to give the control group sexuality education and give the experimental group sexuality education plus assertiveness training. The assertiveness training would differentiate the groups and allow an experimental design. All the suggestions were discussed with school officials, and it was decided to offer a traditional sex education class to half the 10th-grade students (the control group); the remaining students (the experimental group) would get the traditional sex education material but would also receive classes on assertiveness training and values clarification. This design will not allow for the evaluation of traditional sex education classes versus no information, but it will provide all students with the health information (an ethical compromise) and allow for the evaluation of a traditional program on sexuality versus that traditional program plus assertiveness and values clarification information (an approach to reduce teenage pregnancies that is supported in the literature).

 Take Note

Notice that the decision to offer information on assertiveness and values clarification as part of teen sexuality classes was based on documentation from the literature. Rosemont is not the first community to offer health promotion programs. Many communities have assessed the health status and perceived health needs of the residents and have followed up with planned and implemented programs that have been evaluated, with the results reported in the literature. One contribution that the community health nurse can make is to review and synthesize the results of similar programs and present this information to the community for use in decision making. After the program topics have been decided, you should begin a literature review to study the ways in which other communities have addressed and evaluated similar programs.

Usefulness to Evaluation

An experimental design can yield data on whether a program has produced the desired *outcomes* when compared with the absence of such a program or, alternatively, whether one program strategy has produced better results with regard to the desired outcomes than some other strategy. However, the experimental design is not useful for the evaluation of program progress or program cost-efficiency.

Monitoring (Process)

Monitoring measures the difference between the program plan and what has actually happened. Monitoring focuses on the sequence of activities of the program, specifically, how the program is to be implemented (the activities), by whom (the personnel and other resources), and when (the timing of activities). Monitoring is usually done with a chart, and, although there are several different styles of charts, all arrange activities in a sequence and specify the time allotted to complete each task. Figure 15.1 shows an example of a monitoring chart.

Monitoring Charts

To construct a monitoring chart for your program plan, information is needed on the *inputs* (resources necessary to carry out the program such as personnel, equipment, and finances), the *process* (the program activities, their sequencing, and timing), and *outputs* (the expected results of the program, including immediate and long-term health effects). It is helpful to make a list of inputs, processes, and outputs.

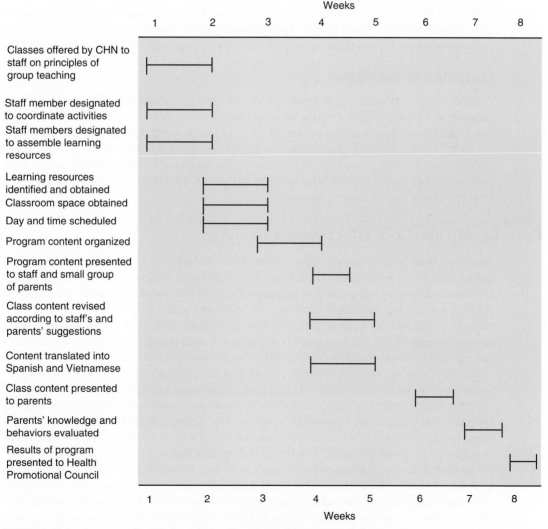

FIGURE 15.1   Sequence of events for program: Common health problems of children.

Take Note

You have already recorded this information as part of your program plan. Refer to Chapter 13 and note that resources, program activities, and learning objectives were listed for the proposed class on common health problems of children. Resources are the same as inputs; program activities correspond to processes; and learning objectives designate expected outputs. So all that remains is to place the data into a chart for monitoring.

Figure 15.1 lists the inputs, processes, and outputs for the proposed program in Rosemont, along with a time sequence for beginning and completing each event. It is difficult to decide on the amount of time that will be needed to complete any task. After assessing the organizational structure and management methods of the agency, you can determine the approximate amounts of time that will be needed to complete the activities of the program. Monitoring charts are easy to formulate, and provide useful information for measuring program evaluation if the chart is realistic. The Further Readings list at the end of this chapter includes references to several other types of monitoring charts, including the Gantt, Program Evaluation and Review Technique (PERT), and Critical Path Method (CPM). These provide a slightly different variation of the basic time-sequencing, activities-monitoring chart that appears in Figure 15.1.

Usefulness to Evaluation

A monitoring chart measures progress and can be used to evaluate whether a program is on schedule and within budget. Perhaps no other evaluation method is as perfectly suited to *process evaluation* as the monitoring chart. In addition, monitoring can provide information on the *cost-efficiency* of the program by measuring the average cost of the resources required per client served. The effectiveness of the program can be measured by monitoring the chart if the chart records outputs achieved. Monitoring charts cannot determine program relevance or the long-term impact of a program, however.

Cost–Benefit and Cost-Effectiveness Analyses

Much has been written and discussed about the escalating cost of health care services and ways that cost can be reduced. The turmoil over health care reform in the United States and the intense debate regarding the pros and cons of various alternative approaches to health care delivery, such as the Affordable Care Act, are testimony to the need to contain cost and yet increase access and maintain quality. Every program has a dollar price both in terms of the resources needed to offer the program (e.g., personnel and equipment) and the dollar benefits to be gained from improved health (such as increased worker productivity).

Two of the most common methods of analyzing the economic costs and benefits of a program are cost–benefit analysis (CBA) and cost-effectiveness analysis (CEA). Both CBA and CEA are formal analytic techniques that list all costs (direct and indirect) and consequences (negative and positive) of a particular program. The distinction between CBA and CEA is based on the value that is placed on the consequences of a program. In CBA, consequences or benefits of a program are valued in terms of dollars; this makes it possible to compare different projects, because all measurement is made in dollars. Therefore, the worth of a project can be judged by asking if dollar benefits exceed dollar costs and, if so, by how much. In contrast, CEA does not place a dollar value on either the consequences or the costs of a project. Another outcome is used for programs whose benefits or costs are difficult to measure (e.g., how could a dollar value be placed on each suicide prevented by a primary prevention program to decrease teenage suicide?). Therefore, CEA, unlike CBA, does not determine if total benefits exceed total costs.

However, CEA can be used to compare programs with similar goals and objectives (e.g., two different primary prevention approaches to decrease the incidence of teenage suicide share the same benefits, so only costs need be compared—a CEA). A CEA can also be used if the costs of alternative programs are the same or if only a given amount of money exists and the objective is to select the program with the greatest benefits (not measured in dollar terms). The decision is obvious; select the program that produces the most effectiveness (i.e., the most benefits per dollar spent or the least cost for each unit [individual, family, or community] benefited).

The choice between CBA and CEA depends on the type of questions and programs considered. Neither technique is superior to the other. Both techniques can be used in planning for future programs or as an evaluation strategy of present or past programs. The actual procedures for completing a CBA or CEA are beyond the scope of this book; however, several references that include the procedural steps are listed in the Further Readings list. Obviously, both CBA and CEA are strategies for measuring program cost-efficiency and do not address the issues of relevancy, progress, effectiveness, or impact.

Summary

Several methods of evaluation have been presented and discussed. No one method will evaluate the components of relevancy, progress, cost-efficiency, effectiveness, and outcome equally well. It is important to be knowledgeable about different methods of program evaluation and to discuss the benefits and limitations of each with the community as the program is being planned and before program implementation occurs. Table 15.5 presents a summary table of appropriate evaluation methods for program components. Once evaluation methods are selected, the methods (case study, experimental design, or monitoring charts) become part of the program plan.

You may be wondering which evaluation methods were used to evaluate the health promotion programs in Rosemont. A variety were used. To evaluate the relevancy of the health promotion programs (crime-prevention and effective-parenting classes), nominal group meetings were scheduled, and both health care providers and consumers attended. In addition, the use of rates and demographics of the participants using the health promotion programs was assessed, as were the participants' perceptions of the value of the information. Program progress was evaluated with monitoring charts such as the one presented in Figure 15.1. The effectiveness and impact of individual programs were evaluated with knowledge, attitude, and behavioral intent surveys (i.e., questionnaires, interviews, and tests) given to participants before the program, immediately after the program, and at predetermined follow-up times (6 weeks and 3 months after the program). As often as was feasible, an evaluation research

TABLE 15.5 Examination of the Appropriateness of Different Evaluation Methods for Program Components

Components	Method			
	Case Study	Survey	Experimental	Monitoring
Relevancy	Yes	Yes	No	No
Progress	Yes	Yes	No	Yes
Cost-efficiency	No	No	Yes	Yes
Cost-effectiveness	Some	No	Yes	Some
Impact	No	No	Yes	No

design was followed, such as a one-group pretest–posttest. Additional measures of effectiveness and impact were community statistics on crime, child abuse, and teenage pregnancies before as compared to after the program, as well as health policy changes that affected the residents of Rosemont (e.g., access of minors to contraceptives, disciplinary practices in the public schools, and financial eligibility requirements for health services). CEA was completed on several of the programs.

You are ready now for program implementation and the reinitiation of the nursing process; namely, assessment of the program's effects. As you implement the planned program, data will be added to the community assessment profile, which will demand addition, deletion, and revision of the community nursing diagnoses and the associated program plans and interventions. Let us take a final look at the community-as-partner model (see Fig. 10.4) and ask: Will the planned programs assist the community to attain, regain, maintain, and promote health? Strengthen the community's ability to resist stressors? Enhance the community's competence and self-reliance?

 Take Note

It is fitting that the final chapter of this section on the application of the nursing process in community health nursing ends with questions. Community health nursing is the constant questioning, prodding, probing, and pondering of the health status of a population. Although individual and family health are always important, the uniqueness of our field is the application of nursing techniques to the health of a community. Each community is unique and special. No other community is quite like the one in which you are practicing community health nursing. We have enjoyed sharing the uniqueness of Rosemont with you and the application of the nursing process to community health nursing.

Critical Thinking Questions

Describe an evaluation plan for your intervention chosen in Chapter 14:

1. Which program evaluation type (process, impact, outcome) will you use? Why?
2. What method will you use? Provide rationale.
3. Who will be involved in the evaluation?
4. How will you collect data that are sensitive to your target audience?
5. How credible will your evaluation be? Describe your rationale.

REFERENCES

Green, L. W., & Lewis, F. M. (1986). Measurement and evaluation in health education and health promotion. Palo Alto, CA: Mayfield.

World Health Organization (2005). The Bangkok Charter for Health Promotion in a Globalized World. Accessed March 17, 2014 http://www.who.int/mediacentre/news/releases/2005/pr34/en/index.html

W. K. Kellogg Foundation. (1998). Evaluation handbook. Battle Creek, MI: Author.

FURTHER READINGS

Aronson, R. E., Wallis, A. B., O'Campo, P. J., Whitehead, T. L., & Schafer, P. (2007). Ethnographically informed community evaluation: A framework and approach for evaluating community-based initiatives. *Maternal and Child Health Journal, 11*(2), 97–109.

Baatiema, L., Skovdal, M., Rifkin, S., & Campbell, C. (2013). Assessing participation in a community-based health planning and services programme in Ghana. *BMC Health Services Research*, *13*, 233. Retrieved January 4, 2014, from http://www.biomedcentral.com/1472-6963/13/233

Boulmetis, J., & Dutwin, P. (2005). *The ABCs of evaluation: Timeless techniques for project managers*. San Francisco, CA: Jossey Bass.

Diem, E., & Moyer, A. (2010). Development and testing of tools to evaluate public health nursing clinical education at the baccalaureate level. *Public Health Nursing*, *27*(30), 285–293.

Fatar, K. H. (2007). Enhancing new students' perceptions of nursing using a Healthy People 2010 group project. *The Journal of Nursing Education*, *46*(2), 96.

Gallivan, J., Greenberg, R., & Brown, C. (2008). The National Diabetes Education Program evaluation framework: How to design an evaluation of a multifaceted public health education program. *Preventing Chronic Disease*, *5*(4), 1–8.

Garcia, A. (2011). Cognitive interviews to test and refine questionnaires. *Public Health Nursing*, *28*(5), 444–450.

Griffith, K. N., & Scheier, L. M. (2013, November). Did we get our money's worth? Bridging economic and behavioral measures of program success in adolescent drug prevention. *International Journal of Environmental Research and Public Health*, *10*(11), 5908–5935.

Issel, L. M. (2014). *Health program planning and evaluation: A practical, systematic approach for community health* (3rd ed.). Burlington, MA: Jones and Bartlett Learning.

Joventino, E. S., Ximenes, L. B., Almeida, P. C., & Oria, M. O. B. (2012). The maternal self-efficacy scale for preventing early childhood diarrhea: Validity and reliability. *Public Health Nursing*, *30*(2), 150–158.

Kegler, M. C., Norton, B. L., & Aronson, R. E. (2008). Strengthening community leadership: Evaluation findings from the California Healthy Cities and Communities Program. *Health Promotion Practice*, *9*(2), 170–179.

MacDonald, S. E., Newburn-Cook, C. V., Schop£ocher, D., & Richter, S. (2009). Addressing nonresponse bias in postal surveys. *Public Health Nursing*, *26*(1), 95–105.

Martin, K. S., Wolff, M., Lonczak, M., Chambers, M., Cooke, C., & Whitney, G. (2014). Formative research to examine collaboration between special supplemental nutrition program for woman, infants, and children and head start programs. *Maternal and Child Health Journal*, *18*(1), 326–332.

McMillan, L. R., Smith-Hendricks, C., & Gore, T. (2010). A volunteer citizen-servant pilot program using tailored messages to empower Alabamians to live healthier lives. *Public Health Nursing*, *27*(6), 513–519.

Minkler, M., & Wallerstein, N. (2008). *Community based participatory research for health: From process to outcomes* (2nd ed.). San Francisco, CA: Jossey-Bass.

Mulroy, E. A. (2008). University community partnerships that promote evidence-based macro practice. *Journal of Evidence-Based Social Work*, *5*(3–4), 497–517.

O'Connell, B., Heslop, L., & Fennessy, H. (2010). An evaluation of a wellness guide for older carers living in the community. *Public Health Nursing*, *27*(4), 302–309.

Prochaska, J. M., Mauriello, L., Dyment, S., & Gokbayrak, S. (2011). Designing a health behavior change program for dissemination to underserved pregnant women. *Public Health Nursing*, *28*(6), 548–555.

Rew, L., Hoke, M. M., Horner, S. D., & Walker, L. (2009). Development of a dynamic model to guide health disparities research. *Nursing Outlook*, *57*(3), 132–142.

Rossi, P. H., Lipsey, M. W., & Freeman, H. E. (2004). *Evaluation: A systematic approach* (7th ed.). Thousand Oaks, CA: Sage.

Roy, K., Haddix, A. C., Ikeda, R. M., Curry, C. W., Truman, B. I., & Thacker, S. B. (2009). Monitoring progress toward CDC's health protection goals: Health outcome measures by life stage. *Public Health Reports*, *124*(2), 304–316.

Walker, L. O., Kim, S., Sterling, B. S., & Latimer, L. (2010). Developing health promotion interventions: A multi-source method applied to weight loss among low-income postpartum women. *Public Health Nursing*, *27*(2), 188–195.

West, G. F., Hayden, M. R., & Benjamin, C. R. (2012). Accuracy of adults' perception of childhood obesity in a military environment. *Public Health Nursing*, *30*(4), 343–350.

Zandee, G. L., Bossenbroek, D., Slager, D., & Gordon, B. (2013). Teams of community health workers and nursing students effect health promotion of underserved urban neighborhoods. *Public Health Nursing*, *30*(5), 439–447.

Practicing With Diverse Communities

Practicing With
Diverse Communities

CHAPTER 16

Promoting Healthy Partnerships With School Communities

Nina M. Fredland

LEARNING OBJECTIVES

After studying this chapter, you should be able to:

1. Design programs that are specific to the specialized school setting at the primary, secondary, and tertiary levels of prevention.

2. Design culturally relevant, developmentally appropriate, environmentally responsible and sustainable programs that appeal to school-aged youth and are congruent with the goals of Healthy People 2020.

3. Implement creative programs that nurture healthy relationships and model healthy behavior to school-aged children, their parents, school faculty, and staff.

4. Utilize the community resources of the school's geographic community, and involve the local residents in program planning and implementation.

5. Create a safe school climate that is conducive to learning and promotes healthy development.

Introduction

Most health care professionals would agree that a major goal for the 21st century would be to create a nation of children who are optimally well so they can lead long, happy, productive lives. This goal is congruent with the overarching goals of the Healthy People 2020:

1. Eliminate preventable disease, disability, injury, and premature death.
2. Achieve health equity, eliminate disparities, and improve the health of all groups.
3. Create social and physical environments that promote good health for all.
4. Promote healthy development and healthy behaviors across every stage of life (US Department of Health and Human Services, Healthy People 2020, n.d.-a).

How do we as nurses achieve this goal? This chapter focuses on strategies and partnerships within the community setting of the school. The school nurse or the public health nurse, depending on the community, is ideally situated to provide health care to school-aged children. Nurses with advanced preparation in child health, such as pediatric nurse practitioners and family nurse practitioners, are also well prepared to initiate partnerships with schools. An ideal model is one in which the school nurse or public health nurse collaborates with the advanced practice nurse. In this way, health promotion, risk reduction, disease prevention, and health maintenance are important components included within the delivery of health care. School-aged children are a captive audience, and their parents/guardians are closely connected to the school community. This situation makes the school community an ideal center for health promotion activities for the entire family.

The health of our nation's children has been an area of concern for some time. Casual observations at any school reveal a high percentage of overweight children, youngsters easily fatigued while running around the playground, and children choosing nonnutritious snacks. Obviously, these children are at a disadvantage; their health is compromised. One has only to observe adult role models to understand why children are making unhealthy choices. Recently, there seems to be a backlash against healthy food choices, as evidenced by fast food meal options that continue to promote large portions of high-fat/high-calorie foods. A sticker prominently displayed on a car bumper captured this notion with the slogan: *My Dad Can Eat More Than Your Dad.* Therefore, health-education approaches must be comprehensive and include the children as well as all groups of individuals involved in their care and nurturing. For the purposes of this chapter, these key adults, together with the children and adolescents they serve, are referred to as the school community. The school community encompasses:

- School-aged children and adolescents
- Parents and guardians
- School personnel (faculty, staff, and administrators)
- Neighborhood residents, business owners, and service providers.

Healthy People 2010 started as a grassroots initiative in the 1990s following the Surgeon General's Report of 1979 (U.S. Department of Health and Human Services, n.d.; U.S. Department of Health and Human Services, Office of Disease Prevention and Health Promotion, n.d.). Healthy People 2020 builds on the 10 priority areas of Healthy People 2010 for health education for school-aged children/adolescents: unintentional injury, violence, suicide, tobacco use and addiction, alcohol and other drug use, unintended pregnancy, HIV/AIDS and sexually transmitted infection, unhealthy dietary patterns, inadequate physical activity, and environmental health. (More information about the development of the Healthy People Initiative is available at http://www.healthypeople.gov/2020/about/history.aspx.) There is a Healthy People Coordinator in each state or territory. For regular updates on the collaborative campaign, webinars and events or to get involved visit http://www.healthypeople.gov/2020/GetInvolved/ UpcomingEvents.aspx and/or subscribe to Healthy People Listserv (US Department of Health and Human Services, Healthy People 2020, n.d.-b).

In addition to promoting optimal health and preventing illness through the education of all members of the school community, school health programs must strive to identify and resolve existing health problems. Therefore, comprehensive school health programs should focus on delivering health services mandated by state laws and the individual school system as well as on health education. Additionally, both internal and external environmental issues are critical areas of assessment and intervention for school nurses. Advanced Practice Nurses and Community Health Nurses are well educated in Public Health issues and ideally suited to participate in health policy decisions affecting our nation's children. The Affordable Care Act is an opportunity to promote health through prevention strategies, discussed later in this chapter. Twenty-six areas for prevention are identified under the law related to children, and many insurers are now covering these programs at no cost to the consumer, including hearing screening for all newborns, autism assessment for toddlers 18 to 24 months, and depression and substance abuse assessments for adolescents, to mention a few. More information is available at http://www.hhs.gov/healthcare/prevention/children/index.html.

DELIVERING HEALTH SERVICES FOR HEALTH PROMOTION

Each state mandates certain requirements to maintain the health of school-aged children. Vision and hearing screening programs are required. Measurements of height, weight, and blood pressure are also usually part of these health services. Spinal, nutritional, dental, and developmental screening may also be required in the school setting. Some states now require school nurses to screen for Acanthosis Nigricans (AN), a skin condition that is associated with high levels of insulin in the body and the development of type 2 diabetes mellitus later in life. Initiating preventive measures early on such as nutrition counseling and exercise regimens may be enough to delay or even prevent diabetes from occurring in these individuals. Texas is one such state where AN is mandated, and certification of school nurses is implemented through the Border Health Office (The University of Texas-Pan American Border Health Office, 2011). Check out this website to learn more: http://www.utpa.edu/bho/PDF_Documents/TRAT2DC_Legislative_Report_2011. pdf. To find out about screening requirements in your state, contact your local state health department. The following list outlines some common state requirements:

Vision: Screen all new students within 120 days of enrollment. Screen students in kindergarten, 1st, 3rd, 5th, 7th, and 9th grades by May of each school year.
Hearing: Screen all new students within 120 days of enrollment. Screen students in kindergarten, 1st, 3rd, 5th, 7th, and 9th grades by May of each school year.
Spinal: Screen all 6th- and 9th-grade students.

Certification is required to perform vision and hearing screening. Certification training is available through state health departments or through individuals the state has designated with this authority. To find out how to receive certification training, contact your state health department. Certification for registered nurses is not usually required for spinal screening, yet ancillary personnel or volunteer assistants are required to have attended an approved educational program. Therefore, it is important that student nurses be taught a thorough procedure for assessing spinal deformities as part of their health assessment curriculum. Some argue that owing to limited resources and a low yield related to identifying spinal deformities that actually progress to require surgical intervention, school-based spinal screening is unnecessary. Some states have moved to eliminate this requirement. Nurses and many orthopedic physicians would agree that the potential to prevent severe cardiac and respiratory complications in even a few children is worth the effort. Therefore, nurses should adopt a holistic approach, using the preferred terminology of "spinal screening" and not "scoliosis screening," which focuses on only one condition and medicalizes the entire process. Spinal screening, a more positive term, is an opportunity to assess a child's overall health as well as the condition of the spine. In addition, the nurse can take advantage of brief teaching moments that can be individualized.

When screenings are conducted privately and confidentially, the nurse can assess for many things, such as nutritional status, dermatological conditions, the AN marker, bruising, etc. During the process, the nurse has an opportunity to engage the child in health-related conversation. This may be a follow-up to a previous visit to the health room. A question such as *What did you have for breakfast this morning?* can lead to a discussion reinforcing the importance of a nutritious breakfast. What barriers might prevent the child from eating a healthy breakfast, and what self-responsibility measures can the child take toward the goal of getting adequate nutrition in the morning? A few simple suggestions can empower even a very young child, and this health education can occur within the context of "spinal screening."

Immunizations are required by state law to be current and on file before or on the first day of school, although a school district can establish a short grace period, usually 30 days. Immunization requirements must be strictly supported by the school administration. Each state sets a standard for immunizations; a school district can increase the requirements but must include the minimum standard. For example, tuberculosis (TB) screening for school-aged children may not be required by state law; however, school districts can set a higher standard and require new students to have an approved skin test for TB screening at the time of initial enrollment. Furthermore, school districts can require school personnel to be tested annually. Some institutional systems are now requiring titers for selected immunizations. The Centers for Disease Control and Prevention (CDC) is the best source for recommended immunization schedules for children and adults. It would be helpful to familiarize yourself with the CDC website (http://www.cdc.gov) and the current recommended immunization schedule for school-aged children because these requirements change frequently.

Although most parents are vigilant about immunizing their children in a timely manner, some parents question the need for or safety of some vaccines or the practice of receiving multiple vaccines at one visit. They may have concerns about immunizing in general, or they may have specific questions related to select vaccines, the combinant forms, or the recommended timing. Nurses in school settings are well positioned to respond to such concerns, and provide parents and guardians with accurate information to make informed choices about immunizing their children. The CDC provides reliable information in both English and Spanish to help health care professionals and consumers better understand vaccine issues and maintain "herd immunity." These resources, including parent information sheets, can be easily accessed at www.cdc.gov/vaccines or 800-CDC-INFO (232-4636).

In addition to conducting mass screening programs, a nurse in the school setting identifies and monitors existing health problems, both acute and chronic, such as common respiratory infections and asthma. The school nurse is a referral agent and case manager, and offers education within the scope of nursing practice. For many economically disadvantaged families, the school nurse is the first line of defense.

HEALTH EDUCATION FOR HEALTH PROMOTION

Major issues affecting children in the United States can be categorized under headings of nutrition; interpersonal violence; substance abuse; mental health issues; safety; sexuality; and environmental hazards such as lead, asbestos, and air pollution. Specific topics from which you might select health-education programs are listed in Box 16.1. Some of these topics are more appropriate for children, parents, or teachers. As you are thinking of the topic, consider the audience you are targeting. For example, healthy food choices might be geared toward easy recipes that children can prepare. There are a number of cookbooks written with children in mind; a favorite is the American Heart Association's (AHA) *Healthy Recipes Kids Love Cookbook*. Alternatively, have students compile their own cookbook with simple healthy recipes. This activity can be conducted at grade level or as a schoolwide fundraiser. Box 16.1 is not exhaustive; it is designed to promote ideas. Consider how you might assess interest for any of the programs. Contrary to grocery store displays (which emphasize unhealthy choices by devoting whole aisles to soda pop or front aisle displays of unhealthy snacks and processed foods), children's museums often have displays and play areas that challenge children to make healthier food choices. Children can be taught to recognize devious marketing techniques at an early age as a counter measure.

Health Promotion Programs for School-Aged Children

Programs for children and adolescents in the school setting must be age-appropriate. For example, breast self-examination and testicular self-examination are most likely not appropriate material for elementary school children. It is critical to assess the developmental and maturity level of the children before deciding on the educational content of a program or a strategy.

Box 16.1 Health Education Program Ideas

Nutrition
Healthy food choices
Healthy recipes for busy families
Healthy lunches children can prepare
Disordered eating (such as anorexia, bulimia, and compulsive eating)

Violence
Domestic violence—effects on children and sources of help for the whole family
Discipline versus child abuse
Anger management/impulse control
Bullying behaviors
Dating violence
Date rape/acquaintance rape
Gang behavior
Signs of child abuse/incest

Substance Use
Cigarettes and chewing tobacco
Underage drinking
Illicit drugs (marijuana, crack, cocaine, inhalants, speed, ecstasy, heroin, and so forth)

Mental Health Issues
Self-esteem
Attention deficit disorder/hyperactivity disorder
Depression
Suicide

Personal Safety
"Latchkey" kids
Problem-solving/decision-making skills

Recreational Safety
Bicycles, in-line skates, sports
Vehicle safety (seat belts, booster seats, riding in open vehicles)
Water safety (swimming, boating, skiing)

Sexuality
Personal hygiene
Teenage pregnancy
Teen parenting
Sexually transmitted diseases

Environmental
Internal (air, water, space), external (pollution, noise)
Psychological (grade stress, parent–child discord, parent–teacher and teacher–teacher conflicts, peer harassment)

Societal Influences
Changing family structure
Peer pressure
Media influences (video games, films, television)

Even if you think you know how to relate to a certain age group, each class is different. The children may be in a very young class for their grade level, or they may be a very advanced group. The students may or may not be well socialized. Several may have attention deficit disorder or exhibit hyperactivity. Students are sometimes mainstreamed despite having considerable behavioral issues that can affect the class group dynamics. Risky behaviors may be more likely to emerge earlier in such instances.

Important information is gained from observing the student population before planning programs. Always visit the classroom and observe how the students and teachers interact. Classroom management skills are essential. It is difficult to manage the classroom successfully when the nurse's contact with the youngsters is only occasional. Relying on the regular classroom teacher for assistance always works best. Unfortunately, the amount of time that classroom teachers have to devote to programs beyond the prescribed curriculum is limited. They may not feel that they can assist with programs beyond the prescribed curriculum duties. Therefore, it is critical to involve key people such as the teachers, counselors, school nurses, and parents from the very beginning of the planning phase of health programs and to choose programs that are well developed and require minimal preplanning. For example, the AHA has a program called Healthier Kids, and many resources are available on the following website: http://www.heart.org/HEARTORG/GettingHealthy/HealthierKids/Healthier-Kids_UCM_304156_SubHomePage.jsp. Outlining the expectations of the key people will contribute to the overall success of the program and help them become vested in the outcomes of the project. Such an approach is usually well received by students, administrators, teachers, and parents. Programs that are research based can provide evidence of successful outcomes. These data can be shared with faculty, staff, and parents to further the buy-in for implementing the specific program.

Another consideration is marketing your program. It may be a great idea, but if no one attends or follows through, it will be a waste of time and resources. Use flyers, bulletin boards, and public address announcements to reach your audiences. Try various strategies to pique interest. For example, brightly colored signs and charts; guessing games; poster contests; door-decorating competitions; and age-appropriate, healthy food rewards (e.g., juice bars, fruit) are a few suggestions. Involving the students in the promotion of the program is ideal. The following are examples of health promotion ideas for school-aged children:

- Red Ribbon Week
- Breast self-examination/Testicular self-examination (teens)
- Muscle Mover Club, Triathlon or Walk-a-Thon, Swim to Bermuda or Ride to Alaska
- Monthly health bulletin board
- Make a cookbook or start a vegetable garden
- Pet responsibility
- Arts-based interventions

The following sections discuss a few of these health promotion programs.

Red Ribbon Week

The Red Ribbon Campaign was established in 1988 by the U.S. Congress. Each year a week in October is set aside to celebrate being drug free. Red Ribbon Week has now become a standard in many schools. The goal is to increase the awareness of the dangers associated with the use of tobacco, alcohol, and other drugs. The internet has many examples of how different schools across the nation celebrate the week. See Box 16.2 for a sample agenda for a week's program focusing on drug abuse prevention, which can be incorporated into the curriculum of an elementary school. Each student recites a promise to stay away from drugs and wears a red ribbon for the week.

Box 16.2 Sample Agenda for Red Ribbon Week

Monday: Hold a flag ceremony and have the student body recite the drug-free pledge.

PLEDGE:
I pledge to be drug free and support the *(state)* Red
Ribbon Campaign by taking a stand against alcohol and drug abuse

---

Signature
Designate a place for pledge signing for the students, faculty, and staff.
Display the pledge cards in a central location.
Have a group of children, parents, and school staff deliver the signed pledge cards to an official person in city government (e.g., the mayor). Have red ribbons delivered to all classes by 5th graders (or oldest students in school). Ask that each student wear a red ribbon. Decorate school grounds with red ribbons.

Tuesday:	Wear red to school on this day.
	Hold a drug-free poster contest in art classes.
Wednesday:	Have a classroom door-decorating contest.
	Display finished posters in halls.
Thursday:	Hold drug prevention programs per grade levels.
Friday:	Judge posters and doors.
	Gather for an assembly and drug-free pep rally.
	Listen to a motivational speaker.
	Perform drug-free songs and cheers.
	Announce contest winters.
Saturday/Sunday:	Have a community parade.

For more ideas check out the many red ribbon week websites. Search via www.google.com and insert the words *red ribbon week.*
http://www.imdrugfree.com is a good one!

The community should be involved in the program along with the students. Parents can be invited to some programs. The parents' organization can be asked to decorate the school with red ribbons. Community leaders (e.g., church, civic, and police) can judge contests. The police and fire departments can facilitate a parade route and provide security. Media coverage, such as local newspapers and radio and television stations, is an important strategy that schools should use. (Often, worthwhile events are not covered by the media simply because media personnel have not been notified. Why not highlight good news?) Older students and campus leaders can influence younger students by positive peer pressure, such as wearing their ribbons, participating in all activities, and having a major role in organizing and implementing the activities.

It is very important to give clear messages to young people, particularly on the subject of drugs. The nurse should select speakers very carefully. Recovering drug abusers should not be used to speak to groups of students who are not users. It is also risky to choose high-profile role models, such as well-known sports or media individuals, who may be positive non–drug users one day, but may appear in the news media at a later time for using drugs or for violent behavior. Invite ordinary community members to come to the school and share their success stories of living a drug-free life. Consider asking the students to give 1-minute talks on why they are not going to use drugs. Have a poem or "smart saying" contest. Get the speech or debate club involved.

Muscle Mover Club, Triathlon, or Walk-a-Thon

The Muscle Mover Club encourages physical activity by rewarding aerobic exercise, such as walking, running, swimming, and biking. Each child receives a badge and adds stickers for city blocks or track laps completed. Healthy competition can be encouraged by racing to a goal either individually or as a team or classroom. Another strategy is to include parents by having them sign off on triathlon or walk-a-thon mileage sheets. Encourage parents to do the activity with their children. A parent/teacher bulletin board recognizing athletic achievement, such as running a 5-mile race or marathon, highlights adults leading healthy lifestyles. Elementary school-aged children are very proud to have their parents and teachers value their achievements. They are also delighted when healthy behaviors their parents engage in are acknowledged and appreciated by their teachers and school administrators. In addition to health promotion, these strategies reinforce positive adult role modeling, which is so important in a child's formative years. Although research has typically focused on preventing risky behaviors, a recent emphasis has been on increasing protective factors—such as school connectedness, parental presence, and having a meaningful relationship with at least one caring adult—which are essential elements to support positive child outcomes. The CDC (2009) has developed six strategies designed to improve school connections; they are available at http://www.cdc.gov/healthyyouth/adolescenthealth/connectedness.htm.

Health Promotion Programs for Parents and Relatives

The following are ideas for healthy partnerships with parents:

- Parent information sessions
- Parent peer groups
- Late breakfast meetings; "second cup of coffee meeting"
- Grandparents' day
- Breast cancer awareness
- Parents' nutrition committee

The most difficult part of planning health promotion activities that include parents is timing. Most parents are employed and have very little flexibility in their work schedules. Breakfast meetings that are short and occur as children are brought to school may be well attended. Issues must appeal to parents, and it is always a good idea to conduct a "needs assessment" before deciding on topics. In this way, you can include important health information as well as meet parental expectations. Respecting the time constraints of parents and guardians fosters rapport and in turn encourages involvement. Several ideas are presented in the following sections.

Programs to Promote Healthy Habits

Curbing Childhood Overweight/Obesity

Globally and nationally childhood overweight/obesity is considered a major public health challenge for the 21st century. Over the past three decades the rates of childhood overweight/obesity have increased steadily and dramatically, with approximately 170 million children worldwide deemed overweight (WHO, 2012). Industrialized nations have had the highest prevalence rates, but middle and low income nations are catching up. Government, media, communities, schools, and families must continue their efforts to sustain healthy nutrition and support safe, active environments. The WHO has developed population-based policies and initiative aimed at combating childhood by advocating for multicomponent interventions beginning in the day care setting (2012). Suggested areas to address include topics such as nutrition labeling, marketing of unhealthy foods and beverages to children, food taxes and subsidizations, and funding for health promotion and physical activity campaigns.

An alarming fact is that one in eight (12%) of preschoolers qualify as obese according to the Centers for Disease Control and Prevention (CDC, 2013). Recent progress has been noted, with 19 states reporting a decrease in preschool obesity rates between 2008 and 2011. However, this highlights the fact that a comprehensive strategy is needed to reverse the trend among all children, especially because children who are obese in preschool are five times more likely to be overweight or obese in adulthood. Excess weight is recognized as a potential risk factor for chronic conditions and has been associated with heart disease, hypertension and stroke, type 2 diabetes, some types of cancer (CDC, 2012a, http://www.cdc.gov/obesity/causes/health .html). In addition to chronic disease risks, there is the more immediate concern of social discrimination. This experience could lead to mental health problems such as poor self-esteem or depression. Some children become targets of bullies because of their weight (Robinson, 2006).

Therefore, it has become essential that school health programs focus on healthy eating and physical activity to promote healthy weight. It is much more effective to address unhealthy childhood weight gain at the primary prevention level than to treat it once it has occurred. There is evidence that school health programs implemented without concurrent family interventions and societal campaigns against overweight/obesity may be ineffective (Muller, Danielzik, & Pust, 2005). This finding is understandable because the determinants of excess weight are also related to socioeconomic factors and living in an environment that permits easy access to food and encourages inactivity. However, programs in the school setting can be effective if enhanced by national efforts and simultaneous family interventions.

One such initiative with governmental backing is *Let's Move,* a comprehensive campaign endorsed by the U.S. first lady, Michelle Obama (www.letsmove.gov). The movement recognizes that children today have lifestyles very different from 30 years ago when the norm was to walk to school, to have active recess time, and to participate regularly in gym classes. Today most children ride to school, physical education is often not prioritized, and resources are not available for extracurricular programs. For safety reasons, sometimes recess is indoors or eliminated. The *Let's Move* initiative hopes to curb childhood obesity within one generation and offers factual information about the health implications of obesity, as well as resources for parents and educators. The campaign encourages consuming more fruits and vegetables, eating a healthy breakfast, and drinking more water. Links to *My Plate Kid's Place*, a new feature of the *Choose My Plate* website, suggests kid-friendly solutions to eating healthier and increasing physical activity. (See Box 16.3 for resources dedicated to reducing Childhood Overweight/Obesity.)

Box 16.4 provides an example of an agenda for a parent information session on nutrition. Marketing strategies for this evening program include: credit for parent volunteer service hours, a cooking demonstration with samples, and prizes such as a 1-year subscription to a parenting magazine or a healthy fruit or vegetable basket. Always try to involve the community merchants in the donation of prizes. Perhaps the local grocery store will donate a fruit or vegetable basket, or the beauty salon will donate a free hair styling. The more involved community businesses are in school activities, the better the community health nurse can promote the health of all citizens.

Parent Peer Groups

Establishing a parent peer group in which parents agree to certain rules of behavior for the children or teens, such as curfews and party rules, is helpful to parents and school personnel. Parents can agree not to allow drinking of alcohol, use of tobacco, or drugs at their houses. Parents in the group can then feel comfortable when their children/teens are in the company

---

Box 16.3 Resources to Reduce Childhood Overweight and Obesity

Let's Move
First Lady's nationwide initiative to combat childhood obesity in the current generation of children.
http://www.letsmove.gov/

Let's Move Child Care
Focus is on starting healthy habits early in a child's life.
http://www.healthykidshealthyfuture.org/welcome.html

Choose My Plate
U.S. Department of Agriculture educational initiative has lots of helpful tips starting with pregnant women and breast-feeding.
http://www.choosemyplate.gov/

We Can!
A collaboration with NIHLBI to promote eating right, getting active, and reducing screen time.
http://www.nhlbi.nih.gov/health/public/heart/obesity/wecan/

---

of peers whose parents subscribe to the same rules. A consistent approach sets limits for youth while providing an atmosphere of positive peer pressure. Parents also feel comfortable consulting with each other and form a support system.

Grandparents' Day

Grandparents' Day is a day in which the school actively involves grandparents, many of whom may not have been in an educational setting for a long time. Activities of the day can include classroom visitation, a healthy lunch, and blood-pressure screening. Seventh-grade (or higher grade) students can be taught to measure blood pressure in science, physical education, biology, math, or health class. Nurses can work with the respective teacher and conduct the practice sessions together. Youth take the elders' blood pressure under the supervision of a health professional such as a community health nurse, parent volunteers who are nurses, or other trained adults. This activity provides a service for the elderly guests and also increases the

---

Box 16.4 Sample Agenda: Healthy Habits, Healthy Kids! (An Evening for Parents)

Register, sign up for door prizes, complete survey related to nutritional knowledge
Welcome and panel introductions
Healthy Habits, Healthy Kids overview
Effects of cholesterol, sugar, and salt on our daily diet
Making sense of food labels
Making good choices in the grocery store
Making good choices in the restaurant
Making your family recipes healthy
Healthy heart discussion
Door prizes awarded

students' awareness of the importance of preventing heart disease and monitoring blood pressure. If elevated blood pressures are noted, have a referral plan complete with name and phone numbers of clinics, the local health department, or private medical care providers to which the person with an elevated blood pressure can be referred if he or she does not have a primary health care provider. Also follow up on elevated blood pressure measures, and offer all participants written information on elevated blood pressure and its association with poor health.

Mother–Daughter and Father–Son Programs

Cancer-prevention programs for mothers and daughters can promote breast self-examination and mammography. Culturally appropriate programs can be designed to attract women of various ethnic backgrounds. For example, if it is not culturally acceptable to discuss breast matters in public meetings, perhaps you can involve the local worship centers or other culturally acceptable agencies where the information could be hosted. (Those centers may also be able to provide bilingual presentations for women not fluent in English.)

Equally important is awareness for fathers and sons about testicular cancer and the correct technique for testicular self-examination. Perhaps mother–daughter talks can be scheduled at the same time as father–son talks. This program can be beneficial for the whole family, regardless of age, and, again, can involve the whole community. Girl Scout and Boy Scout troops or local FFA chapters (Future Farmers of America) might be interested in sponsoring a family awareness day because these groups usually meet at a school and are interested in hosting activities that contribute to the development of students and the good of the community.

HEALTH PROMOTION STRATEGIES FOR THE SCHOOL

The following are ideas for health promotion strategies that can be used with groups such as teachers or staff in the school setting:

- Blood pressure screening on the same day each month
- Cancer awareness programs
- Stuffing payroll envelopes with health promotion material
- Healthy heart lunches, such as salad day once a week
- Referral and resource information
- TB skin testing

Again, this list is not exhaustive, but is meant to generate ideas for viable strategies. Have an in-service day to assess the school climate and create a more social school atmosphere. Many other health issues for members of the school community are particular to the school environment. The following sections discuss some specific health promotion strategies.

Nutrition Awareness

If the school meal program is not healthy, form an ad hoc committee to study the problem. The committee should consist of students, parents, the public health/school nurse, cafeteria personnel, representatives of the faculty and administration, and a dietitian, if available. (Hint: Seek consultation from parents. Frequently, a professional dietitian is among the parents.) Action steps would include the following:

1. Conduct a survey to assess parental interest and areas of concern. What would parents like to see happen? What are they willing to do to make change happen?
2. Conduct a survey to assess student opinion and food preferences.
3. Do a plate waste study to determine what children are actually eating (Box 16.5).

Box 16.5 Plate Waste Study

1. Recruit parent volunteers, cafeteria staff, and teachers to help you.
2. Choose at least two days of the week to conduct the study.
3. Place volunteers next to the tray return and trash containers.
4. Record types and amount of food put into the trash.
5. Look into lunch bags for types of discarded, uneaten food.
6. Record all information (perhaps onto form with different food types).
7. You now have important information, such as nutritious food waste and the amount of soft drinks and candy consumed (from the wrappers).
8. Write a one-page report.
9. Give the report to parents, staff, and students.
10. Present the results to school administration along with suggestions to decrease food waste.

---

4. Form a committee, remembering to include the students.
5. Based on what you learned in steps 1, 2, and 3, identify other options to evaluate the present menu, such as hiring a nutritionist to study the present food service. You may also want to organize a committee to visit other schools to sample food, look at menus, and talk to those students about satisfaction.
6. Make recommendations to the school administration.
7. Make a presentation to the school board.
8. Pilot alternatives.

Bullying Prevention Programs

Bullying has become a topic of much concern in the United States. Research has focused on trying to understand the phenomenon. The word *bully* or *boele* can be traced to Dutch roots; however, the most common definition, first articulated by Olweus, includes three elements: aggression, repetition, and a power imbalance (Fredland, 2008). Repetition and power inequality are central to the concept of bullying. Two main types of bullying behavior are described in the literature: direct bullying and relational bullying (Woods & White, 2005). Different characteristics of behavior can be identified within each type. For example, there are pure bullies and pure victims as well as a mixed type (i.e., one who is a victim of bullying but also behaves as a bully). In addition, there are always neutral individuals or bystanders who watch the behavior but do not intervene in any way. The silent onlooker or bystander exemplifies indirect bullying behavior. Girls are said to engage more than boys in indirect bullying behavior. This latter, more subtle form of bullying may be just as devastating to childhood development. Both direct and indirect bullying must be addressed with age-appropriate, effective intervention programs.

A number of antibullying programs have been implemented; however, more information is needed to ascertain what interventions work best to prevent bullying behavior and to curtail instances of bullying when they do occur. What is known is that the problem is a public event (i.e., bullying usually occurs in the presence of others). Solutions must target the bullies, those bullied, children who fall into the category of bully-victims, and the bystanders. Most bullying takes place on or near school grounds in classrooms, hallways, bathrooms, and playgrounds during school hours and after dismissal while the children are still on school property. Bullying can also take place on school buses. Nansel et al. (2001), in a landmark study in the United States, reported that 29% of 6th to 10th graders were involved in some form of bullying behavior. Olweus (1994) reported that students with a bullying history were four times more likely to engage in criminal behavior in their twenties. Bullying may escalate to dating violence and later adult intimate partner violence. The most recent data from the Youth Risk Behavior Surveillance Survey revealed that 16% of high school students were bullied during the previous year (Centers for Disease Control and Prevention, 2012b).

Bullying has also been associated with a variety of physical, psychosomatic, and mental health effects such as colds, poor appetite, and fear of going to school. Recently, researchers have focused on understanding the effects of bullying on health. School nurses should consider bullying as a possible contributory factor when children come to the school clinic complaining of sore throat, colds, respiratory problems, and gastrointestinal ailments (Wolke, Woods, Bloomfield, & Karstadt, 2001). Bullying behaviors have been linked to physical and psychological symptoms in a comparative cross-sectional survey of 28 countries (Due et al., 2005). Students aged 11, 13, and 15 who had been bullied weekly were almost twice as likely to experience headaches, stomachaches, and sleeping problems compared with students who were not bullied. These youth were also two to four times as likely to admit feeling "low," "lonely," "irritable," and "nervous" when compared with the students who were not bullied. Violent youth frequently admit to perceived feelings of loneliness and being disliked by classmates (Thomas & Smith, 2004). Improving school connectedness and individual social skills may reduce negative behaviors and symptomology and should be studied further. For these reasons, it is important to address bullying behavior in its early stage with young students. Students should be encouraged to know what their personal boundaries are and to articulate when someone is crossing the line. Standing up for themselves and learning to be an active bystander when others are being victimized nurtures healthy social development.

Changing the school atmosphere to promote prosocial behavior and to not accept antisocial behavior such as bullying and other forms of aggression including electronic aggression may be the most important strategy. A systemic, rather than an individualistic, approach is important to guard against glorifying or passively accepting the bullying behavior. A multifaceted, multicomponent approach that includes students, administration, teachers, staff, and parents is necessary. Legal actions have been taken against school personnel and school districts that failed to intervene in situations of "hostile and abusive learning environments." Federal law requires schools to have a sexual harassment policy (Cavendish, 2001). Check on your school policy. Perhaps you could be involved in developing and implementing an antibullying policy.

There are a number of ways a nurse working in a school setting can address the problem of bullying. On March 10, 2011, the White House Summit on Bullying focused the nation's attention on the problem. The following conference highlights summary can guide adult stakeholders in their efforts to curb bullying:

- Strive to teach the Golden Rule—Do the Right Thing!
- Insist on a respectful school environment.
- Keep in mind what childhood was like.
- Incorporate ways to encourage empathy in day-to-day interactions.
- Focus on the behavior, not the technology.
- Success depends on a multifaceted approach.

The Department of Health and Human services supports the stop bullying website in partnership with the CDC, the Department of Education, Health Resources and Services Administration (HRSA), and Substance Abuse and Mental Health Services Administration (SAMSHA). You can visit the site at www.stopbullying.gov. There is a kids' section, and the site includes the topic of Cyber Bullying. Now it links to a Spanish website, "En Espanol." The following sections suggest additional steps to implement primary, secondary, and tertiary prevention programs modeled after Olweus' Bullying Prevention Program, one of the earliest evidence-based programs (Olweus, 1994, 2001).

Primary Prevention

A core component of any antibullying intervention program is the awareness and involvement of key adults in the school community. Implementing primary prevention may include the following steps:

1. Conduct a teacher/staff in-service program to educate the members of the school community about the problem of bullying.
   a. Discuss the prevalence of bullying in the United States.
   b. Discuss the various roles that are pertinent to the bullying issue, such as the bully, the victim, the bully-victim, and the bystander role.
   c. Determine if bullying/sexual harassment policies are in place in the school system.
   d. Include content about various forms of electronic aggression and cyberbullying, such as disclosures made in a public forum of personal information, embarrassing photos, rumors, lies, etc. See CDC (2010), http://www.cdc.gov/violenceprevention/pub/ea-tipsheet.html for more information on electronica aggression.
2. If no policies exist, assist school administration to develop a school policy for handling bullying/peer sexual harassment situations.
   a. If a policy exists, formulate a plan to increase awareness.
   b. Have a parent meeting to discuss preventing school violence and explain that addressing and stopping bullying is an important component of violence prevention. (Parents are very concerned about this issue because of media coverage about school shootings and the threat of terrorism. With careful planning, you could get a sizeable turnout.)
3. Formulate a coordinating group of teachers, staff, school nurse, administration, parents, community members, and students.

Secondary Prevention

Screen for bullying behaviors to determine the prevalence of both victimization and perpetration of bullying. An assessment of school climate (i.e., tolerance of such behaviors and bystander attitudes) is also indicated. Schoolwide/classroom measures include:

1. Assess for bullying and cyberbullying behaviors using a student questionnaire such as the Peer Relations Questionnaire. Definitions and questionnaire available at http://www.kenrigby.net/prq-child.pdf and cyberbullying http://www.stopbullying.gov/cyberbullying/what-is-it/
2. Having a school conference day to disseminate the results of the survey and launch a multicomponent plan to tackle the problem.
3. Implementing effective adult supervision during recess, lunchtime, and classroom/bathroom breaks. Monitoring hallways and other congregating areas, especially before and after school, should be part of the plan.
4. Teacher–student discussion groups to reinforce antibullying messages and contribute to changing the school culture. In other words, students must believe that the adults in the school community will not tolerate bullying behavior and that victims can comfortably report such behavior.
5. Implement steps to block cyberbullying using technology.
6. Developing classroom rules based on respect.

In addition to schoolwide and classroom measures, the problem of bullying must be addressed on an individual level. Special consideration must be given to how to handle bullies and their victims. Individual measures include:

1. Separate counseling of bullies and victims.
2. Involve parents of bullies and victims in the discussions.

3. Develop individual care plans for students, both bullies and victims, addressing physical, mental, and behavioral health needs.
4. Make referrals to health care providers as appropriate.

Tertiary Prevention

Once the policy and plans have been implemented, it is necessary to monitor the progress, particularly the school climate and bystander behavior. A maintenance program aimed at reducing the prevalence of future bullying is crucial and includes the following:

1. Have regular meetings of the coordinating committee.
2. Formally assess for bullying behaviors on an annual basis.
3. Continue school meetings and teacher–student discussion groups.
4. Encourage parental involvement in a variety of school activities.

AIR QUALITY, WASTE MANAGEMENT, AND RECYCLING

Teaching youth about the importance of protecting the environment has become more important than ever in recent years. Aided by the media focus on environmental issues, a conscientious, environmentally responsible generation is emerging. There are numerous ways to involve youth through environmentally friendly educational programs and field trips. Lessons on air quality and waste management and recycling can be embedded within the school curricula and involve administration, faculty, staff, facility managers, parents, and students. Here are some ideas: Involving teachers, staff, and parents, the school nurse can lead the campaign to improve the indoor air quality (IAQ) for all students, especially those diagnosed with asthma. Such efforts promise to keep all students healthier, improve attendance and in turn school performance. The following resources are available from the American Lung Association:

- Prepare to Go Back to School with Asthma (Available at http://www.lung.org/about-us/our-impact/top-stories/prepare-to-go-back-to-school-with-asthma-2013.html).
- IAQ School Action Kits (Available at http://www.epa.gov/iaq/schools/actionkit.html).
- *The Magic School Bus Gets Cleaned Up* (Available at http://www.epa.gov/cleanschoolbus/msb-book.htm).

Field trips can be arranged for students to visit a recycling or reuse center. There is nothing as effective as actually observing piles of refuse, bales of plastic bags, and blocks of aluminum cans to demonstrate to youngsters the monumental scale of the waste that would occur without reusing and recycling.

HEALTH PROMOTION STRATEGIES FOR THE COMMUNITY

Involving the neighboring community in health promotion programs can benefit school-aged children and their families, as well as members of the surrounding community. Health promotion strategies involving the community may include the following:

- Involve the elderly in school activities such as reading programs, mentoring, and monitoring lunch.
- Collaborate with the local civic association.
- Establish a drug-free zone.
- Have a community parade celebrating being drug free.
- Establish a safe traffic pattern.

- Publicize a smoke-free environment for all who work at or visit the campus.
- Contact radio and television stations, and newspapers and ask them to report health promotion events.
- Plan immunization programs.
- Provide school-based family clinics.
- Use the community forum to address neighborhood alcohol availability/consumption.
- Collaborate with local law enforcement to conduct a gun safety awareness program, including handgun issues.

Summary

This chapter focused on health promotion strategies that are congruent with the *Healthy People Initiative* and that can be implemented in the school community setting to achieve the goal of optimum wellness for school-aged children. We have reviewed the components of health services, health education, and environmental issues, and we have suggested ways to incorporate parents, teachers, staff, and the neighboring community in health promotion efforts. We have included community resources specific to the school setting. Now, we hope you will have fun promoting healthy partnerships with schools and school districts.

Critical Thinking Questions

1. Bullying at school is an increasingly common problem that can affect a child's physical and psychological health. As part of your community assessment, it is important to ascertain whether the school climate hinders bullying behaviors or promotes them. Pick a school in your geographic area. Does the school have an antibullying policy? If yes, how was it formed? Explain the policy and how it is implemented.

2. Some schools have adopted a zero-tolerance policy related to bullying. What are the advantages and disadvantages (if any) of having a zero-tolerance policy against bullying in the schools? What are the pros and cons of such a policy from the school administration perspective and from the student perspective? Discuss the impact of expulsion on students, the school, the community, and society.

3. Do antibullying policies tend to curtail deviant behaviors or lump relatively minor incidents, such as name calling, in with more serious aggressive behaviors? Does such a policy tend to trivialize sexual harassment? Discuss a legal situation that involves bullying or sexual harassment in the school setting. (Consult the literature for real case scenarios.)

4. Examples of several advocacy campaigns related to clean air and the prevention of respiratory conditions are listed below. Check out the American Lung Association website (http://www.lungusa.org) for information about these campaigns and educational resources. Pick one and develop an action plan for the school community. Be sure to note applicable federal regulations.
   - What is the State of Your Air? (Available at http://www.stateoftheair.org/).
   - Making the Connection: Asthma and Air Quality (Available at http://www.lung.org/about-us/our-impact/top-stories/making-the-connection-asthma-and-air-quality.html).
   - Fight for Air Climb (Available at http://www.lung.org/donate/events/fight-for-air-climb/).

5. To date, schools are not required to report student injuries to the Department of Education (Kaldahl & Blair, 2005). Frequently, injury and violence prevention programs

are sporadic and limited in scope. Do you think injuries should be reported? What are the advantages and disadvantages of reporting injuries? Develop a standardized checklist that can be used for schools to inspect environmental hazards. How might such a list be customized to individual schools?

6. School violence is an increasingly distressing phenomenon. What are the warning signs that might identify a student with problems? What schoolwide steps can be implemented to address the issue of school violence? Can social media be a positive influence to address these issues?

REFERENCES

Cavendish, R. S. C. (2001). Bullying and sexual harassment in the school setting. *The Journal of School Nursing, 17*(1), 25–31.

Centers for Disease Control and Prevention. (2009). *School connectedness: Strategies for increasing protective factors among youth.* Atlanta, GA: U.S. Department of Health and Human Service. Retrieved from http://www.cdc.gov/healthyyouth/protective/pdf/connectedness.pdf

Centers for Disease Control and Prevention. (2010). *Technology and youth: Protecting your child from electronic aggression.* Retrieved from http://www.cdc.gov/violenceprevention/pub/ea-tipsheet.html

Centers for Disease Control and Prevention. (2012a). *Causes and consequences: What causes overweight and obesity.* Retrieved from http://www.cdc.gov/obesity/causes/health.html

Centers for Disease Control and Prevention. (2012b). Youth risk behavior Surveillance-United States, 2011. *Morbidity and Mortality Weekly Report, 61*(4), 1–162.

Centers for Disease Control and Prevention. (2013). *Progress in childhood obesity.* Retrieved from www.cdc.gov/VitalSigns/ChildhoodObesity/

Due, P., Holstein, B. E., Lynch, J., Diderichsen, F., Gabhain, S. N., Scheidt, P., & Currie, C. (2005). Bullying and symptoms among school-aged children: International comparative cross sectional study in 28 countries. Health Behaviour in School-Aged Children Bullying Working Group. *European Journal of Public Health, 15*(2), 128–132.

Fredland, N. (2008). Sexual bullying: Addressing the gap between bullying and dating violence. *Advances in Nursing Science, 31*(2), 95–11.

Kaldahl, M. A., & Blair, E. H. (2005). Student injury rates in public schools. *Journal of School Health, 75*(1), 38–40.

Muller, M. J., Danielzik, S., & Pust, S. (2005). School- and family-based interventions to prevent overweight in children. *Proceedings of the Nutrition Society, 64,* 249–254.

Nansel, T. R., Overpeck, M., Pilla, R. S., Ruan, W. J., Simons-Morton, B., & Scheidt, P. (2001). Bullying behaviors among US youth: Prevalence and association with psychosocial adjustment. *Journal of the American Medical Association, 285*(16), 2094–2100.

Olweus, D. (1994). Annotation: Bullying at school: Basic facts and effects of a school based intervention program. *Journal of Child Psychology and Psychiatry, 53*(7), 1171–1190.

Olweus, D. (2001). Bullying at school: Tackling the problem. Research Center for Health Promotion, University of Bergen, Norway.

Robinson, S. (2006). The victimization of obese adolescents. *Journal of School Nursing, 22*(4), 201–206.

Thomas, S. P., & Smith, H. (2004). School connectedness, anger behaviors, and relationships of violent and nonviolent American youth. *Perspectives in Psychiatric Care, 40*(4), 135–148.

The University of Texas-Pan American, Border Health Office (2011). *Texas risk assessment for type 2 diabetes in children: A report to the governor and the 82nd legislature of the state of Texas.* Retrieved from http://www.utpa.edu/bho/PDF_Documents/TRAT2DC_Legislative_Report_2011.pdf

The White House. (2011). President Obama and the First Lady: Conference on bullying prevention. Retrieved from http://www.whitehouse.gov/blog/2011/03/10/president-obama-first-lady-white-house-conference-bullying-prevention

U.S. Department of Health and Human Services. (n.d.). *The Surgeon General's call to action to prevent and decrease overweight and obesity.* Retrieved from http://www.surgeongeneral.gov/library/calls/obesity/index.html

U.S. Department of Health and Human Services, Healthy People 2020. (n.d.-a). Retrieved from http://www.healthypeople.gov/2020/default.aspx

U.S. Department of Health and Human Services, Healthy People 2020. (n.d.-b). Retrieved from http://www.healthypeople.gov/2020/GetInvolved/UpcomingEvents.aspx

U.S. Department of Health and Human Services, Office of Disease Prevention and Health Promotion. (n.d.). *Healthy People 2010.* Retrieved from http://www.healthypeople.gov

Wolke, D., Woods, S., Bloomfield, L., & Karstadt, L. (2001). Bullying involvement in primary school and common health problems. *Archives of Disease in Childhood, 85*(3), 197–201.

Woods, S., & White, E. (2005). The association between bullying behavior, arousal levels and behavior problems. *Journal of Adolescence, 28,* 381–395.

World Health Organization. (2012). *Population-based approaches to childhood obesity prevention.* Geneva, Switzerland: WHO Document Production Services.

FURTHER READINGS

Journals

Journal of School Health—Official monthly journal of the American School Health Association focusing on health issues from pre-K to 12th grade.
Journal of School Nursing—Bimonthly publication
NASN School Nurse—The official clinical bimonthly publication of the National Association of School Nurses

Books and Articles

Fredland, N. (2008). Nurturing hostile environments: The problem of school violence. *Family and Community Health, 31*(1S), s32–s41.

Great Resources

Guidelines/health manuals/continuing education programs for school nurses developed by local school districts
State and local health department guidelines and laws
State associations for school nurses. Websites: access through state associations
Volunteer agencies such as the American Heart Association, American Lung Association, American Cancer Society, and American Diabetes Association.

CHAPTER 17

Promoting Healthy Partnerships With Faith Communities

Nina M. Fredland

LEARNING OBJECTIVES

After studying this chapter, you should be able to:

1. Define a faith community.

2. Relate the goals of the *Healthy People* initiative to the faith-based movement.

3. Discuss the roles of the nurse in promoting the health of faith communities.

4. Design and implement health promotion programs in partnership with faith communities.

5. Identify potential sources of collaboration, funding, and resources to assist the faith community nurse in planning and implementing health programs.

Introduction

In the face of the changing health care environment, congregations of worshipers are increasingly forming partnerships with nursing for health promotion programs. This movement of nursing in faith communities is based on the principles of holistic nursing that recognize the dynamic relationship between spirituality and health of mind and body throughout the life span (Solari-Twadell, 1999). Factors such as an increasing concern for disparities in health care; access to health care and insurance coverage; dissatisfaction with the disease-focused medical model; recent emphasis on bioethics and genetics as evidenced by institutions devoted to the interface of medicine and health; and church-based 12-step and meal programs have historically contributed to the movement (Evans, 1999). Other influencing components are self-responsibility for health care, increasing autonomous roles in nursing, increasing lay ministry responsibilities in faith-based communities, and limited health care system resources. Congregational nursing, parish nursing, faith-based organizations (FBOs), and faith community nursing are descriptive terms found in the literature and apply equally to the concept of nursing in faith communities. Faith community nursing refers to "a model of care that uses nurses based within faith communities (e.g., churches, synagogues, etc.) to provide health services to the other members of those communities, including health promotion and disease prevention programs, chronic disease management, and culturally sensitive services" (McGinnis, 2009, p. 173). For the purposes of this chapter, faith community will be used to describe the setting, and the term *faith community nurses* (FCNs) will denote nurses working in such settings. People in these faith communities are referred to as "participants."

Although faith community nursing programs have been in existence for some time, attention has focused on these types of programs as alternative methods of delivering services, through the establishment of the White House Office of Faith-Based and Community Initiatives (Executive Order 13199, 2001). In the policy statement of this executive order, faith and neighborhood communities are deemed vital to meeting the health services needs of low-income and underserved groups. Within this Office, domestic policy councils and advisory boards address contemporary issues. Two councils salient to this chapter are the Office of Faith-based and Neighborhood Partnerships and the White House Council for Community Solutions. The latter council delivered its Final Report on June 4, 2012, recommending cross-sector community collaboratives to search for innovative, data-driven solutions and best practices capitalizing on strong community leadership, and youth input. Researchers found that one in six youth, ages 16 to 24 are not engaged in education or the workforce. This wasted talent has a tangible societal cost as well as a generational loss. (Visit the website for details on key recommendations and strategies at http://www.serve.gov/sites/default/files/ctools/12_0604whccs_recommendations_factsheet.pdf.)

Amendments to Executive Order 13199 in 2009 expanded the mission and renamed the Office. Faith communities and secular initiatives are now eligible to apply for support from the Office of Faith-based and Neighborhood Partnerships. The Office has recently issued new guidelines for federal agencies on how to form partnerships and best implement Executive Order 13199 while adhering to the nation's laws and at the same time respecting religious liberty (Office of Faith-based and Neighborhood Partnerships, 2013). The advisory council researches, evaluates, reports, and recommends to the White House administration best practices and procedures for coordinating and delivering social services through community partnerships. In April of 2013, the council issued a report titled *Building Partnerships to Eradicate Modern-Day Slavery*; i.e., human trafficking. (Read the report at http://www.whitehouse.gov/sites/default/files/docs/advisory_council_humantrafficking_report.pdf)

Clearly, the notion of delivering health care through faith communities has been acknowledged and encouraged. The understanding that healthy people are interrelated with healthy communities has been affirmed by the Healthy People (HP) initiative.

HP 2020 calls for collaborations across community sectors. Its overarching goals are consistent with the philosophy of faith community nursing. The goals are to (1) "attain high quality longer lives free of preventable disease, disability, injury, and premature death"; (2) "achieve health equity, eliminate disparities, and improve the health of all groups"; (3) "create social and physical environments that promote good health for all"; and, (4) "promote quality of life, healthy development and healthy behaviors across all life stages" (Healthy People 2020, 2012, http://healthypeople.gov/2020/about/default.aspx). Twelve topic areas and 26 leading health indicators (LHI) have been updated and determined to be critical areas for keeping communities healthy. Use them to assess communities and as a model for planning health programs (Healthy People 2020, 2013a, http://www.healthypeople.gov/2020/TopicsObjectives2020/pdfs/HP2020_brochure_with_LHI_508.pdf). (See Box 17.1 for LHI topical areas.)

In sum, faith community programs fit the vision of the White House initiative and meet the objectives of the grassroots initiative of HP.

Box 17.1   Healthy People Leading Health Indicators: Topical Areas

Access to Health Services
Clinical Preventive Services
Environmental Quality
Injury and violence
Maternal, Infant and Child Health
Mental Health
Nutrition, Physical Activity, and Obesity
Oral Health
Reproductive and Sexual Health
Social Determinants
Substance abuse
Tobacco

Source: http://healthypeople.gov/2020/LHI/default.aspx

INITIATING HEALTHY PARTNERSHIPS WITH FAITH COMMUNITIES

The role of the nurse with faith communities is dictated, as always, by the needs of the people and includes, but is not limited to, health educator, health counselor, referral agent, advocate, facilitator, and liaison between the dimensions of spirituality and health (Watts, 2007). Frequently, FCNs are licensed professional nurses, with varied educational backgrounds and areas of expertise, who share their nursing skills as a means to give something back to their community of spiritual support. Frequently, the professional nurses donate their time and expertise as well as their own equipment (e.g., stethoscopes or sphygmomanometers). In some settings, however, the faith community may employ the nurses. Some are advanced practice nurses specializing in critical care, trauma, or ambulatory care, or are nurse practitioners with adult or family certification. Some are professional nurses with expertise in home health, rehabilitation, nursing home administration, hospice and acute care. Other volunteers are retired professional nurses. This group of FCNs is rich with varied experiences. As the nursing workforce ages along with the baby boomer generation, creative ways to maintain an adequate cadre of nurses to meet the health needs of the population are needed. It will be important to restructure health care delivery by innovative opportunities to keep the most experienced nurses in the workforce (McGinnis, 2009). The Affordable Care Act will require more health care professionals to deliver quality care to individuals formerly ineligible for routine and preventative clinical services. Older nurses are likely to want or need more flexibility in their schedules and work situations that are less physically demanding. Faith communities are ideal settings to gain from the vast experiences of this group of nurses, who may be able to contribute in new and important ways.

From the very beginning, faith community nursing has embodied the holistic approach to health care with an understanding of the dynamic relationship of human needs (physical, psychological, spiritual, emotional, social, and economic) to a person's health (Solari-Twadell, 1999). Nurses in faith communities are recognized members of the ministerial team. Home health care and invasive treatment procedures are usually not in this nursing practice; however, these procedures could be included should the faith community and the nurse so agree. In fact, these options may become necessary components to meet the demands under the Affordable Care Act. Nursing within faith communities is not intended to compete with public or private health service organizations. However, faith community programs may be the most expeditious way to increase access to the health care system and reduce health care costs for individuals and society in general.

Research has documented that health care costs may rise more from delayed access to care rather than overuse or misuse of the health care system by the worried well (Rydholm, 2006). It is time to put this debate to rest and be proactive in encouraging consumers to seek preventative care. Educating consumers related to quality versus quantity care is an important role for modern FCNs. FCNs can intervene by encouraging participants in faith communities to seek care earlier. Infected wounds, confusion related to medications, allergic reactions, shortness of breath, ignoring dental decay, and urinary tract infections are just a few examples of instances where conditions could deteriorate and end up costing much more to resolve. FCNs through health counseling/education, advocacy for the vulnerable, referrals, brokering for services, and providing resources can prevent the exacerbation of many conditions.

If nursing within faith communities is based on a model such as the community nursing assessment, intervention, and evaluation model presented in this textbook, then the continuous growth and evaluation of programs are ensured. Assessments (monthly screenings), annual surveys, and analysis of the components of participants' needs dictate what intervention programs need to be implemented (e.g., healthy eating classes, exercise classes, walking clubs, or diabetes management instruction). These programs are implemented in a timely fashion that is most supportive of the participants. Evaluations of the programs lead us to expand or to minimize programs, depending on their effectiveness. Effectiveness is measured by the number of participants in the individual programs, as well as individual goal accomplishment and overall satisfaction with the health outcomes (e.g., weight loss, increased feelings of fitness, decreased fatigue, better perceived control of stress with lowered blood pressure, and actual control and direction of one's lifestyle choices).

The following are some strategies for identifying faith community needs:

- Distribute an educational needs survey to various groups within the faith community, such as the women's auxiliary, the young mothers' support group, the young adult group, the elder group, the men's organization, and the non-English-speaking community. A helpful tool appears in Box 17.2.
- Attend meetings for the different groups.
- Form focus groups to discuss options to increase health or join an initiative already in progress, such as prayer groups or faith renewal groups.
- Provide a suggestion box.
- Form an ad hoc committee to study the health ministry, and include key people such as clergy, lay ministers, school principal, social and health agency personnel, and so forth. Be sure that both formal and informal leaders are included.
- Remember to only make decisions with input from the faith community.

The educational needs survey in Box 17.2 could be distributed at worship meetings to maximize the number of people reached. Of course, the survey should be available in all appropriate languages. It is helpful to have pencils available so that surveys can be completed and collected at this time. After the information has been gathered and synthesized, concerns and topics are prioritized. If an English version and non-English version are used, respective priorities are noted.

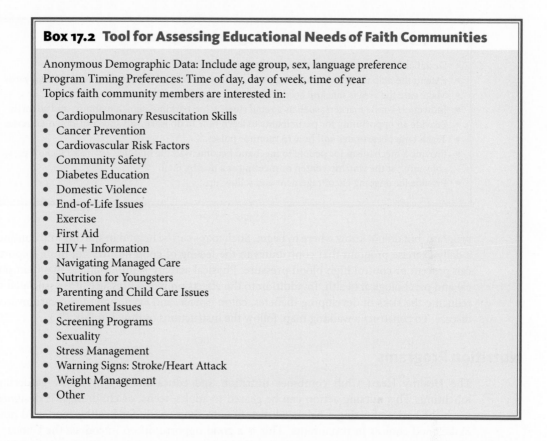

Box 17.2   Tool for Assessing Educational Needs of Faith Communities

Anonymous Demographic Data: Include age group, sex, language preference
Program Timing Preferences: Time of day, day of week, time of year
Topics faith community members are interested in:

- Cardiopulmonary Resuscitation Skills
- Cancer Prevention
- Cardiovascular Risk Factors
- Community Safety
- Diabetes Education
- Domestic Violence
- End-of-Life Issues
- Exercise
- First Aid
- HIV+ Information
- Navigating Managed Care
- Nutrition for Youngsters
- Parenting and Child Care Issues
- Retirement Issues
- Screening Programs
- Sexuality
- Stress Management
- Warning Signs: Stroke/Heart Attack
- Weight Management
- Other

HEALTH PROMOTION PROGRAMS FOR FAITH COMMUNITIES

After assessing the community's educational preferences, the nurse plans intervention programs based on the results. Here is a list of classes that may be of interest to faith community members:

- Exercise group
- Nutrition classes
- Cardiopulmonary resuscitation (CPR) and emergency cardiovascular care
- Positive parenting
- AIDS/HIV information sessions
- Planning for a healthy retirement
- Immunization program
- Health fair
- Stress-reduction and coping strategies
- Emergency preparedness
- Navigating the Health Care System

Walking Programs

If the community is interested in an exercise group, suggest a walking map. A walking map is a self-directed exercise tool that is popular particularly with the elderly. These maps have mileage-marked routes in each neighborhood. Many participants may be trying to begin an exercise

> **Box 17.3 Instructions for Creating a Walking Map**
>
> - Design a 1-mile map around the worship center.
> - Extend the map to include shopping malls, a recreational park, or neighborhood school yards.
> - Make sure the area is safe and accessible.
> - Indicate 1/4-mile markers, such as a retail store, a "no parking" sign, a mailbox, and so forth.
> - Provide an opportunity for participants to learn how to do warm-up and cool-down exercises.
> - Teach target heart rates and how to monitor pulses.
> - Provide a mechanism for people to meet and become walking buddies, such as a kickoff party, convening at the worship center, or meeting at a nearby mall.
> - Provide for ongoing encouragement and follow-up.

program, but do not know where to begin. Such maps can be helpful in starting and continuing a daily exercise program that contributes to the feeling of good health and, more important, can prevent or control high blood pressure. Physical activity is important to maintain physical and psychological health. In addition to the effects on blood pressure, it is associated with reducing the risks of developing diabetes, colon cancer, and even dying from cardiovascular disease. To construct a walking map, follow the instructions outlined in Box 17.3.

Nutrition Programs

The Healthy Heart Club combines nutrition and education in a monthly gathering at lunchtime. This nursing action can be geared to adults, teens, or children. It is designed to teach the basics of eating a balanced diet, how to shop wisely for healthy food, and how to make good choices in restaurants. This is a good opportunity to introduce the Choose My Plate, a broad initiative based on the 2010 U.S. Department of Agriculture (USDA) *Dietary Guidelines for Americans*. This food guidance system has replaced MyPyramid and is user-friendly. For example, the *10 Tips Educational Nutrition* series covers many interesting topics for adults and for parents to use to instill healthy food habits in their growing children. These tips can be downloaded and printed in color and put on the refrigerator or in the office coffee room. (See Box 17.4 for *10 Tips to a Great Plate*.) This is an easy, fun way to address the national problem of overweight and obesity and prevent cardiac disease. Box 17.5 offers a plan for Healthy Heart Club activities and incorporates the Choose MY Plate initiative.

This heart-healthy eating idea can be expanded to include children. Try starting a "Healthy Tots" or "Kids' Club" focusing on healthy food choices for healthy kids. How about serving

> **Box 17.4 10 Tips for a Great Plate**
>
> 1. Balance Calories.
> 2. Enjoy your food, but eat less.
> 3. Avoid oversized portions.
> 4. Foods to eat more often
> 5. Make half your plate fruits and vegetables.
> 6. Switch to fat-free or low-fat (1%) milk
> 7. Make half your grains whole grains.
> 8. Foods to eat less often
> 9. Compare sodium in foods.
> 10. Drink water instead of sugary drinks.
>
> Available at: http://www.choosemyplate.gov/food-groups/downloads/TenTips/DGTipsheet1ChooseMyPlate.pdf

---

Box 17.5 Healthy Heart Club Activities

- Gather in the faith community center at a convenient time once a month.
- See if a faith community member who is a dietitian is available; this tends to attract people to the session.
- Identify content to be explored, such as healthy food recognition and preparation, economic purchases, eating out, and celebrating with healthy food choices.
- Assist class in personalizing their healthy eating and activity plan using the http://www.choosemyplate.gov website technology.
- Include cooking demonstrations with healthy nonalcoholic drink or smoothie recipes that can be made in a blender and then sampled by participants.
- Initiate recipe sharing that includes multicultural traditions; this is always popular for the young and old alike.
- Offer tips on how to maintain favorite tastes in family recipes and still eat healthy (e.g., substitution of 1% milk for full cream milk, egg substitute for eggs, or oil for lard).
- Schedule field trips to ethnic restaurants and grocers.

---

chicken or tuna salad in an ice cream cone? Toss a banana, a peach (without the pit), some orange juice, and plain yogurt in a blender. Serve it over crushed ice. Challenge the children to come up with their own healthy, fruity concoction. Finally, celebrate with a heart-healthy party. Box 17.6 shows a healthy lifestyle program for children that reinforces the notion that healthy choices can be incorporated into celebrations.

Emergency First Aid Programs

A trustworthy site for health information is the American Heart Association (AHA). They offer CPR training, and emergency cardiovascular care classes are other healthy lifestyle primary prevention activities. The AHA (n.d.-a) offers numerous online products and classroom programs that can be extended to the community. For example, popular programs include *Family and Friends CPR Anytime, Hands Only CPR, HeartSaver First Aid, CPR, and AED* (Automatic External Defibrillator), *CPR in Schools, HeartSaver-Pediatric* to mention a few. (See the AHA website for details and how to arrange for a program or find an event such as Heart Walk in your area; AHA, n.d.-b). These AHA resources are invaluable tools for the FCN. Many public facilities now have an AED in a prominent area. Faith communities should

---

Box 17.6 Pear and Apple Party Time Activity for Kids

- Pick a time when children are assembled (perhaps after the worship service).
- Equipment you will need: pears, apples, toothpicks, little plates, napkins, a chalkboard (for tallying votes), cutting board, and knife.
- Have a variety of apples on hand (Red Delicious, Jonathan, McIntosh, Granny Smith, Golden Delicious).
- Have a variety of pears on hand (Anjou, Bosc, Comice).
- Cut the apples and pears into cubes.
- Have children taste each kind.
- Take a vote on what kind of apple and pear they liked most.
- Tally the votes on a scoreboard.
- Decorate the apple and pear with the most votes.
- Take a picture of everyone (and the pears and apples, of course).
- Celebrate and enjoy!

consider purchasing an AED. A fundraiser can be dedicated for the purchase of an AED, or a local business may want to donate one. Many businesses and organizations have already installed these units in their facilities. Perhaps the faith community has a unit and needs ongoing training of its members. This can be an important annual event to train a cadre of responders in both CPR and the use of AEDs. Together these strategies can significantly reduce death from sudden cardiac arrest.

Health Fairs

If a faith community undertakes the project of a health fair, timing is very important. One theory is that it should have its own special time of year; another view is that it can coincide with an annual bazaar or fundraiser. Because the community usually supports the annual fundraiser, a captive audience is present. On the other hand, sometimes people would rather take health more seriously and not try to focus on fun and games and screening or health-education activities at the same time. Also, if immunizations are provided, sometimes this is an unpleasant association for children who set out for a fun time. Both situations can work with proper planning and marketing, depending on the commitment and support of the faith community. Let the community decide. Box 17.7 lists steps to consider when setting up a

---

Box 17.7

- Organizing a Health Fair for a Faith Community
- Contact the clergy and lay council.
- Set the date (try to allow at least 6 to 8 weeks to prepare).
- Decide what health promotion areas to cover, depending on the audience (adults only, families, elders).
- Invite identified organizations to participate.
- Invite health care providers, health service vendors, and community resources from the geographic area.
- Solicit prizes from local merchants.
- Offer incentives for attendance, such as door prizes and coupons for free services (e.g., mammograms, heart scans).
- Collaborate with other professionals, such as a dental school, pharmacy school, or optometrist.
- Offer free immunizations.
- Have a women's health booth, a men's health booth, a teen's health booth, and a children's health booth.
- Include screening stations, such as vision, hearing, blood glucose, blood pressure, lead, tuberculosis skin testing, depression, HIV testing, and counseling.
- Have a plan for referral and follow-up.
- It may be a good idea to have an HIV-positive ministry booth providing information about HIV, as well as providers from treatment centers.
- Have stations that focus on environmental health, including booths on mosquito control and water safety. People from rural areas can bring in water samples for testing.
- A home safety booth sponsored by the utility company and/or fire department can address indoor air quality, electrical hazards, and gas appliances.
- A Crime Watch booth sponsored by the police can address self-defense and home security.
- Set up computers for health risk appraisal programs.
- Assign booth areas considering flow pattern. Provide for privacy if breast self-examination is demonstrated or skin cancer checks are done.
- Invite the media.
- Include fun activities, such as craft booths for the children and adults.

TIP: Visit the Family and Consumer Services website for a Health Fair Planning Guide that offers national resources for health fairs including forms you can customize at http://fcs.tamu.edu/health/hfpg/index.php

health fair. This outline is not meant to be exhaustive, but to provide ideas and some direction. Although the faith community is a church, synagogue, mosque, or temple, it is important to include the greater community in its health ministry. A health fair is a wonderful opportunity to open the boundaries of the faith community.

Additional Programming Considerations

Additional health promotion strategies for faith communities include:

- Blood pressure screening
- Glucose screening
- Vision and glaucoma testing
- Bereavement program
- Weight-management programs—how about "Weigh to go!" for a title?
- Smoking cessation programs
- Diabetic education classes
- Caregiver support groups
- Asthmatic support group
- Respite care programs
- Healthy Aging

Involving nursing volunteers from the community ensures that the multicultural diversity of the community can be mirrored in the nursing team. The problem of language is thereby mitigated by the volunteers, who speak the same language as the participants. Cultural practices that contribute to healthy lifestyle (e.g., Vietnamese and Chinese cultures' heavy use of vegetables in the diet) are emphasized at social and educational activities. Importance is placed on cultural recognition and adaptation of health-supporting behaviors.

Economic factors as well as cultural factors are essential concerns of problem identification and solution. The faith community is a microcosm of the larger economic pattern of the city. Services should be accessible to all members of the faith community as appropriate. The affluence of the community will affect the type of programs that can be implemented. It is an accepted fact that families with more discretionary income are more able to engage in health promotion activities. This fact will impact the overall health of the community. Economics also influences how members of the community access health services. The faith community for an increasing number of participants may be the only consistent source of health care.

ESTABLISHING A LASTING PARTNERSHIP WITH FAITH COMMUNITIES

Now that background information and program strategies have been explored, let us focus on the essential elements of establishing a nursing partnership with a faith community. Building a healthy community will take time, careful planning, and a great deal of organization. The HP initiative suggests a formula for this process, MAP-IT (Healthy People 2020, 2013b). MAP-IT stands for Mobilize, Assess, Plan, Implement, and Track (Box 17.8). These are essential components the nurse working with a faith community should follow. Here are some suggestions:

- Obtain support from the clergy and administration.
- Identify a core of health professionals willing to participate. Ideally, they will be participants in the faith community.
- Establish a marketing system.

Box 17.8 MAP-IT Strategy for Creating a Healthy Community

Mobilize	individuals that care about the faith community's health into a coalition.
Assess	the areas of greatest need in your community, and the resources and strengths you can tap into to address those areas of need.
Plan	your approach: Start with a vision of where you want to be as a community; then add strategies and action steps to help you achieve that vision.
Implement	your plan using concrete action steps that can be monitored and will make a difference.
Track	your progress over time.

Source: http://healthypeople.gov/2020/implement/MapIt.aspx

- Find a school of nursing or a community college to assist you in developing the ministry.
- Identify sponsor support through faith community members and neighborhood establishments. (Local businesses are usually supportive because they recognize that their clients are of the faith community. Check advertisements in the neighborhood gazette or church bulletin.)
- Acquire supplies, such as cotton swabs, disposable gloves, stethoscopes, blood pressure cuffs, glucose meters, and so forth, from various sources.
- Recruit additional volunteer health professionals to participate.
- Recruit high school and/or college volunteers to help with organizational details. Many are required to do service hours as a condition for graduation. They may be waiting to find just such an opportunity.
- Have a team meeting and plan nursing actions. Probably the first action would be to conduct a needs assessment. Be sure it is conducted in languages that reflect the constituency.

It is acceptable to start small or to have volunteers who are only able to give a little time. The nature of the ministry is that it builds on itself as time and community needs dictate. A successful marketing strategy is critical to starting and maintaining an active program. Several approaches can be implemented. Depending on resources and community contacts, some approaches may be more feasible than others. Local newspapers, radio and television spots, and civic association bulletins are possibilities. Posting on the faith community marquee or other community billboards is usually a very effective way of notifying the community about activities. Another effective strategy is pulpit announcements during or immediately after regularly scheduled services. Surveys completed at this time usually yield excellent response. A nurse column in the faith community's weekly bulletin announcing scheduled health-screening activities and health-education programs can be a regular feature. Catchy names such as "Positively Healthy Choices," "Nurse's Notes," or "Here's to Healthy Choices" will focus attention on the health information, which should be published in all languages commonly spoken. Remember to partner with nearby or affiliated schools, community stores, and fast-food restaurants. Ask to market the faith community "nursing news" and events in their flyers and newsletters and on their marquees.

Partnerships between faith communities and schools of nursing, though challenging, can be mutually beneficial (Otterness, Gehrke, & Sener, 2007). FCNs should consult with nursing faculty at area community colleges or universities to assist with establishing health promotion programs and health services. Faculty members may be willing to assist with the writing of a needs assessment survey. Then, the faith community can be assessed annually with a tool, an invaluable part of the process. Graduate student nurses can be lead players in the community assessment. They can work with lay members of the faith community and guide the actual assessment. Student help would be a tremendous asset to the FCNs because, most often, they are volunteering and such needs assessments can be very time consuming. Reciprocally, the students would have an opportunity to gain cultural awareness and competence and hone critical thinking and communications skills, while participating in a valuable and realistic clinical experience. Another benefit to colleges is the opportunity for sharing research data. Government funding sources are available to pilot projects that address health and social issues. Partnerships between university academics and faith communities should explore such funding opportunities.

Health care provider systems (hospitals, Health Maintenance Organization (HMO), Preferred Provider Organization (PPO)) have come to realize the importance of outreach and collaborating with faith community health programs as a valuable model. Frequently, faith communities will sign agreements of support with health-management systems such as hospitals, private clinics, or group medical practices. The collaborator may be a local public health department who partners with the faith community. Activities may include sharing information among health care professionals, disseminating information to the community at large, setting community health goals, sponsoring community health activities, conducting community assessments, coordinating and delivering direct services to community clients, and implementing specific state health agendas (Zahner & Corrado, 2004). The collaborating health care system can be a referral option for faith community participants. Fast-food restaurants, retail shops, businesses, colleges and universities, as well as civic and public service organizations (e.g., Lions Clubs, women's organizations, League of Women Voters), as well as national and local foundations, such as the March of Dimes, may be receptive to being a sponsor, thus providing needed money for supplies, brochures, and other essential items. Because space on faith community property is usually limited, the program is totally portable. Many volunteers bring their own equipment (e.g., stethoscopes and sphygmomanometers). Representatives from drug companies and medical supply companies who are members of the faith community may supply the program with other needed equipment.

An example of how important this program is concerns a "healthy-feeling" parishioner who, because of his spouse's urging, had his blood pressure and glucose checked. The results were abnormal for age and gender. He was given the written test results, counseled, and referred to a health provider of his choice. A month later, the spouse reported that her husband was recuperating splendidly from coronary bypass surgery and learning to manage his newly diagnosed diabetes.

Registered nurses, who are the diabetic management experts, and the nurse practitioners, with the support of the sponsor agent, can be the usual blood glucose screeners. Participants feel comforted and assured when their screening data are within normal range. The participants who regulate their Type 2 diabetes without monitoring at home, usually because of limited income, can use the screening program for self-management evaluation and further education.

Although not well adopted nationally yet, Acanthosis Nigricans screening can lead to early intervention for young children and adolescent at risk to develop Type 2 Diabetes Mellitus. By identifying these youngsters and instituting primary prevention measures, these individuals may avert chronic illnesses, and costly health care dollars will be saved.

Classes that are age or content specific are popular and well attended. For example, a nurse with a background in men's health issues can speak to the men's organization. A male nurse can make a particular contribution speaking to the group about testicular self-examination, prostate and colon cancer, and penile erection issues. Nurses also have an opportunity to discuss domestic violence and abuse. Presentations focus on defining abusive situations, identifying community resources available to victims and perpetrators of abuse, and especially teaching skills for relationships without violence. A special meeting of teen or youth groups should address the subject of adolescent relationship violence.

A goal should be to establish the faith community nursing program as a valuable ministry. Visibility is key to gaining rapport with participants and credibility for health programs. FCNs should seek opportunities to support other ministries of the faith community in diverse ways such as assisting with emergencies at services, providing health coverage during retreats or scout outings, organizing back-to-school immunization programs, creating multilanguage health literature displays, and offering to speak at meetings.

Role of Faith Communities during Extraordinary Circumstances

Churches, synagogues, and other places of worship have historically been recognized as focal points of care during natural disasters, large-scale accidents, and terrorist attacks. A faith community with a nurse ministry system in place could provide immediate holistic care and quickly coordinate services with federal agencies. Since the tragedy of September 11, 2001, our nation realizes how important it is to have extensive community-based emergency plans in place. Horrific, devastating storms such as Katrina and Sandy have also highlighted the need for emergency preparedness. Faith communities can be part of the short- and long-term plans to deliver health services to communities suffering from injuries and traumatic stress. Schools and churches are often the designated emergency shelter in a community. Community Education Response Teams (CERT) work with professional responders should a disaster occur. See if your community has such a program.

Closing the Gap on Health Disparities

Faith communities are ideal places to deliver health services to minority populations and thus contribute to closing the gap between majority and minority populations in relation to health disparities. For a variety of reasons, minority groups often fall through the cracks when it comes to health care. These same groups are often socially connected through a faith community. By valuing the environmental context, participants who worship together and share common interests and beliefs are more likely to accept behaviors that enhance physical and mental health (Drayton-Brooks & White, 2004).

AN EMERGING MODEL

Nursing in faith communities has made great strides in recent years; yet it is still in the development phase. It has an enormous potential to grow and evolve into an enhanced health care delivery system especially in this era of economic uncertainty, high unemployment rates, and limited health care resources. The Affordable Care Act may afford a window of opportunity for creative ways to improve the health care of Americans. Nurses are singularly well equipped to use their multifaceted skills and their extensive body of knowledge to improve the health status of individuals, families, and communities in the changing health care arena.

Through the expansion of the nurse role—specifically the nurse practitioner role—more services can be brought to the faith community. Faith community nursing can be expanded to include primary care services across the life span. Annual faith community surveys can expand to the wider neighborhood. Nursing students can assist with this activity. Analyzing databases to identify community assets as well as problem focuses will provide important information for prioritizing programs.

One of the most crucial steps will be acquiring physical space for the nurse ministry to provide services. Clergy and administrative personnel, who are supportive of the program and eager for it to advance, will see this as a necessity. If renovation plans are under way, space for the nurse ministry should be incorporated. Although the program can be entirely mobile, it is more practical to have a designated space for storage and to render services. To maintain focus, ensure quality, and preserve the volunteer and multicultural components of the faith community, both short- and long-term goals are required. Identify a variety of health promotion strategies and health-education needs to be addressed in the future. Then set realistic, short-term goals that focus on the specific areas identified, such as enhancing diabetic education, restructuring the weight-management classes, or offering stress-reduction methods (e.g., aromatherapy, realistic relaxation techniques, caregiver support). Because members of the team are often managing careers, professional commitments, and family and personal responsibilities, limiting the focus at the beginning stage of development is the best strategy to ensure continued success of the program.

An important aspect to working with faith communities is related to the delivery of culturally competent care. Cultural competence is very important in terms of religious beliefs. It is likely that the FCNs will be of the same faith as participants. However, public health nurses may be employed by a collaborating sponsor such as a public health department and may not share the same religious beliefs. Therefore, nurses working with faith communities should educate themselves in the values and beliefs of the members of the faith community. They should also recognize that there are often a number of variations within each faith.

Summary

Partnerships between local health departments and faith communities potentially can do much to deliver services and reduce health disparities experienced by vulnerable groups (Zahner & Corrado, 2004). More exploration is needed to determine how these collaborations can work best under the Affordable Care Act. Information is emerging related to the cost-effectiveness of such partnerships. This type of articulation between health departments and faith communities should be explored and developed further. Public health nurses and other providers should pursue this opportunity.

The practice model of nursing partnerships with faith communities described in this chapter is still evolving. Nurses need to be proactive in this era of continuous health care reform. We must participate in and help shape future decision making for health care delivery. This nurse ministry, whether volunteer or reimbursed service, is a cost-effective enhancement of health care delivery systems. Nursing partnerships with faith communities are part of the solution.

Critical Thinking Questions

1. Several members of the faith community have come to you to voice concerns and frustrations associated with balancing caregiving duties for elderly family members and maintaining their own family integrity. Often, these responsibilities are overwhelming and impact the woman in the family to the greatest extent. As the FCN, you decide to create a support system for this group.

   a. How would you begin to address the concerns of the faith community members? What methods could you use to identify specific issues? What strategies could be implemented to educate, support, and alleviate some of the extra burden care giving creates? How would you advocate making needed services available through the faith community? Who should be included in the planning and decision-making phases?

   b. Visit the internet and identify sources available to address this issue. How would you incorporate this information in your plan?

2. Faith communities have belief systems that may reflect commonalities as well as differences. It is important to consider how different processes influence health outcomes. Pick two faith communities and explain how their belief system may affect their health choices, including access to care. What specific methods would you use to identify concerns?

3. Several residents from the retirement home within the geographic area of your faith community have learned about PAD (public access defibrillator) programs. They are interested in obtaining an AED for the premises. Make a case for implementing such a program at the retirement home. How would you go about gaining approval? What requirements would be necessary? Plan an educational approach for implementation of the unit.

REFERENCES

Amendments to Executive Order 13199 and Establishment of the President's Advisory Council for Faith-Based and Neighborhood Partnerships. (2009). Retrieved from http://www.whitehouse.gov/the_press_office/ObamaAnnouncesWhiteHouseOfficeofFaith-basedandNeighborhoodPartnerships/

American Heart Association. (n.d.-a). Retrieved from www.heart.org

American Heart Association. (n.d.-b). *Heart walk*. Retrieved from http://www.heartwalk.org/site/c.flKUIeOUIgJ8H/b.8939141/k.BD45/Home.htm

Drayton-Brooks, S., & White, N. (2004, September/October). Health promoting behaviors among African American women with faith-based support. *The ABNF Journal, 15*(5), 84–90.

Evans, A. R. (1999). *The healing church: Practical programs for health ministries*. Cleveland, OH: United Church Press.

Healthy People 2020. (2012). *About Healthy People*. Retrieved from http://healthypeople.gov/2020/about/default.aspx.

Healthy People 2020. (2013a). *Healthy People 2020 brochure: Updated with LHI*. Retrieved from http://www.healthypeople.gov/2020/TopicsObjectives2020/pdfs/HP2020_brochure_with_LHI_508.pdf

Healthy People 2020. (2013b). *Implementing Healthy People 2020; Map-IT and guide to using Healthy People 2020 in your community*. Retrieved from http://healthypeople.gov/2020/implement/MapIt.aspx

McGinnis, S. L. (2009). The emerging role of faith community nurses in prevention and management of chronic disease. *Policy, Politics, & Nursing Practice, 9*, 173–180.

Office of Faith-based and Neighborhood Partnerships. (2013). *Partnerships that reflect our laws and values*. Retrieved from http://www.whitehouse.gov/administration/eop/ofbnp

Otterness, N., Gehrke, P., & Sener, I. M. (2007). Partnerships between nursing education and faith communities: Benefits and challenges. *Journal of Nursing Education, 46*(1), 39–44.

President's Advisory Council on Faith-based and Neighborhood Partnerships. (2013). *Building partnerships to eradicate modern-day slavery: Report of recommendations to the President*. Retrieved from http://www.whitehouse.gov/sites/default/files/docs/advisory_council_humantrafficking_report.pdf

Rydholm, L. (2006). Wanda Alexander builds bridges to better care. *Creative Nursing, 12*(2), 10–12.

Solari-Twadell, P. (1999). *The emerging practice of parish nursing*. In P. Solari-Twadell & M. McDermott (Eds.), Parish nursing: Promoting whole person health within faith communities (pp. 3–24). Thousand Oaks, CA: Sage.

Watts, J. M. (2007). Faith community nursing. *Virginia Nurses Today, 15*(1), 11.

White House Council on Community Solutions. (2013). *White House Council on community solutions-recommendations*. Retrieved from http://www.serve.gov/?q=site-page/white-house-council-community-services

Zahner, S. J., & Corrado, S. M. (2004). Local health department partnerships with faith-based organizations. *Journal of Public Health Management, 10*(3), 258–265.

FURTHER READINGS

American Nurses Association. (2012). *Faith community nursing: Scope and standards of practice* (2nd ed.). Silver Spring, MD: Author.

Smucker, C. J., & Weinberg, L. (2009). *Faith community nursing: Developing a quality practice*. Silver Spring, MD: ANA.

Solari-Twadell, P. A., & Hackbarth, D. P. (2010). Evidence for a new paradigm of the ministry of parish nursing practice using the nursing intervention classification system. *Nursing Outlook, 58*, 69–75.

U.S. Department of Health and Human Services and Department of Agriculture. (n.d.). *Choose my plate*. Retrieved from http://www.choosemyplate.gov

Journals

Creative Nursing, quarterly; based on values, issues, experiences, and collaboration, nurses are encouraged to think creatively and take risks

International Journal for Human Caring; published quarterly and focuses on the knowledge of care and care giving within the discipline of nursing and in collaboration with other disciplines

Journal of Holistic Nursing, quarterly; integrates holistic health concepts of body, mind, emotions and spirit within the context of a changing environment

CHAPTER 18

Promoting Healthy Partnerships With Marginalized Groups

Nina M. Fredland

LEARNING OBJECTIVES

After studying this chapter, you should be able to:

1. Discuss what it means for a group to be "marginalized," "vulnerable," or "disadvantaged."

2. Identify groups that society has marginalized.

3. Discuss commonalities of marginalized groups.

4. Discuss barriers to health care specific to marginalized groups.

5. Adapt a program for a vulnerable or marginalized population, such as homeless persons, migrants, or persons with chronic disabilities.

Introduction

Nurses throughout history and in modern times have been concerned about "vulnerable populations" (Nyamathi, Koniak-Griffin, & Greengold, 2007). Public health nurses, particularly, are committed to remain focused on the health needs of populations who, for various reasons, have been relegated to the margins of society. These groups may be impoverished, discriminated against, or functionally impaired in some way.

The word *marginalize* means to treat someone or something as if he or she is of no consequence or is unimportant. Marginalization conveys a process in which individuals in certain groups seem not to matter or to be of little concern to the rest of society, thus falling beyond the margins (Vasas, 2005). To marginalize or be marginalized may be more accurate terminology than the concept of vulnerability, which may imply a degree of "blaming the victim." "Vulnerable" stems from the Latin word *vulnare*, which means "to wound." This terminology implies that the wounded or the "less than perfect" are not particularly valued and easily marginalized. By using the terminology of marginalization instead, the emphasis is societal.

Flaskerud and Winslow define vulnerable populations as "social groups who experience limited resources and consequent high relative risk for morbidity and premature mortality"

(Flaskerud & Winslow, 1998, p. 69). Vulnerable groups in a review of five decades of nursing research included people of color; the poor; and those individuals marginalized by sexual preference, immigrant/refugee status, and religious beliefs (Flaskerud et al., 2002).

Although progress has been made in some nations, others are falling behind. As a result of the global economic slump, war and civil unrest, education for individuals in the poorest nations has suffered. The World Health Organization (WHO, 2008) advocates making disparities more visible so that any given society can create objectives and mobilize resources for change. This supports focusing on health disparities, rather than on race or ethnicity, as a more productive approach. National agendas, therefore, should have action plans to identify and monitor health disparities among all groups and increase awareness when these inequities exist in marginalized or vulnerable groups. The U.S. government addressed health disparities by establishing the Healthy People initiative, the Office of Minority Health, and the National Institutes of Health's National Center on Minority Health and Health Disparities (Stone, 2002).

Healthy People 2020 has renewed its commitment to reduce health inequities by "identifying, measuring, tracking, and reducing health disparities through a determinant of health approach" (Healthy People 2020, 2013a). The Rio Declaration identified the place where a person is born, grows, lives, works, and ages as being critical areas and determinants of health (World Health Conference on Social Determinants of Health, 2011). Consistent with world policy, the Healthy People 2020 initiative has established five critical areas or determinants of health, including economic stability, neighborhood and the built environment, health and health care, social and community context, and education. The goal is "to create social and physical environments that create health for all." (Healthy People 2020, 2013b).

The National Institute for Nursing Research (NINR), in keeping with national and international recognition that health is negatively affected by factors of race, ethnicity, gender, economic disadvantage, geography, and culture, has adopted a strategic plan focused on reducing health disparities. NINR supports research designed to increase understanding of the determinants of health disparities and culturally appropriate strategies and interventions to reduce and eliminate health disparities in underserved and vulnerable populations (National Institutes of Health, U.S. Department of Health and Human Services, 2006). Health disparities seem to disproportionately affect ethnic minority populations to a greater degree than nonethnic minority populations, especially in conjunction with economic disadvantage. Blacks and nonwhite Hispanics in the United States received worse quality care than the white reference group based on 2008, 2009, and 2010 data from the National Healthcare Disparities Report (NHDR) (National Healthcare Disparities Report, 2012). Further, persons categorized as poor, low income, and middle income frequently experience worse health care than the majority white populace on 40% to 60% of the quality measures. Disparities in access to health care were also found for American Indians, Alaskan Natives, Hispanics, and the poor. In addition, poor whites have below-average health. Vulnerable groups, including minorities, women, children, and those with disabilities, are more susceptible to infectious diseases, especially HIV/AIDS and sexually transmitted infections (STIs) (Peragallo & Gonzalez, 2007).

WHO ARE THE MARGINALIZED?

Individuals or groups who live on the fringes or margins of society lack key resources and are most often underserved or not served at all, particularly in health care systems. Included among marginalized groups are:

- Persons with chronic disabilities
- Persons who are experiencing homelessness
- Immigrants, refugees, and migrants

These marginalized groups are discussed in the sections that follow. Furthermore, gender, ethnicity or race, education or income, geographic location, or sexual preference may account for group differences that lead to marginalization and subsequent health inequities (Healthy People, 2020). The comprehensive report by the Institute of Medicine (2002) in its review of more than 100 studies found that minorities were less likely to obtain health care than were whites. The review also documented inequities related to cancer, heart disease, diabetes, HIV/ AIDS, and mental illness.

The annual NHDR gives evidence of such inequities and serves as a regularly updated source for health care professionals to use as a guide to identify health disparities and plan strategies to improve health care (NHDR, 2012). The purpose of NHDR is to monitor health care quality and health disparities in the United States, note changes from the previous report, and determine where the greatest emphasis should be placed. The NHDR 2012 reported that despite overall improvement in the quality of health care, access to quality health care for minority and economically disadvantaged groups had not improved. Particular areas of concern centered around diabetes and cancer care, and care of persons living in the southern regions of the United States.

Persons With Disabilities

More than 37 million people or 12.1% of those individuals in the United States are estimated to be living with a disability, according to the American Community Survey (Erickson, Lee, & von Schrader, 2013). The American Disabilities Act (ADA) Public Law 101-336 enacted July 26, 1990, by the 101st Congress ensures that persons with disabilities are not discriminated against in employment opportunities and public services, including public accommodations, recreation, and transportation. The ADA Amendments Act of 2008, effective January 1, 2009, ascribes to the basic ADA definition: "an impairment that substantially limits one or more major life activities, a record of such impairment, or being regarded as having such impairment" (The U.S. Equal Employment Opportunity Commission, 2009a). However, the amendment revises the regulations defining "substantially limits" and amends the definition of the term *disability* by expanding the list of activities specifically identified, such as walking. For example, reading, bending, and communicating are now identified. Bodily functions (immune system, bowel/bladder, etc.) are now also identified as potential disabilities. The notion is that the definition of disability should be interpreted in a broad sense. Further standards for accessibility have also been added to the ADA Act for new or altered construction effective as of March 15, 2012 (Department of Justice, 2010). (For a full report of the ADA Act and the Amendment of 2008 made effective January 1, 2009, see The U.S. Equal Employment Opportunity Commission, 2009b.)

Nurses keeping the broader terminology for what constitutes a disability in mind should assess for disability because it may not always be obvious. Two simple questions can begin the conversation: (1) Are you limited in any way in activities because of physical, mental, or emotional problems? (2) Do you now have any health problem that requires you to use special equipment, such as a cane, a wheelchair, a special bed, or a special telephone? (CDC, 2006).

The ADA home page provides information and technical assistance related to the provision and spirit of the law at http://www.ada.gov/. Another useful resource is the free ADA information line 800-514-0301 (voice) or 800-514-0383 (TTY). In addition to the ADA homepage, the Department of Justice website maintains a *Disabilities Rights Section* to assist with the implementation of the ADA as well as opportunities to stay connected through social media (Department of Justice, 2013, http://www.justice.gov/crt/about/drs/).

Because the definition of disability is evolving, it is difficult to report the prevalence of persons with disabilities in general. It depends on how the data are collected and for what purpose. For example, the limitation may relate to a sensory, physical, mental, self-care, or a work disability. The National Center for Health Statistics (NCHS) reports that 34.4 million (11.8%) of noninstitutionalized individuals have a limitation in usual activities due to a chronic condition (NCHS, n.d.). For specific disability information, the reader is directed to the U.S. Census Bureau disability main page at http://www.census.gov/hhes/www/disability/disability.html.

The WHO, in its 66th assembly, focused on reducing disparities for persons living with disabilities, recognizing that compared with nondisabled individuals, persons with disabilities have less access to health care and poorer health in general (WHO, 2013a). Specifically, the WHO is advocating for more inclusive national action and treatment plans to address the disparities, better data collection procedures, and, perhaps most importantly, increased support for informal caregivers with the goal of improving overall functionality for persons with disabilities.

Persons Who Are Experiencing Homelessness

Individuals who make up the US homeless population are among the most marginalized and vulnerable to disabilities and disease. Although it is impossible to accurately report prevalence rates for those individuals lacking permanent housing due to methodological and funding issues, two trends have emerged over the past 20–25 years that have increased the number of those lacking housing: the reduced number of affordable rental units and the growing number of individuals living in poverty (National Coalition for the Homeless, 2009a).

The economic crisis, foreclosures, the collapse of the housing market, job shortages, and devastating natural events have affected individuals who are homeless and those at-risk for homelessness, despite efforts over the last decade to end homelessness (National Coalition for the Homeless, 2009b). Affordable housing, defined as housing that costs no more than 30% of income, exceeds the means of many families, rendering them at-risk of becoming homeless (Cunningham, 2009).

According to the Stewart B. McKinney Act, 42 USC 11301, et seq. (National Coalition for the Homeless, 2009a), the definition of a homeless person is one who "lacks a fixed, regular, and adequate night-time residence." Those people whose primary night residence is a supervised temporary shelter, an institution that provides temporary shelter for those intended to be institutionalized, or a public place not intended for sleeping would be considered homeless under the McKinney Act, 42 USC 11302. Homeless people who live in shelters, abandoned buildings, or other public areas are considered literally homeless. The McKinney definition is consistent with the literally homeless view, including those people who face imminent eviction (i.e., within 1 week). Marginally homeless people live doubled up in places they do not own or rent and consider their situation to be temporary. These people may be an illness, an accident, or a paycheck away from eviction and usually depend on utility assistance. When hospitalized, they often have no place to go after discharge.

The annual homeless assessment report to Congress (U.S. Department of Housing and Urban Development, 2012) estimates for the first time in 4 years the numbers of homeless persons decreased overall and in all subpopulations. For example, the Point In Time (PIT) estimate performed on a single night in January 2011 revealed that 1,502,196 persons used an emergency shelter or transitional housing. This reflects a decline of 5.7% from 2010 and a 5.4% decline since 2007. Policy changes responsible for this downturn include the Homeless Prevention and Rapid Re-Housing Program (HPRP), the HUD-Veterans Affairs Supportive Housing Program (HUD-VASH), and the Permanent Supportive Housing (PSH) initiative. However, this hopeful trend may be challenging to continue owing to the current financial climate and the temporary nature of funding streams such as the HPRP. Since 2007, homeless families increased by 13.5% and children comprised 341,040 of sheltered persons in 2011. Although numbers of homeless veterans decreased by 6% since 2009, a 2% increase in this group was noted between 2010 and 2011, with current estimates reported at 141,449 in 2011. More than half of the homeless individuals were counted in five states: California, New York, Florida, Georgia, and Texas, according to the PIT estimate in 2011.

Some individuals are not counted because they may be doubled up in temporary housing, living in cars, abandoned buildings, and on the street. In fact, the decrease in homeless counts may be in part due to families doubling up with relatives. Clearly, demographics of the homeless have changed in recent years. The alcoholic or illicit drug user is no longer the typical homeless person. Demographic profiles of homeless persons show that women with children comprise an exceedingly large portion of this marginalized group. The lack of affordable housing continues to be one of the primary causes of homelessness in the United States, with many Americans paying close to 50% of their disposable income for housing (Cunningham, 2009). Short-term solutions such as sheltering are not the ultimate answer. A multifaceted approach that focuses on affordable housing and resources that help people who are homeless or at-risk for homelessness deal with the complex issues that affect their lives, whether they stem from abuse, unemployment, or the sequelae of war or natural disasters, is essential. In light of this continuing public health problem, nurses must explore how effective, healthy partnerships with people who are homeless or at-risk can be initiated and sustained.

HEALTH PROMOTION STRATEGIES FOR PEOPLE WHO ARE HOMELESS

Primary Prevention

Primary prevention measures to prevent people who are at-risk for homelessness from becoming homeless are the first steps in health promotion for this population. Short-term solutions must be coupled with strategies to assess and care for the health needs of those vulnerable in our society. Affordable housing is crucial if the goal is to keep people in their homes. Some short-term measures are

Emergency financial assistance—Frequently, utility companies have an emergency fund that can be used to prevent utilities, such as water and electricity, from being discontinued. To find out if such an emergency fund exists, call the local utilities and ask. Inform at-risk homeless people how to apply for this assistance, and advise them of the information they will need to have handy when they call.

Legal assistance, such as consultation or mediation to prevent eviction—Is there a volunteer group of lawyers in the community? Find out where no-cost or sliding-scale legal assistance is available. Call the organization and learn about waiting time for an appointment, required documentation, and so forth.

Financial advisement—Free financial counseling programs are available in most communities. These programs can help inform people about money management. If instituted early enough, this strategy can effectively prevent homelessness. It is important that people at-risk for homelessness not be disconnected from the social support that they currently have. Sometimes, a small, one-time loan (i.e., money that is paid back) or grant (i.e., money that is not paid back) is all that is needed to pay the rent, thus preventing homelessness. Some state welfare programs have added a "one-time" emergency financial grant for housing and basic needs (water, electricity) in lieu of ongoing welfare assistance. Inquire about present assistance programs in your community. Such emergency financial aid for rent, security deposits, utility bills, and moving expenses can maintain an at-risk person in his or her residence during a critical period until a paycheck is received.

However, with high unemployment rates continuing, many will need more than short-term or a one-time type of assistance.

Political Advocacy—Nurses, as the group most trusted by the public, must recognize their role as political advocates for the vulnerable. The most effective measure may be to lend their voice in support of programs that support affordable housing and permanent solutions to prevent homelessness.

Secondary Prevention

Secondary prevention focuses on people who no longer have stable housing. Begin by listing all their perceived needs. It is helpful to categorize needs as housing needs, health care, or employment. Health care needs must be addressed first. Identify the barriers homeless people encounter in receiving health care and how these barriers might be eliminated. Many times, homeless people cannot access the health care system because they do not have a permanent address or adequate identification forms, such as a valid driver's license. Perhaps the person is a military veteran entitled to health care and other benefits, such as financial support associated with a disability. Frequently, waiting at hospitals and clinics for health care can interfere with obtaining shelter for the night. Often, there are a limited number of beds at homeless shelters, and, once the beds are filled, no additional people are admitted.

To promote the health of persons who are homeless, assess and evaluate community resources for serving this population. How many shelter beds are available? Are there shelters for families, for teens, for pregnant women, and for people with special dietary needs (e.g., diabetics or those with lactose intolerance)? Are emergency shelters available on a "walk-in" basis? What is available in terms of social and psychological support? Once in a shelter, rehabilitation may be necessary for medical or substantive problems such as alcohol or drug addictions. Is a counselor available to the shelter, and is a nurse or physician available for emergency medical needs?

The ultimate goal is exiting homelessness and counteracting the effects of being homeless. To reverse homelessness, transitional housing is important. Transitional housing needs to be free or very low cost. Frequently, homeless people are allowed to live in such housing units for extended periods of time to save up to afford permanent housing. In addition to shelter, social support is usually available (and always essential) at transitional housing.

A common concern for homeless people is following medication and treatment regimens. The following is a list of common conditions that require your constant awareness as you promote healthy partnerships with homeless people:

- Frequently, medications cannot be easily refrigerated.
- It is difficult to follow special dietary restrictions when meals are eaten at a shelter. Food is often very salty, high in fat, with limited fruits and vegetables. It is important for nurses to learn about food served at shelters and day centers. Ask if you might stay for a meal.
- Food may not be allowed in the sleeping areas at the shelter, so taking medication along with food may not be possible.
- Sometimes, medicine is swapped or sold for cash or people are assaulted for the medicine. Counsel those in the shelter as to where medicines may be safely stored.
- Often people who are homeless will request vitamins to compensate for nutritional deficits. Understand that they are usually trying their best to follow treatment regimens. Acknowledge this fact.

Part of a healthy partnership with homeless populations is further assessment of health and social service resources. See the list below for additional community assessment information. (This is a good time to refer to your general community assessment and evaluate it in terms of information specific to individuals and families who are homeless.)

- Do shelters offer clinic services? Is the service daily or weekly? What services are on-site and what services are referred? Unfortunately, funding sources for many of these health services have been eliminated. What alternative sources of community support can be mobilized to assist homeless individuals to access health services?
- Are local health departments and county hospitals within walking distance? Are bus tokens available for medical appointments? How long are the waits?
- Do mobile health vans operate in the area? Are they consistent in their delivery of health care (i.e., do they come the same day of the week to the same street corner)? What services do they offer? Some services are key to treating people who are homeless (e.g., laboratory services, including HIV testing and counseling, x-ray, and dental services).
- Are services linked to a religious group? There may be expectations associated with receiving services that may or may not be acceptable to the person who is homeless.

Overcoming Barriers Related to the Education of Youth Who Are Homeless

Education is a critical area and social determinant of health (World Health Conference on Social Determinants of Health, 2011). The McKinney-Vento Homeless Education Act of 2001 legislated the reduction of barriers to enrollment, attendance, and success in school. Under the reauthorization, each homeless child/youth is ensured equal access to an appropriate public education, including public preschool. The Act also stipulates that homelessness alone is not a reason to separate children from mainstream education. See the full text of the legislation at the National Center for Homeless Education website (http://www.serve.org/nche/), a clearinghouse for information and resources on the educational rights of homeless children and youth. To escape the cycle of adult poverty, it is imperative that children and youth who experience homelessness stay in school. Furthermore, school may be the only stable factor in their lives. Unfortunately, some well-meaning school personnel may be unaware of or insensitive to the educational system barriers faced by parents and their children without stable housing. See Box 18.1 for an outline of these barriers.

Box 18.1 Education System Barriers for Homeless Individuals

Enrollment Barriers
- Transportation
- Lack of immunizations/medical records
- Lack of previous school records
- Guardianship/residency issues
- School fees

School Success Barriers
- Frequent mobility
- Inability to complete assignments
- Poor health/inadequate medical care
- Lack of food/clothing
- Teacher/staff unawareness/insensitivity
- Isolation or stigma associated with being homeless
- Difficulty accessing services (psychological, special education, English as a second language [ESL] instruction, and so forth)

PROMOTING THE SEXUAL HEALTH OF ADOLESCENTS WHO ARE HOMELESS

Adolescents, particularly young women, constitute one of the most vulnerable groups within the homeless population. In one study by Rew, Chambers, and Kulkarni (2002), these young women reported the need for more instruction in self-care and stated that access to health care was less than adequate. The women claimed that they were routinely treated with a lack of respect and often not even called by name. These claims are particularly alarming in relation to a study of the National Cancer Institute that reported increased rates of cervical cancer in certain groups such as southern African American women, Latinas on the Texas–Mexico border, European American women in Appalachia, Native American women in the northern plains, Vietnamese American women, and Alaskan Natives. These increased rates are in sharp contrast with rates of the general US population, which have decreased substantially, suggesting that cervical cancer may be an indicator of a larger issue—access to health care. Transportation and lack of financial resources were additional barriers to health care identified in Rew's study. The young women preferred to seek care in designated homeless outreach clinics, where their situation was understood and nonjudgmental medical care was usually dispensed; however, this was not always possible.

The following points are important to consider when designing a sexual health education and health care program for homeless adolescents or adolescents in general:

- When possible, conduct focus groups to allow adolescents to have a voice in planning for their sexual health needs.
- Establish trust with a respectful and nonjudgmental attitude.
- Maintain confidentiality and privacy.
- Use small media, such as brochures, to deliver health information.
- Provide sexual health information that is broad in nature and not narrowly focused on HIV (Ensign & Panke, 2002; Rew et al., 2002).

PROMOTING HEALTHY PARTNERSHIPS WITH PEOPLE EXITING HOMELESSNESS

Most people will exit their homeless state. To prevent recurrence of homelessness, it is imperative that a strong support system be in place. It is not enough merely to provide transitional housing. Preventing recurrence requires a commitment to support those exiting homelessness for long periods of time (usually several years). Health promotion strategies to support people exiting homelessness include

- Coordination of services, such as health, social, substance abuse, and mental health
- Continuity of care
- Case management services
- Transportation
- Job training
- Child care options
- Sources for funding programs

Public health nurses working in the community can lobby for changes in legislation that can prevent homelessness at the primary prevention level. Supporting legislation to raise the minimum wage is one example. The National Coalition for the Homeless formulates annual priorities related to the plight of the homeless. Current priorities relate to the Housing Trust

Fund, Medicaid Expansion in Affordable Care Act, and disputing criminalization of homeless individuals. (For full details, see National Coalition for the Homeless, n.d.).

Recognizing that measures to raise the minimum wage and create adequate, affordable housing are harder to accomplish in difficult economic times, yet such initiatives must be prioritized to continue the downward trend in homelessness. Lastly, one must recognize that some people choose to remain on the streets and continue their homeless existence. However, most people without housing do not want to remain homeless, but are caught in a desperate situation. It is the responsibility of public health nurses to promote healthy partnership with homeless populations.

IMMIGRANTS, REFUGEES, AND MIGRANTS

Marginalization experienced by persons who are homeless or live with disability is also experienced by those who come to live in America from foreign lands, including immigrants, refugees, and migrants. These individuals and families have commonalities, but their differences are significant and central to their health status and access to care. The first step for nurses who care for these groups is to understand those differences with the objective of adapting health care to meet specific needs.

Although aliens in the United States are commonly called *immigrants*, there are important legal distinctions. The Immigration Act (INA) of 1990 excludes noncitizens living in the United States under legally recognized circumstances from the term *immigrant* (U.S. Citizenship and Immigration Services [USCIS], n.d.). A noncitizen recognized and documented is known as a *permanent resident alien, lawful permanent resident, resident alien permit holder,* or *green card holder.* Conversely, someone who enters the United States without proper authority or inspection is called an immigrant under the INA. Most permanent residents come to the United States for economic or social benefit. However, a person unable or unwilling to return to his or her country of origin out of fear of persecution for religious, racial, ideological, or political beliefs qualifies as a refugee. For example, the USCIS has redesignated Syrians as eligible for Temporary Protected Status (TPS) through March 31, 2015 due to extraordinary and temporary dangerous conditions that continue to plague their country or origin, Syria (USCIS, 2013). The President with Congress set annual quotas for admission of refugees. Some nonimmigrants seek temporary residence or transit through the United States for a specific purpose, and they can be accompanied by family members. International students fit this category. Migrant workers or temporary agricultural workers come to the United States to perform services or labor of a temporary or seasonal nature. Some migrants obtain permanent residence status in the United States, but travel seasonally to different *colonias* in search of work. Childhood arrivals, that is, those children who arrived in this country as children and who meet guidelines, are granted a deferred status without threat of removal (USCIS, 2012). See the U.S. Department of Immigration Services for more information and resources at http://www.uscis.gov/.

The circumstances surrounding the motivation for leaving one's country of origin vary. Personal experiences have an impact on health. For example, the health needs of immigrants, refugees, or migrant workers are likely to be different, and access to health services will also differ. These groups frequently hesitate to object when health care services have been denied or to contact authorities when their human rights have been violated. Language barriers often add another layer of complexity and misunderstanding between health care providers and these marginalized groups.

Consider this true scenario of an immigrant hospitalized in four-point traction for 2 weeks. Only when a student nurse engaged a translator, did his distressing story unfold. When the young man asked for wages due after several weeks of work, he was thrust out of a moving van on a major interstate. He had no family in the United States. He had family in Mexico, but no one had been contacted. Ethical arguments could focus on limited health care resources and the absence of legal authority in this case. The reality is that nurses and other health care professionals will encounter similar situations in health care settings across the nation and must understand the complexities and differences of each situation to develop and implement culturally relevant humane plans of care.

Refugees and immigrants typically experience three phases as they assimilate into the country of destination, with each phase having specific health care implications. The phases are an acute period (the immediate arrival in the new country), followed by a time of transition, and a resolution or chronic phase (Kemp, 2008). Acute health problems, such as tuberculosis, parasites, or hepatitis, may stem from conditions in the country of origin or result from travel to the new country. For example, one refugee who left Vietnam in a crowded small boat stated it was 14 days before the evacuees were rescued. Food and fresh water were scarce and nutritional concerns immediate. In addition, she was distraught at the time because several of her brothers had been killed in the war. Boat People SOS (BPSOS, n.d.) is a Vietnamese organization whose original mission began as to rescue boat people escaping oppression in Viet Nam. It has grown into a national organization designed to empower and create strong ethical leaders among Vietnamese Americans, former refugees and their offspring. Visit their website to learn more about this intriguing community (BPSOS, http://www.bpsos.org/mainsite/en/about-us.html).

History taking is an important step in planning care. Once the acute health needs have been identified and resolved, chronic conditions may emerge, including post-traumatic stress disorder (PTSD). The resolution phase is connected to how well the immigrant or refugee assimilates into the American culture. This includes identifying with mainstream politics and communicating in English. A special report, *Building an Americanization Movement for the 21st Century,* addresses this process, while recognizing that America was built as a nation of immigrants. It can be found at http://www.uscis.gov/files/nativedocuments/M-708.pdf (U.S. Department of Homeland Security, Task Force on New Americans, 2008).

PROMOTING HEALTHY PARTNERSHIPS THROUGH EDUCATION

As previously stated, education is an important determinant of health. This is a particularly critical area for the vulnerable populations discussed in this chapter. Various educational strategies are discussed in the following sections. As you read the different sections, consider how you might change, modify, or combine the different educational programs to accommodate various marginalized populations.

Educating About Chronic Conditions

Having a chronic condition presents many challenges. The following is an educational program for diabetics who are homeless. You may choose to adapt this model to meet the specific needs of another marginalized group. You can make the necessary changes for another chronic condition, such as hypertension. The program can be presented in a cultural center for recent immigrants, a colonia for migrants, or the local health clinic for an impoverished community. Be sure to do a needs assessment and ask members of the community to participate in the planning phase.

- Arrange with shelter administration to have a diabetic teaching class in the main waiting area of the shelter.
- Emphasize the importance of foot care using posters written at the 3rd-grade level.

- Demonstrate proper foot care by having homeless people in attendance soak their feet in basins. Inspect feet with attention to any red, swollen, cracked, or infected areas. Be sure to discuss the importance of properly drying the feet.
- Discuss the importance of shoes that fit properly and dry, clean socks.
- Offer attendees socks, perhaps donated from local merchants or collected by neighborhood schoolchildren. A letter of solicitation to merchants for socks can be drafted from the educational institution with which student nurses are affiliated and with the shelter's name.
- Gather shoes in advance by placing receptacles in city or suburban fitness clubs encouraging runners to donate slightly used athletic shoes. (Runners often replace shoes every 2 to 3 months. Although the shoes may no longer be suitable for running, there is usually a lot of wear left for day-to-day use.)
- Distribute incentives in a fair, organized manner. Doing so requires detailed advance planning. Distribution is best done at the end of the program.
- Provide referrals for health needs (e.g., foot infections, ingrown toenails, fungal conditions, circulatory concerns); follow-up mechanisms must be in place.
- Offer blood pressure and glucose screening in conjunction with the educational program.

Offering Positive Parenting Sessions

To assist women and men in shelters learn better strategies for coping with children, parenting classes can be offered. Suggested topics to include are

- Advantages of breast-feeding
- Normal behaviors for developmental ages
- Behaviors that indicate a child is ill
- Normal height and weight for age
- Nonviolent ways to discipline (e.g., time-out, consistency, clear rules)
- Healthy, low-cost food choices (fruit, peanut butter, cheese, eggs)
- Assertiveness and empowerment training

Organizing a Health Fair

A health fair is another way to cover a number of health promotion and education areas at once. Screening procedures such as dental, blood pressure, cholesterol, blood glucose, vision, hearing, and lead poison can be included in the agenda. Steps for organizing a health fair are listed below:

- Contact the shelter administrator.
- Set the date well in advance (6 months to 1 year, if possible).
- Decide what health promotion areas to cover, depending on the audience (e.g., families versus only adult males).
- Invite identified organizations to participate.
- Solicit prizes from local merchants.
- Offer incentives for attendance, such as educational hours (most shelters require participation in self-help programs). Other ideas to consider when planning a health fair include the following:
  - Collaborate with other professionals, such as a dental school.
  - Offer immunizations.
  - Include screening stations, such as vision, hearing, blood glucose, acanthosis nigricans, blood pressure, lead, tuberculosis skin testing, HIV testing, depression, and intimate partner violence.

- Assign booth areas, considering flow pattern.
- Include fun activities, such as a magician for children or massage therapy for adults.
- Have a plan for referral and follow-up.

Visit the Family and Consumer Services website (http://fcs.tamu.edu/health/health_fair_planning_guide/objectives_and_planning.php) for a Health Fair Planning Guide that offers national resources for health fairs for more ideas (Family and Consumer Sciences, 2011).

Summary

Poverty impacts health. It potentially contributes to the marginalization of certain groups more than any other factor. Often these marginalized groups are underserved or not served at all. They are likely to be uninsured or underinsured. Americans must realize that this is a societal problem that requires multiple strategies to decrease and eventually eliminate disparities in health care.

Several marginalized groups were discussed in this chapter. More research is needed to identify marginalized populations and their particular problems. Persons with disabilities comprise a substantial portion of the US population. The number of people who are homeless or at-risk for homelessness continues to increase, although the demographics are changing. Immigrants, refugees, and migrant workers are entering the United States by legal and illegal methods. To embrace the goal of Healthy People 2020, aimed at achieving health equity, eliminating disparities, and improving the health standards for all groups, a concerted effort should target and model already successful programs. Furthermore, the most important strategies are probably politically based. Nursing is well positioned to address disparities as related to the health of marginalized groups, and should work diligently to move health care for these groups into the mainstream.

Critical Thinking Questions

When working with marginalized groups, it is important to consider how different processes influence outcomes.

1. Identify political, economic, legal, cultural, and access to health care realities for a marginalized group in your community, and explain how these factors may lead to positive or negative health outcomes.

2. Adherence to medical regimen is often very difficult or impossible for the homeless. As a nurse working in the health department clinic of a homeless shelter, you have noticed a high prevalence of hypertension among the residents of the shelter. Routinely, you advise your clients to modify their daily sodium intake. Is this a realistic expectation for someone living in a homeless shelter? What questions need to be answered? How is the food prepared? Who prepares the food? Is bulk food received from a government source? Do the residents have input into the meal planning? What steps or solutions would you implement to address this issue? Be sure to consider strategies at different levels of prevention. Who should be involved in the plan? What are some other conditions that might pose problems with adherence to a medical regimen?

3. What is the role of bias, stereotyping, and discrimination in relation to unequal treatment of marginalized groups? First, define the terms. How do these concepts impact ethnic/racial or otherwise marginalized groups in our society? What historical or contextual

factors might be influential? Think of examples that have occurred in your community or health care setting. What strategies can you identify to increase awareness of health care providers?

4. Optional: Visit a homeless shelter in your town and observe or sample the food served. What did you learn?

5. Optional: Visit a community home for the disabled. What are some of the barriers the disabled face in the course of daily living?

6. Consider the scenario of the young hospitalized immigrant discussed in this chapter. What were the shortcomings of the health system in that case? What other situations can you think of that affect the care of immigrants? Refugees? Migrants? What steps can nurses delivering health services to these groups take to increase the quality of care? Visit the internet to find advocacy groups specific to immigrant issues.

REFERENCES

Boat People SOS. (n.d.). Retrieved from http://www.bpsos.org/mainsite/en/about-us.html

Centers for Disease Control and Prevention. (2006). *Disability and health*. Retrieved December 5, 2009, from http://www.cdc.gov/ncbddd/dh/hp2010.htm

Cunningham, M. (2009). *Preventing and ending homelessness—next steps*. Washington, DC: The Urban Institute. Retrieved February 27, 2009, from http://www.urban.org/UploadedPDF/411837_ending_homelessness.pdf

Department of Justice. (2010). *2010 Standards for Accessible Design*. Retrieved from http://www.ada.gov/regs2010/2010ADAStandards/2010ADAstandards.htm#titleIII

Department of Justice. (2013). *Disabilities Rights Section*. Retrieved from http://www.justice.gov/crt/about/drs/

Ensign, J., & Panke, A. (2002). Barriers and bridges to care: Voices of homeless female adolescent youth in Seattle, Washington, USA. *Journal of Advanced Nursing, 37*(2), 166–172.

Erickson, W., Lee, C., & von Schrader, S. (2013). *Disability Statistics from the 2011 American Community Survey (ACS)*. Ithaca, NY: Cornell University Employment and Disability Institute (EDI). Retrieved September 1, 2013, from www.disabilitystatistics.org

Family and Consumer Sciences. (2011). *Health fair planning guide*. Retrieved from http://fcs.tamu.edu/health/health_fair_planning_guide/objectives_and_planning.php

Flaskerud, J. H., Lesser, J., Dixon, E., Anderson, N., Conde, F., Kim, S., . . . Verzemnieks, I. (2002). Health disparities among vulnerable populations. *Nursing Research, 51*(2), 74–85.

Flaskerud, J. H., & Winslow, B. J. (1998). Conceptualizing vulnerable populations health-related research. *Nursing Research, 47*(2), 69–78.

Healthy People 2020. (2013a). *Understanding and improving health*. Retrieved from http://www.healthypeople.gov/2020/about/new2020.aspx

Healthy People 2020. (2013b). *Social determinants of health*. Retrieved from http://www.healthypeople.gov/2020/topicsobjectives2020/overview.aspx?topicid=39

Institute of Medicine. (2002). *Unequal treatment: Confronting racial and ethnic disparities in health care*. Washington, DC: National Academics Press.

Kemp, C. (2008). *Promoting healthy partnerships with refugees and immigrants*. In J. McFarlane & E. Anderson (Eds.), *Community as partner* (pp. 357–367). Philadelphia, PA: Lippincott.

National Center for Health Statistics. (n.d.). *Summary health statistics for the U.S. Population*. Retrieved from http://www.cdc.gov/nchs/fastats/disable.htm

National Coalition for the Homeless. (2009a). *Who is homeless?* Retrieved from http://www.nationalhomeless.org/factsheets/who.html

National Coalition for the Homeless. (2009b). *Why are people homeless?* Retrieved from http://www.nationalhomeless.org/factsheets/who.html

National Coalition for the Homeless. (n.d.). *Advocacy*. Retrieved from http://www.nationalhomeless.org/advocacy/index.html

National Health Disparities Report. (2012). Retrieved from http://www.ahrq.gov/research/findings/nhqrdr/nhdr12/nhdr12_prov.pdf

National Institutes of Health, U.S. Department of Health and Human Services. (2006). *Strategic plan: National Institute for Nursing Research (NINR), 2006–2010*. Retrieved December 5, 2009, from http://www.ninr.nih.gov/NR/rdonlyres/9021E5EB-B2BA-47EA-B5DB-1E4DB11B1289/4894/NINR_StrategicPlanWebsite.pdf

Nyamathi, A., Koniak-Griffin, D., & Greengold, B. A. (2007). Development of nursing theory and science in vulnerable populations research. *Annual Review of Nursing Research, 25*, 3–25.

Peragallo, N., & Gonzalez, R. M. (2007). Nursing research and the prevention of infectious diseases among vulnerable populations. *Annual Review of Nursing Research, 25*, 83–117.

Rew, L., Chambers, K. B., & Kulkarni, S. (2002). Planning a sexual health promotion intervention with homeless adolescents. *Nursing Research, 51*(3), 168–174.

Stone, J. (2002). Race and healthcare disparities: Overcoming vulnerability. *Theoretical Medicine, 23,* 499–518.

U.S. Citizenship and Immigration Services. (2012). *USCIS begins accepting requests for consideration of deferred action for childhood arrivals.* Retrieved from http://www.uscis.gov/portal/site/uscis/menuitem.5af9bb95919f35e6 6f614176543f6d1a/?vgnextoid=450a5b0325a29310VgnVCM100000082ca60aRCRD&vgnextchannel=c94e6d26 d17df110VgnVCM1000004718190aRCRD

U.S. Citizenship and Immigration Services. (2013). *DHS announces re-designation and 18-month extension of Temporary Protected Status for Syria.* Retrieved from http://www.uscis.gov/portal/site/uscis/menuitem.5af9bb95919f35e 66f614176543f6d1a/?vgnextoid=70045815fd15f310VgnVCM100000082ca60aRCRD&vgnextchannel=68439c77 55cb9010VgnVCM10000045f3d6a1RCRD

U.S. Citizenship and Immigration Services. (n.d.). Retrieved from http://www.uscis.gov

U.S. Department of Homeland Security, Task Force on New Americans. (2008). *Building an Americanization Movement for the Twenty-first Century: A Report to the President of the United States from the Task Force on New Americans.* Washington, DC 2008: Author. Retrieved December 11, 2009, from http://www.uscis.gov/files/ nativedocuments/M-708.pdf

U.S. Department of Housing and Urban Development. (2012, November). *The 2011 annual report on homelessness to Congress.* Retrieved from http://www.iaced.org/2011/06/ahar-homeless-congress-201/

U.S. Equal Employment Opportunity Commission. (2009a). *Notice concerning the Americans with Disabilities Act (ADA) Amendments Act of 2008.* Retrieved December 5, 2009, from http://www.eeoc.gov/ada/amendments_ notice.html

U.S. Equal Employment Opportunity Commission. (2009b). *The ADA Amendments Act of 2008.* Retrieved from http://www.eeoc.gov/laws/statutes/adaaa.cfm

Vasas, E. B. (2005). Examining the margins a concept analysis of marginalization. *Advances in Nursing Science, 28*(3), 194–202.

World Health Conference on Social Determinants of Health. (2011). *Rio political declaration of social determinants of health.* Retrieved from http://www.who.int/sdhconference/declaration/Rio_political_declaration.pdf

World Health Organization. (2008). *The World Health Report: Primary health care now more than ever.* Retrieved from http://www.who.int/whr/2008/whr08_en.pdf

World Health Organization. (2013a). *66th World Health Assembly adopts resolution calling for better health care for people with disabilities.* Retrieved from http://www.who.int/disabilities/media/news/2013/28_05/en/

World Health Organization. (2013b). *What are the social determinants of health?* Retrieved from http://www.who.int/ social_determinants/sdh_definition/en/index.html

FURTHER READINGS

U.S. Department of Health and Human Services. (2008). The Secretary's Advisory Committee on National Health Promotion and Disease Prevention Objectives for 2020. *Phase I Report: Recommendations for the framework and format of Healthy People 2020.* Retrieved January 6, 2010, from http://www.healthypeople.gov/hp2020/advisory/ PhaseI/sec4.htm#_Toc211942917

U.S. Department of Health and Human Services. (2012). *National Healthcare Disparities Report 2012.* Retrieved from http://www.ahrq.gov/research/findings/nhqrdr/nhdr12/nhdr12_prov.pdf

CHAPTER 19

Promoting Healthy Partnerships in the Workplace

Ann T. Malecha

LEARNING OBJECTIVES

After studying this chapter, you should be able to:

1. Assess health promotion needs in the workplace.

2. Discuss strategies for successful primary, secondary, and tertiary health promotion programs.

3. Plan, implement, and evaluate programs that teach healthy behaviors to diverse groups of employees and their families.

Introduction

Health promotion, disease prevention and control, wellness, risk factor reduction, and preventive health care are some of the terms applied to workplace health programs. In this chapter, the term *health promotion* is used to denote a process by which employees learn about primary, secondary, and tertiary prevention strategies to improve their health and quality of life. A partnership between employer and employee to promote the safety and health of the workers benefits both parties. The *Occupational Safety and Health Act of 1970* created the Occupational Safety and Health Administration (OSHA) to assure the safety and health of all American workers via partnerships and alliances with employers and other agencies (U.S. Department of Labor, Occupational Safety and Health Administration, 2013a). OSHA establishes and enforces standards to help employers and employees reduce injuries, illnesses, and deaths on the job. In 1970, an estimated 14,000 workers were killed on the job—about 38 every day. For 2010, the Bureau of Labor Statistics reports this number fell to about 4,500, or about 12 workers per day, with US employment increasing to over 130 million workers at 7.2 million worksites (U.S. Department of Labor, Occupational Safety and Health Administration, 2013a). Workplace health promotion programs have been developed and refined over the past 30 years and have achieved long-term behavior change and risk reduction among employees. Workplaces are ideal settings in which to implement health promotion programs because they contain groups of people usually in one location who share a common purpose and culture (Woolf et al., 2009).

Occupational and environmental health nursing is the specialty practice that focuses on preventive health care, health promotion, and health restoration within the context of a safe and healthy environment (American Association of Occupational Health Nurses, 2012). The process of promoting health in the workplace involves providing information and developing health-education programs that encourage employees to take responsibility for their health to lower risk of disease and injury (American Association of Occupational Health Nurses, 2012). New knowledge and new skills implemented in daily life followed by sustaining the learned behaviors results in healthier workers.

The occupational health nurse is often responsible for health promotion programs at the worksite and is an excellent resource person for establishing a community partnership. If the organization does not have an occupational nurse, health programs may be the responsibility of the safety officer or an employee in the company's human resources or benefits department. Ask who coordinates health activities. For businesses with 2 to 100 employees, health promotion efforts can be facilitated by partnering with other local businesses, county extension or agricultural agents, state departments of health, or national awareness campaigns. The nursing processes for promoting health at the workplace focus on the entire workforce of the company and may even extend to the employees' dependents (spouses and children).

Most American businesses employing 50 or more workers are involved in health promotion activities. Companies integrate health promotion into employee recruitment (e.g., membership at a health club), job training (e.g., back care), safety (e.g., hearing conservation), health (e.g., risk profiles and screenings), and recreation efforts (e.g., fun runs and sports teams). Employers are interested in promoting the health and safety of their employees for multiple reasons, including increasing productivity, reducing absenteeism, maintaining safety standard requirements, improving employee morale, and lowering workers' compensation and insurance claims.

Health promotion activities at the workplace begin with assessing the health needs of the entire workforce, including management. The next step is creating an awareness of the health issues through companywide education, screening, and interventions that focus on behavior or lifestyle changes. This chapter discusses strategies for successful health promotion and safety programs, describes the steps used in implementing various programs, and lists several available resources.

TYPES OF HEALTH PROMOTION ACTIVITIES FOR THE WORKPLACE

Common workplace activities that promote health or prevent injury and disease are exercise, smoking cessation, back care, and stress-management programs. Frequently, companies offer employee health newsletters; health risk appraisals (HRAs); health fairs; and screenings, such as blood pressure checks and blood lipid levels. HRAs and employee health-focused newsletters can be made available to employees via purchased printed materials or online subscriptions. Some web-based programs allow the employee to connect with discussion forums, encourage personalized goal setting and outcomes tracking, and provide the employer with confidential aggregate reports. Web-based programs are a particularly well-matched method to serve small businesses and telecommuters.

Health promotion in the workplace typically falls within three basic program types:

- *Awareness programs* increase the employees' level of knowledge and interest (e.g., flyers, seminars, and newsletters).
- *Behavior change activities* help participants develop healthier behaviors (e.g., smoking cessation, regular exercise, and healthy nutrition).
- *Supportive environments* create work opportunities that encourage healthy lifestyles (e.g., low-fat foods in the cafeteria, on-site aerobic classes, release time for health screenings, sunscreen dispenser by walking trail).

When deciding on the type of health promotion program to offer, it is important to determine how consistent that program is with the company's mission and goals. Also consider the costs and benefits of the activity for both the employer and the employee. Whereas employers are aware of the potential for financial benefits, such as reducing absenteeism or improved work output, most employees participate in health promotion programs for personal reasons (weight reduction, increased physical fitness). The worker desires to look and feel better or to have an improved quality of life. Meeting the needs of both the organization and the employees will support wide employee participation and a highly successful health program.

PLANNING A HEALTH PROMOTION PROGRAM

Needs Assessment

Questionnaires and HRAs are commonly used to identify employees' interest in educational topics and to describe present health and safety behaviors. Ideas for health and lifestyle survey topics to include on a questionnaire appear in Box 19.1. To include all these topics on one questionnaire would be overwhelming. However, if a plan for the year were developed with a different focus each month that began with a brief questionnaire to establish interest, then one could be assured of success.

Employee health and insurance records can also be used to identify prevalence of chronic illnesses of the employees that need to be addressed. Safety records, workers' compensation

---

Box 19.1 Ideas for Health and Lifestyle Survey Topics

Exercise and fitness
Overweight and obesity
Nutrition and eating well
Vitamins and natural remedies
Smoking cessation
Weight management
Vision and hearing care
Men's health
Women's health
Pregnancy and care of the newborn
Pediatric fever and pain management
Menopause, osteoporosis, and estrogen replacement therapy
Safety (bicycle, motorcycle helmets, safety belts, and car air bags)
Safely traveling abroad
Violence (women, children, older adults, disabled persons, and workplace)
Depression and anxiety
Stress management and relaxation
Adult pain management (back, neck, and wrists)
Heartburn and indigestion
Heart health (blood lipid levels, hypertension, heart attack, and stroke)
Chronic disease management
Cancer (prevention, treatment, and survivors)
Allergies and asthma

forms, or employee and manager interviews are additional resources for determining employee and company health promotion needs.

Once the needs have been identified, you may assist the occupational nurse or planning advisory committee in securing management support for a health promotion program. A proposal presentation or executive report is often one of the first steps in convincing management of the value of the project. A feasibility or business plan approach to communicating your program is used to establish a common language and understanding of the project by everyone in the organization. A sample business plan might include the following:

- *Executive summary:* A short summary of the health promotion plan, which includes the purpose (e.g., to decrease lower back strain); methods (e.g., three 30-minute classes); expected benefits (e.g., fewer work days missed, increased productivity); and costs (e.g., program costs, such as brochures, flyers, teaching time, and incentives, as well as avoidance costs, such as averted absenteeism and decreased insurance and workman's compensation claims).
- *Methods:* How, when, and where the plan will be put into action. List each task to be completed (e.g., brochure and flyer design and dissemination). Who is the responsible person(s)? Develop a timeline for task completion. Outline the content of the program, including use of guest speakers, demonstrations, return demonstrations, and methods to increase employee participation and adaptation of the taught behaviors. Include program goal and objectives in this section of the proposal. *A program goal might be*: Eighty percent of employees completing the back care program will report a decrease in the number of sick days related to low back pain. *A program objective could be*: After lectures and demonstrations on correct lifting procedures, 90% of participating employees will demonstrate correct lifting techniques.
- *Expected benefits:* List outcomes of program (e.g., fewer work days missed due to low back pain). This is a good point in the proposal to note the number of days missed in the last year and by what percentage the proposed program will decrease that absenteeism. This is also a place in the report to cite other companies that you have found in the literature that have implemented similar programs and the results these companies experienced.
- *Costs:* An accurate projection of program costs (materials, teachers' time, incentives), as well as profits expected due to decreased absenteeism and increased productivity.

Health Risk Appraisals

A HRA is an easily administered, confidential instrument used to determine life expectancy based on current risk behaviors. The HRA can also calculate the amount of risk that could be avoided if lifestyle behaviors were changed. Some HRAs determine the person's readiness to change behavior. An HRA can be used as a teaching tool that gives positive feedback for healthy behaviors and encouragement and information for changing those unhealthy behaviors. An HRA is often completed on an interactive computer program and provides an accurate individualized report to each employee in a timely manner (within 2 weeks). Anonymous aggregate data are provided to the company. The usefulness of the information to the employer depends on a significant proportion of the employee population participating (hopefully at least 70% to 80% of employees). Confidentiality of HRA information and publicizing highlights of the aggregate summary may boost future participation levels.

Specific HRAs exist to assess nutritional status, weight, and general fitness status. If you are ready for a study break, stop and check out these HRAs on the internet. (When you get the website, search for HRA). Consider how each could be used for a health promotion program at the worksite.

- Sample HRA—http://www.nationalwellness.org/TestWell/index.htm
- Centers for Disease Control and Prevention—http://www.cdc.gov/nccdphp/dnpa/hwi/program_design/health_risk_appraisals.htm

USING STAGES OF CHANGE IN HEALTH PROMOTION PROGRAMS

Because most health promotion programs involve lifestyle behavioral change, Prochaska's change process (Prochaska & DiClemente, 1983), Pender's Health Belief Model (Pender, Murdaugh, & Parsons, 2010), or your chosen model/theory can guide the process from planning through evaluation. A brief review of the stages of the change process follows.

- *Precontemplation:* In this stage, the employee is not even thinking about changing his or her behavior. The goal is to make the person aware of the benefits of change and to get him or her to start thinking about the possibility of change.
- *Contemplation:* In this stage, the employee is at least considering making an effort to change behavior. The employee is weighing the pros and the cons. The employee may not know how to change and may consider the change to be almost impossible. The attempt to change is not worth the effort if failure is to occur. The goal is to help the employee identify the benefits and to decide that putting forth an effort to change is worthwhile.
- *Preparation:* A person at this stage has decided to try and change a behavior(s). This employee desires help in making the change and is ready for information and skills to maintain the behavioral change.
- *Action:* At this stage, the employee is practicing the new behavior; however, it is not yet incorporated into his or her lifestyle. The new behavior requires lots of effort, which leaves the employee at risk for relapsing to the old behavior. The employee needs support, incentives, and sincere encouragement.
- *Maintenance:* The new behavior is ingrained in the lifestyle behaviors. A crisis or major stressor at work or personal life can become the impetus to revert to the previous behavior. The employee needs reinforcement, support, and opportunities to practice the new behavior. The employee benefits by sharing the newly learned behavior.

PROGRAM IMPLEMENTATION

Marketing is an essential part of successful program implementation. Some strategies for marketing include:

- *Must be professional looking.* Catchy words and titles are essential (e.g., "Weigh to Go" for a weight reduction program). Change posters frequently to keep attention focused.
- *Electronic mail messages.* Count down to event; offer a related health quiz question, and give the answer and rationale the following day.
- *Health newsletter.* Detail a success story, such as early detection of malignant melanoma, weight loss regimen using a walking program, or not knowing a person had high blood pressure until participating in a screening program and how simple lifestyle changes helped control the disease (without medication).
- *Letter from the company's president or benefits manager.* Offering company time for health screening, announcing that the company will pay for all or a portion of smoking cessation program/health screening test, or allowing a trade-in of 2 hours of sick time for wellness program attendance would be appropriate messages.
- *Incentive gifts.* Offer incentive gifts to participating employees, such as T-shirts, hats, sunscreen samples, a healthy fruit snack, or water bottles.

PROGRAM EVALUATION

The evaluation process provides an opportunity to determine the outcomes derived by the health promotion program and directs improvement of employee health services. Evaluating the structure of the program, the process by which the program was delivered, as well as the outcomes of the program is a three-pronged approach common to quality assurance reviews.

Structural evaluation involves (1) reviewing the mechanism for reporting to management and the support given to the health promotion program; (2) determining if the physical facilities were adequate for the program; (3) identifying equipment and supplies used; (4) identifying staffing requirements and their qualifications; (5) analyzing employee demographics and their health status needs; and (6) determining if the program mission, goals, and objectives were formulated to meet both the health needs of the employee and the business needs of the employer.

Process evaluation addresses (1) whether the health promotion activity was appropriate for the setting; (2) whether the health promotion program was designed to meet workplace needs (you can measure against the initial needs assessment); and (3) whether there was documentation and record keeping.

Outcome evaluation focuses on (1) were expected goals and objectives achieved; (2) did the program lead to positive outcomes; (3) did health outcomes demonstrate prevention of illness/injury, increase compliance, increase employees' self-care knowledge, restore function, or relieve discomfort; (4) how did program benefits compare with program costs; and (5) satisfaction (of employees, employers, dependents) with the quality of health promotion services received.

Common methods for evaluation are postprogram rating scales, observation, and interviewing of employees about their opinions, attitudes, and satisfaction with the program. Chart-and-record reviews can be used to determine morbidity and mortality differences.

TIPS FOR MAINTAINING A HEALTH PROMOTION PROGRAM

To sustain a health promotion effort, always design the program according to the goals of the organization. Include from the beginning an identified, key workplace employee or manager. As part of the health promotion program, teach employees where, when, and how to use community resources. Include short- and middle-range evaluation of the program. If possible, give projections of long-range success, savings, health benefits (e.g., morbidity and costs of finding early-stage disease and averting possible surgery, pain, hospitalization, workman's compensation, and so forth). Always propose to incorporate health promotion into the employee benefits plan.

EXAMPLES OF HEALTH PROMOTION PROGRAMS

Skin Cancer Prevention

This Skin Cancer Prevention Program easily incorporates primary, secondary, and tertiary prevention strategies into the activities planned for the company's annual fun run, summer picnic, or sports event. Here is a schedule and accompanying prevention level:

- *Two weeks before event*—Add visual graphics to the event advertising that depict a runner with a hat on, a volleyball player putting on sunscreen, or other sun-appropriate activity. (*Primary prevention*)
- *Ten days before the event*—Give a brown bag lecture or have a guest "expert" speaker from the American Cancer Society discuss skin cancer (incidence, prevalence, types of skin

cancer, risk factors, warning signs, and prevention). Announce at the lecture that there will be skin cancer screening as part of the company event. (*Primary prevention*)

- *Seven days before the event*—Set up a table-top poster display on types of sun protection describing the amount of protection offered by each product (broad-brimmed hat vs. cap, white T-shirt vs. tightly woven shirt, sun block vs. sunscreen) or multiple types and forms of sunscreens (alcohol-based, creams, waterproof, water-resistant, gels, sprays), and have samples for testing. (*Primary prevention*)
- *Five days before the event*—Distribute an email announcement that a dermatologist or skin cancer specialist will be conducting skin cancer screenings at the picnic. Have employees reserve a 5-minute time slot for each member of their family by phoning the "appointment hotline" number that you staff. (*Secondary prevention*)
- *Four days before the event*—Distribute an email quiz regarding a fact about skin cancer prevention. Have the employees respond by the end of the work day. Place the prize and a flyer of congratulations on their desks or in their mailboxes the following morning. Continue the marketing by congratulating for several days. (Award ideas: lip balm with sunscreen, sun visors, sunglasses, sunscreens, and hats). (*Primary prevention*)
- *Event day*—Set up a booth and conduct skin cancer screenings and counseling. Distribute a list of dermatologists within the company's health benefits plan. Set up a station for demonstrating the correct application of sunscreen. Dispense a medicine cup full of sunscreen to each passerby. Give the children red helium balloons imprinted with "Red balloons, NOT red children." (*Secondary prevention*)
- *First day of work after the event*—Send short email evaluation to all employees regarding use of sun-protective products, number of family members sustaining sunburns, and value of the activities to the employee and their family. (*Primary prevention*)
- *Two and 4 weeks after the event*—Follow up on all written referrals given to employees and their families during the skin cancer screening. Determine outcomes and report to management concerning evaluation of the event. (*Tertiary prevention*)

Intimate Partner Violence Awareness and Prevention

Each year in the United States, about 1 million incidents of physical violence occur against women by an intimate partner, such as a current or former spouse or boyfriend. The effects of intimate partner violence spill into the workplace and can impact employment productivity. Working women who are being abused at home have reported being harassed by their abusive partners in person or by telephone while at work, being late, leaving work early, or missing work because of the abuse, and being reprimanded for problems associated with the abuse. Abused women have also reported losing a job because of the violence in their lives. More and more employers are recognizing that domestic violence is a major problem in the workplace and are willing to implement policies and procedures that address domestic violence prevention. The following are elements of a domestic violence awareness program that addresses primary, secondary, and tertiary prevention of intimate partner violence against women.

Primary Prevention

- Support a company policy of zero tolerance against hostility and violence against all persons.
- Support a company policy that rewards collaboration, collegiality, and teamwork, and penalizes controlling behaviors and aggression.
- Maintain a workplace environment in which all employees, regardless of gender, ethnicity, sexual orientation, and religion, are treated with respect and dignity.
- Promote policies that raise the status of women in the company.

- Promote human resource policies that support men as involved coparents, sons, partners, and spouses.
- Display a poster on the "safety bulletin board" about domestic violence awareness and change to a different poster on domestic violence, such as child abuse or elder abuse, several times a year as an effective way to increase knowledge (Coker, 2005).

Secondary Prevention

- Support a company policy with a statement that clearly demonstrates concern and commitment to employees who may be experiencing violence at home. The policy must include nondiscrimination against victims in recruiting, hiring, and promoting, and sensitivity in performance evaluation.
- Offer annual manager and employee educational opportunities, such as brown bag seminars, newsletters, posters, and brochures on domestic violence, to help create a work culture that recognizes and strives to prevent intimate partner violence. October is National Domestic Violence Awareness month, and many national organizations offer resources to raise workplace awareness about domestic violence. Consider having a panel of community experts, such as a police officer, counselor, and nurse; discuss different types of domestic violence, such as stalking, abuse during pregnancy, and sexual assault; and offer available health, social, and legal services. Organizing employees to collect food and clothing for a local battered women's shelter is another way to support prevention efforts. These activities promote and maintain a work environment that supports abuse disclosure.
- Promote employee counseling and intervention. Everyone at the worksite needs to be aware of the signs and symptoms of intimate partner violence. A flexible and empathic work environment allows abused employees to disclose the violence and seek help. A current list of telephone numbers and addresses of community resources and social service agencies specializing in domestic violence should be available at all times. Posting hotline phone numbers and steps of a safety plan in the women's restrooms with a basket or box of business-card-size listing of community resources and telephone numbers (preferably available in individual toilet stalls) is a safe method for dissemination of resource information. Companies that offer an Employee Assistance Program (EAP) need to ensure that counselors are trained to provide appropriate assistance with domestic violence.
- Implement domestic violence screening questions on preemployment and annual health examinations. Information on domestic violence, safety measures, and community resources must be part of every health fair, screening, and health-education event. Examples of domestic violence screening questions are available on the internet.

Tertiary Prevention

- Provide adequate security to employees. All employees need to be reassured of a safe worksite even if an abuser attempts to stalk and harass an employee at work. Procedures must be in place to deal with trespassing, violence in the workplace, harassment, and accessing law enforcement. Safety plans for victimized employees may include advising coworkers of the situation and possibly supplying a photograph of the abuser, temporarily relocating the victim to a secure area, reassigning a parking place, and escorting to and from the worksite.
- Offer flexible work hours. Abused employees may need time off for criminal or civil court proceedings, health care and counseling, and safe housing relocation for themselves and their children.
- Provide financial support to employees. Examples of emergency financial assistance to abused employees include: (1) making changes in benefits at any time during a calendar year to ensure adequate health coverage for the employee and dependents; (2) expediting requests for changing the process of electronic paychecks into different bank accounts; and (3) providing emergency funds for employees in crisis.

Chronic Disease Self-Management in the Workplace

Self-management programs teach problem-solving skills in addition to health education. Self-management programs are successful in helping patients with chronic diseases such as diabetes mellitus and arthritis to make lifestyle behavior changes that improve pain, fatigue, physical function, and emotions. This type of intervention is classified as tertiary prevention; its goal is to maintain or minimize disease progression or to foster rehabilitation. Once a chronic condition has been identified, either for an individual or a subgroup of the worksite population, counseling and plans can be initiated to decrease the disease impact on life and to improve the persons' quality of life and physical functioning. This process is collaborative and often includes assessment, planning, implementation, referrals, coordination, monitoring, and evaluation. Effective chronic disease self-management tasks include:

- Taking care of the disease process—employees self-manage their diseases by knowing their medications, regimens, side effects, reporting changing symptoms to health care providers, healthy eating, and exercising, to name a few.
- Taking care of normal activities—employees self-manage type, amount, and structure of their normal social, work, and home life activities.
- Taking care of their emotions—employees self-manage emotional changes that occur with chronic illness, such as anger, uncertainty, depression, changed role expectations, and goals.

A self-management program for obesity may include group sessions and individual follow-up that includes walking for fitness; healthy eating; setting realistic goals and weekly plans for action; pedometer and activity diary; height, weight, and BMI; community resources.

HEALTH PROMOTION FOR SPECIALIZED WORKPLACES AND WORKERS

Agricultural Workers

More than 2.25 million full-time workers are employed in the agriculture sector in the United States, and there are an estimated 4.5 million additional unpaid farm workers and family members aged 14 years and older. Farming is one of the most dangerous occupations in the United States, with over 700 work-related deaths and another 120,000 agricultural disabling injuries per year (National Safety Council, 2009). Farming is one of the few industries in which the families, who often share the work and live on the premises, are also at risk for injuries, illness, and death. Farmers and their families are exposed to many hazards, which are listed in Box 19.2. Additional factors impacting the risk for farm work–related injuries are discussed in the following sections.

Age

Injury rates are highest among children aged 15 and under and adults over 65. Approximately 1 million children and adolescents under age 15 years reside in a farming household, while another 800,000 children and adolescents live in households headed by hired farm workers. Each year, about 100 children are killed and 100,000 children and adolescents are injured in agriculture-related activities. Most deaths among children on farms result from being innocent bystanders or passengers on farm equipment. Many farm children are working in dangerous environments by the age of 10 (National Institute for Occupational Safety and Health [NIOSH], 2013a). Additional issues of the adolescent worker are presented later in this chapter.

Box 19.2 Potential Hazards for Agricultural Workers

Machinery and Equipment
- Large riding machinery (tractors, combines)
- Entanglement in machinery
- Old equipment lacking safety devices

Chemical Exposure
- Fertilizers, pesticides, fungicides
- Anhydrous ammonia, organophosphates
- Toxic gases
- Cleaning solvents

Livestock
- Unpredictable behavior (crushing, kicking, biting)
- Risk of transferable disease; zoonoses
- Animal health care work
- Exposure to animal excrement
- Cumulative trauma: noise and ergonomics
- Noise exposure
- Repetitive motions; especially hand and wrist
- Excessive stooping, kneeling, twisting
- Vibration exposure; especially with hand tools
- Heavy lifting

Elemental Exposure
- Ultraviolet rays
- Dust and molds
- Heat and cold
- Weather exposure: wind, lightning
- Electricity
- Silos, grain bins, manure pits
- Ponds, mud, ice
- Highway traffic while operating farm equipment

Physical Structures
- Lighting
- Ventilation; especially in silos
- Ladders

Farm Stress
- Weather-related; poor crop yield
- Financial uncertainty
- Fatigue
- Day care facilities rare, expensive

Source: Reed, D. B. (2004). The risky business of production agriculture: Health and safety for farm workers. *AAOHN Journal, 52*(9), 401–409.

Farmers do not usually retire at age 65, and many work well into their 70s and 80s. Senior farmers often take prescribed medications, work with physical disabilities, and may suffer from vision and hearing loss. All these factors may increase senior farmers' risk for work-related injuries and death.

Equipment and Machinery

Most farm accidents and fatalities involve machinery. Proper machine guarding and equipment maintenance according to manufacturers' recommendations can help prevent accidents. Only one half of the farm tractors used on US farms are equipped with life-saving rollover protective structures (ROPSs) with seat belts. Many farm tractors were manufactured before the voluntary installation of ROPSs with seat belts, while some newer tractors have had their ROPSs removed by the owner. Personal protective equipment (PPE) and certain injury prevention activities can reduce the number and severity of farm work-related injuries and illnesses (Table 19.1).

Medical Care

Hospitals and emergency medical care are typically not readily accessible in rural areas near farms. The isolated nature of farms and ranches in our nation's rural areas creates difficult conditions for emergency medical service providers. Farmers and ranchers often work alone and may become entrapped, entangled, or disabled for hours before they receive medical attention.

Health Promotion Activities

Because of the multiple, varied, and serious hazards that exist in the farming community, the types of agricultural safety and health promotion activities are numerous. Box 19.3 provides a list of potential health promotion activities. Accessing and meeting with the farming community is not difficult. Nurses can reach farmers and ranchers by working with the following community partners:

- Local county extension office
- Farm Bureau committees and officers
- State Cooperative Extension Education and Research Service Office (CEERSO)
- Farm organizations
- Farm supply and equipment stores and dealerships
- County fair organizers
- Rural health care providers
- Public health department
- Churches
- Schools (Future Farmers of America, 4-H clubs)

Small Business Employees

A small business is defined as a business that is independently owned and operated, is not dominant in its field of operation, and typically employs fewer than 100 workers. Of the approximately 6.5 million private industries operating in the United States, more than 6.3 million (98%) employ fewer than 100 employees, and more than 5.6 million (87%) employ fewer than 20 employees. Prevention of work-related illness and injury is often difficult in small businesses because they have few safety and health resources, cannot hire staff devoted to safety and health activities, and often lack the ability to identify occupational hazards as well as conduct periodic surveillance (NIOSH, 2013d). The best opportunity to prevent illness and

TABLE 19.1 Personal Protective Equipment and Injury Prevention Objectives for Agricultural Workers

Objective	Health Hazard
Wear respiratory protection (dust masks, cartridge respirators, gas masks, air packs)	Dust, chemicals, gases, pesticides, fertilizers, mold, paint
Wear seat belts on farm machinery	Accidents such as rollovers, collisions, falls
Wear helmets on all-terrain vehicles and when riding horses	Accidents such as rollovers, thrown from horse, falls
Wear hard hats when performing construction work, trimming trees, repairing machinery, and doing other jobs with risk of head injury	Falling and/or airborne debris
Wear skin protection, including sunscreen and sun safety hats (wide brim and neck protection)	Ultraviolet rays
Wear job-matched gloves, barrier creams, and rubber boots	Animal waste products, pesticides, fertilizers, everyday exposure
Wear hearing protection (acoustic earmuffs, earplugs)	Loud and continuous machinery and equipment noise
Use safety eyewear (safety glasses, goggles, face shields)	Chemicals, gases, pesticides, fertilizers, dust, airborne debris, other foreign particles
Keep hair away from machinery by keeping it tied back or under a cap	Power take-off devices and moving machine parts
Do not wear jewelry, scarves, dangling strings, and loose garments near machinery	
Wear safety shoes or boots with nonslip soles and heels	Wet, slippery working environment
Wear impervious garments (long-sleeved shirts, pants, coveralls) when working with irritating or toxic substances	Chemicals, gases, pesticides, fertilizers, paint
Practice safe ergonomics	Heavy lifting; overexertion; excessive stooping, kneeling, and squatting; repetitive hand and wrist work; vibrating tools

injury in small business industries is for the owners, managers, and employees to identify and understand the hazards and risks that workers might encounter on the job.

In 1996, Congress passed the Small Business Regulatory Enforcement Fairness Act (SBREFA) to help small businesses incorporate health and safety prevention into their workplace. Under this act, the Occupational Safety and Health Administration (U.S. Department of Labor, Occupational Safety and Health Administration, 2013b) can help small businesses through a variety of tools, including partnership, consultation, compliance assistance, education and training, outreach, and plain language regulations:

Partnership: The Voluntary Protection Programs (VPP) identify worksites where employers and employees work well together to achieve safety and health excellence. Small firms can be partnered with and mentored by a VPP site that will share its experience and expertise on workplace health promotion programs.

Consultation: Small business owners may also request assistance from the OSHA Consultation Service, a program that provides on-site assistance in finding and fixing potential health and safety hazards before they occur. The consultation service offers workplace safety and health training and technical assistance. This service is completely separate from OSHA's inspection effort; no citations or penalties are issued. The employer's only obligation is to correct serious hazards.

Box 19.3 Agricultural Safety and Health Promotion Activities

- Work with local television and radio programs to feature spots on farm safety and health issues to promote safety throughout the year.
- Organize a safety field day for farmers and farm families that can be used to educate the whole family on farm safety and health issues.
- Organize and conduct a farm safety day camp for youth to educate the children in the community on a variety of hazards found on the farm.
- Make sure any local farm event or gathering has someone on the program speaking about a farm safety topic (e.g., combine safety, hazardous materials handling, respiratory protection, working in confined spaces). Develop a list of local events, desired topics, and possible speakers.
- National Farm Safety & Health Week is the third week of September, an opportunity for special events.
- Sponsor and promote a first responder program for farm families. Familiarize them with what to do in the event an injury occurs on the farm. Train them on farm hazards, how to turn equipment off, rescue procedures (grain entrapment, trenches, manure pit rescues), and how to summon help.
- Sponsor and promote a first aid and a Cardiopulmonary Resuscitation (CPR) course for farm families in your community.
- Sponsor and promote a farm emergency response and rescue training class for emergency medical and rescue personnel in your community.
- Sponsor and promote a Defensive Driving Course for farm and rural residents in your community.
- Organize and promote a farm safety poster or coloring contest at your local grade school or community organization. Offer safety items, farm safety activity books, or coloring books as prizes.
- Work with local businesses to display farm safety and health posters and safety reminders throughout the year.
- Work with rural health professionals to provide free blood pressure and cholesterol testing at farm supply stores, equipment dealerships, etc.
- Develop a farm safety display and use it at farm field days, events and programs, county fairs, etc., to promote farm safety and health.

Source: National Safety Council. (2013). *Agriculture safety*. Retrieved September 18, 2013, from http://www.nsc.org/ resources/issues/agrisafe.aspx

---

Compliance assistance: Small business owners are to contact the OSHA area office closest to them and speak with a compliance specialist. That person can offer advice on training and educating employees on health and safety regulations. A list of offices by region can be found at http://www.osha.gov/html/RAmap.html.

Education and training: OSHA training education centers are located across the United States and provide basic and advanced courses in safety and health. The area offices offer information services such as audiovisual aids, technical advice, and speakers.

Outreach: Computer-based training software developed by OSHA, called *Expert Advisors*, is available on topics such as hazard communication, asbestos, cadmium, confined spaces, fire safety, and lead in construction.

Plain language regulations: A variety of electronic and print materials are available on the OSHA standards, interpretations, directives, compliance assistance materials, and topics specific to small businesses. Additionally, the U.S. Small Business Administration's (SBA) Small Business Development Centers have opened across the country. There are a total of 1,000 centers, with at least one center in every state. These centers provide services to small businesses that include health and safety.

Telecommuting Employees

Telecommuting is a work agreement that allows an employee to perform assigned duties at an alternative site, usually home, during some or all of his or her scheduled work hours. It is a managerial option and not an employee benefit or right, and must conform to all state laws and regulations regarding state employment. Approximately 15% of the total U.S. workforce, 19.8 million Americans, regularly works from home at some point during the work week.

The Occupational Safety and Health Act (OSH Act) does not require inspections of home offices and does not hold employers responsible for injuries sustained while employees are working from home except if an employee is injured while working with job-related hazardous materials. However, because OSHA still requires employers to record all workplace injuries and illnesses, including those that occur in home offices, employers should require telecommuters to immediately report any incident that does occur. Workers' compensation carriers typically will cover occupational injuries that occur in home offices.

Employers are recognizing they have a tremendous investment in their telecommuters' home offices, not only from the standpoint of the equipment the employer might own in those remote locations, but also in terms of safety and security issues. More and more workplaces will develop telecommuting employee guidelines to promote health as well as conduct home visits to promote safety.

The following points should be part of a health and safety checklist for the telecommuter worksite:

- The telecommuter must have a dedicated work space, preferably a room with a door that can be shut or locked, because most alternative work sites are in the employee's home. The space should be large enough to accommodate the office equipment so that the worker can move freely without fear of tripping or falling.
- The work space must have adequate power and power outlets to accommodate the necessary equipment. Power cords, tools, and equipment should be safely arranged and secured.
- The work area must be clean, safe, and free of obstructions and hazardous materials.
- The work area must have ergonomic lighting and seating.
- The employee's home must comply with all building codes, and health and safety requirements, including the presence of functioning smoke detectors.
- The work area has safeguards in place against loss or theft of the employer's proprietary data and equipment.
- The work area has reasonable safeguards in place to protect the confidentiality of matters related to the telecommuter's work.
- If a telecommuter incurs a work-related injury while telecommuting, worker's compensation law and rules apply. Employees must notify their supervisors immediately and complete all necessary or management-requested documents regarding the injury.

Adolescent and Young Adult Workers

In 2010, there were approximately 17.5 million workers less than 24 years of age, and these workers represented 13% of the workforce. Young workers have high occupational injury rates, which are in part explained by a high frequency of injury hazards in workplaces where they typically work (e.g. hazards in restaurant settings associated with slippery floors and use of knives and cooking equipment). Inexperience and lack of safety training may also increase injury risks for young workers. And, for the youngest workers, those in middle and high schools, there may be biologic and psychosocial contributors to increased injury rates, such as inadequate fit, strength, and cognitive abilities to operate farm equipment such as tractors (NIOSH, 2013c).

In 2009, 359 workers less than 24 years of age died from work-related injuries, including 27 deaths of youth less than 18 years of age. For the 10-year period 1998 to 2007, US hospital injury departments treated an annual average of 795,000 nonfatal injuries to young workers. The rate for emergency department-treated occupational injuries of young workers was approximately two times higher than among workers 25 years and older. The U.S. Public Health Service has a Healthy People objective to reduce rates of occupational injuries treated in emergency departments among working adolescents 15 to 19 years of age by 10% by 2020, from the 2007 rate of 4.9 injuries per 100 full-time equivalent workers (NIOSH, 2013c).

The primary federal law governing the employment of workers under age 18 is the Fair Labor Standards Act (FLSA) of 1938 and applies to businesses with gross annual revenues of $500,000 or more. Some state laws extend coverage of child labor laws to all businesses regardless of revenues. However, no federal law covers children working on their parents' or guardians' farms. There are also special regulations that allow children to work in their family's business.

In designing health promotion activities for the adolescent worker, nurses need to partner with various groups and address the following issues (NIOSH, 2013c).

Teen Workers

- All workers must participate in workplace training programs offered by the employer or request training if none is offered.
- All workplace hazards must be identified to the employees before completing a task.
- All workers have the right to work in a safe and healthy work environment free of recognized hazards.
- All workers have the right to refuse unsafe work tasks and conditions.
- All workers have the right to file complaints with the Department of Labor when rights have been violated or safety has been jeopardized.
- All workers are entitled to workers' compensation for work-related injury or illness.
- Know the child labor laws. Visit http://www.youthrules.dol.gov

Employers

- Assess and eliminate hazards in the workplace.
- Make sure equipment used is safe and legal.
- Provide training in hazard recognition and safe work practices.
- Have all young workers demonstrate they can perform assigned tasks safely and correctly.
- Ensure all young workers are appropriately supervised.
- Ensure all supervisors and adult coworkers are aware of tasks teen workers may or may not perform.
- Know and comply with state and federal child labor laws.
- Develop an injury and illness prevention program.

School Educators and Counselors

- Talk to students about workplace hazards and students' rights as workers.
- Ensure all school-based work programs include safety and health training.
- Incorporate worker safety and health into junior and senior high curricula.
- Know the state and federal child labor laws.

Parents

- Know the name, address, and phone number of the child's employer.
- Ask the child about work tasks and equipment used.
- Ask the child about training and supervision.

- Be alert for signs of fatigue or stress as the child tries to balance work, school, home, and extracurricular activities.
- Know the state and federal child labor laws.
- Report unsafe working conditions to the Department of Labor.

PROMOTING A NONVIOLENT WORKPLACE

Workplace violence has emerged as an important safety issue in today's workplace. In 2009, approximately 572,000 nonfatal violent crimes (rape/sexual assault, robbery, and aggravated and simple assault) occurred against persons age 16 or older while they were at work or on duty, based on findings from the National Crime Victimization Survey (Harrell, 2011). (Detailed reports on worksite violence can be found at the Crime Victimization Survey at http://www.bjs.gov/index.cfm?ty=dcdetail&iid=245 with latest data 2011.)

About 700 work-related homicides occur per year, about 15 per week (NIOSH, 2013b). From 2003 to 2010 over half of the workplace homicides occurred within three occupation classifications: sales and related occupations (28%), protective service occupations (17%), and transportation and material moving occupations (13%) (NIOSH, 2013b). Homicide at the worksite is the leading cause of death for female workers and the second cause of death for male workers. It is estimated that workplace violence contributes to 18% of all violent crime in the United States.

The OSH Act of 1970 (U.S. Department of Labor, Occupational Safety and Health Administration, 1970) General Duty Clause, Section 5 (a)(1), requires employers to provide a safe and healthful workplace for all workers covered by the OSH Act. Workplace violence-prevention strategies are currently being developed and tested. However, effective interventions are still lacking as community and public health care providers and researchers learn more about workplace violence.

Defining Workplace Violence

The study of workplace violence is in its infancy stage. A variety of definitions for workplace violence exist, including:

- According to the U.S. Department of Justice, workplace violence is "Nonfatal violence (rape/sexual assault, robbery, and aggravated and simple assault) against employed persons age 16 or older that occurred while they were at work or on duty" (Harrell, 2011, p. 2).
- Physical assaults and threats of assault directed toward employees with two types of workplace violence: (1) coworker initiated violence; and (2) public initiated violence (LeBlanc & Kelloway, 2002).
- According to the Federal Bureau of Investigation (FBI), workplace violence is "a continuum that includes homicide, physical assault, domestic violence, stalking, threats, harassment, bullying, emotional abuse, intimidation, and other forms of conduct that create anxiety, fear, and a climate of distrust in the workplace" (Rugala, 2004, p. 12). The FBI identifies four subtypes of workplace violence:

  Type 1: Committed by criminals who have no connection with workplace
  Type 2: Committed by customers, clients, patients, students, inmates, etc.
  Type 3: Committed by coworkers, supervisors, manager, present or former employees
  Type 4: Committed by someone who does not work at workplace but has a personal relationship with an employee; intimate partner (Rugala, 2004)

The literature on workplace violence presents a continuum of workplace violence including the following, some of which are defined below:

- Incivility
- Horizontal violence
- Harassment
- Verbal abuse
- Threats
- Physical assault

Incivility: The conscious or unconscious behavior that violates workplace norms of courtesy or respect toward others. It may be the subtle, rude, or disrespectful behavior that demonstrates lack of regard for other employees such as interrupting others without care, not listening, disrupting meetings, inappropriate behavior at meetings, speaking with condescending attitude, or using up supplies or breaking equipment without notifying anyone or asking for help (Pearson, Andersson, & Porath, 2004).

Horizontal violence: Nonphysical interpersonal conflict that is manifested in overt and covert behaviors of hostility. This behavior is often associated with oppressed groups and can occur in any arena where there are unequal power relations, and where one group's self-expression and autonomy is controlled by forces with greater prestige, power, and status. Horizontal violence is also referred to as workplace aggression and can be manifested as passive aggression (nondirect, subtle, talking behind a colleague's back, withholding information needed to do a job, ignoring a colleague) or active aggression (criticizing, screaming, physical assault) (Duffy, 1995; Farrell, 2001).

Harassment: Defined as any unwelcome verbal, written, or physical conduct that either denigrates or shows hostility or aversion toward a person on the basis of race, color, national origin, age, sex, religion, disability, marital status, or pregnancy. Harassment can create an intimidating, hostile, or offensive work environment; interferes with an employee's work performance; and affects an employee's employment opportunities or compensation. See Box 19.4 for signs and symptoms of workplace violence.

Addressing Violence in the Workplace

Many companies have policies and procedures on how to address violence perpetrated by strangers, customers, family members, and patients. However, violence between coworkers, supervisors, and employees is rarely addressed by policies and procedures. Workplace policies are needed not only to address physical assault but also to define and address nonphysical aggression, bullying, and harassment. There are 10 steps a workplace can incorporate to prevent workplace violence:

1. Foster a supportive, harmonious work environment. Creating a culture of mutual respect can help reduce harassment and hostility.
2. Train supervisors and employees how to resolve conflicts. Conflict on the job can be reduced by developing employees' skills in negotiating, communicating effectively, team building, and resolving disputes.
3. Develop effective policies to protect employees from harassment. A company policy should clearly denounce harassment and state that it will not be tolerated.
4. Establish procedures for handling grievances. Employees need to be aware of the grievance procedures for reporting complaints of workplace violence and believe the procedures will be followed.
5. Provide personal counseling through an EAP. Family, marital, financial, and personal issues can have a profound impact on employees' work performance, as well as their interactions at work.

Box 19.4 Signs and Symptoms of Workplace Violence

Employee Signs and Symptoms of Being a Victim of Workplace Bullying, Harassment, or Horizontal Violence

- Anxiety, excessive worry
- Loss of concentration
- Disrupted sleep
- Feeling edgy, irritable, easily startled, and constantly on guard
- Stress headaches, migraine headaches
- Increased heart rate
- Body aches in the muscles or joints
- Stress-related fatigue and exhaustion
- Diagnosed depression
- Significant weight change (loss or gain)
- Chronic fatigue syndrome
- Panic attacks
- Skin changes (shingles, rashes, acne)
- Use of substances to cope: tobacco, alcohol, drugs, food
- Suicidal thoughts

Departmental Signs and Symptoms That Workplace Violence May be Present

- A disproportionate turnover rate higher than industry standards.
- A higher rate of absenteeism, paid time off, workers' compensation, or disability insurance claims.
- Employees request transfers from certain departments more than from others.
- A pattern of harassment complaints about particular individuals that do not meet eligibility requirements for illegal violations of civil rights or internal policies.
- When repeated complaints about particular individuals are investigated internally, witnesses routinely refute what the complainant saw, heard, or experienced.

---

6. Implement security programs that protect employees. Security guards, identification badges, monitoring systems, preemployment screening, and safety awareness and training help to ensure safety in the workplace.
7. Provide employee safety education programs.
8. Provide job counseling for employees who have been laid off or fired. Being laid off can be traumatic, and counseling, and support services can help workers develop new skills and ways of coping.
9. Train supervisors how to recognize signs of a troubled employee. Supervisors can be trained on how to recognize signs and symptoms of a potentially violent employee, such as threatening behavior or preoccupation with violence.
10. Set up a crisis plan that addresses violent incidents.

Summary

This chapter discusses many strategies for promoting healthy partnerships with people at the worksite. As you plan worksite health promotion programs, also consider programs discussed in other chapters, such as healthy partnerships with faith communities and schools (remember, many employees have children). Most adults spend about one third of each day at the worksite. This time presents an excellent opportunity for promoting healthy lifestyles. Appendix A provides an occupational and environmental assessment guide.

Critical Thinking Questions

1. An occupational nurse at a chemical and mineral plant is interested in using the results of employee HRAs to assess the need for health promotion programs at this facility.

    a. How would you implement this plan? Identify two potential employee health risk areas, and design an educational and screening program for employees to address the areas.

    b. How would you promote your ideas within management? How would you generate interest among the employees to participate in the prevention offerings?

    c. Discuss several potential barriers to the success of the health screenings. What steps could be taken to counteract the barriers? How would you case-manage the illness of an employee that was first diagnosed during the health screening? What data would you need to evaluate the success of your program?

2. Think of where you live and answer the following questions. How many farms are in your area? What kind of farms are they? What do they produce? What types of machinery do they use? What kinds of chemicals do they use? When are the peak times of farm work? How many people live on a typical farm? How many people work on a typical farm? How many hours per week do they work? Are there any children living or working on the farm? How old are the children? In what types of farm activities do the children participate? What type of schooling do the children receive? What type of health coverage or insurance do the farmers have? Are immunizations current for children and adults? Does anyone have any chronic health problems? Are any existing health conditions exacerbated by farming? What types of recreational and social activities exist? Do the farmers go on vacation? How do the farmers learn about new agricultural information and technology? What other questions would you ask the farmers?

REFERENCES

American Association of Occupational Health Nurses. (2012). *Standards of occupational and environmental health nursing*. Retrieved September 21, 2013, from http://www.aaohn.org.

Coker, A. L. (2005). Opportunities for prevention: Addressing IPV in the health care setting. *Family Violence Prevention and Health Practice, 1*, 1–9.

Duffy, E. (1995). Horizontal violence: A conundrum for nursing. *The Collegian, Journal of the Royal College of Nursing, 2*(2), 5–17.

Farrell, G. A. (2001). From tall poppies to squashed weeds: Why don't nurses pull together more? *Journal of Advanced Nursing, 35*(1), 26–33.

Harrell, E. (2011). *Workplace violence 1993–2009*. U.S. Department of Justice, NCJ 233231. Retrieved September 22, 2013, from http://www.bjs.gov/bjs/content/pub/pdf/wv09.pdf

LeBlanc, M. M., & Kelloway, E. K. (2002). Predictors and outcomes of workplace violence and aggression. *Journal of Applied Psychology, 87*(3), 444–453.

National Institute for Occupational Safety and Health. (2013a). *Childhood agricultural injury prevention initiative*. Retrieved September 21, 2013, from http://www.cdc.gov/niosh/childag/

National Institute for Occupational Safety and Health. (2013b). *Occupational violence*. Retrieved September 22, 2013, from http://www.cdc.gov/niosh/topics/violence/

National Institute for Occupational Safety and Health. (2013c). *Young worker safety and health*. Retrieved September 22, 2013, from http://www.cdc.gov/niosh/topics/youth/#keyresources

National Institute for Occupational Safety and Health. (2013d). *Safety and health resource guide for small businesses*. Retrieved September 20, 2013, from http://www.cdc.gov/niosh

National Safety Council. (2009). *6 ways to help prevent farm fatalities*. Retrieved April 3, 2014, from http://www.nsc.org/resources/issues/agrisafe.aspx

Pearson, C. M., Andersson, L. A., & Porath, C. L. (2004). *Workplace incivility*. In P. Spector & S. Fox (Eds.), *Counterproductive workplace behavior: Investigations of actors and targets* (pp. 256–309). Washington, DC: American Psychological Association.

Pender, N., Murdaugh, C., & Parsons, M. (2010). *Health promotion in nursing practice* (6th ed.). Los Altos, CA: Appleton & Lange.

Prochaska, J. O., & DiClemente, C. C. (1983). Protection motivation theory and preventive health: Beyond the health belief model. *Health Education Research: Theory and Practice, 1*(3), 153–161.

Rugala, E. A. (2004). *Workplace violence: Issues in response.* Retrieved September 18, 2013, from http://www.fbi.gov/publications/violence.pdf

U.S. Department of Labor, Occupational Safety and Health Administration. (1970). *General duty clause.* Retrieved September 15, 2013, from http://www.osha.gov/pls/oshaweb/owadisp.show_document?p_table=OSHACT&p_id=3359

U.S. Department of Labor, Occupational Safety and Health Administration. (2013a). *All about OSHA.* Retrieved September 20, 2013, from http://www.osha.gov/Publications/all_about_OSHA.pdf

U.S. Department of Labor, Occupational Safety and Health Administration. (2013b). *Q's and A's for small business employers.* Retrieved September 21, 2013, from http://www.osha.gov/Publications/OSHA3163/osha3163.html

Woolf, S., Husten, C., Lewin, L., Marks, J., Fielding, J., & Sanchez, E. (2009). *The economic argument for disease prevention: Distinguishing between value and savings.* Retrieved September 22, 2013, from http://www.prevent.org/images/stories/PolicyPapers

CHAPTER 20

Promoting Healthy Partnerships With Community Elders

Teresa L. Maharaj

LEARNING OBJECTIVES

After studying this chapter, you should be able to:

1. Discuss selected health and social factors that impact health status and functional ability of the elderly.

2. Differentiate between individual- and community-based health promotion strategies.

3. Design and implement a health promotion initiative for community elders.

Introduction

Improvements in medicine, science, public health, and technology have enabled older populations to live longer and healthier lives than prior generations. As the "baby boom" population continues to reach retirement age, tremendous challenges of health promotion for elders confront society. Most health care providers agree that a major concern is assisting the elderly to live healthy, independent, and productive lives in their communities. The needs of community elders are as diverse and multifaceted as the elders themselves. Building communities in which elders can live satisfying lives requires a thorough understanding of the issues facing elders as they try to maintain their independence. Elderly populations no longer want to accept disability and chronic illness as inevitable. Health promotion and disease prevention activities are an increasing priority for older adults, their families, and the health care system. This chapter focuses on developing individual-focused as well as community-based health promotion strategies and partnerships with noninstitutionalized elders. The terms *elderly, older adults, aging,* and *senior citizens* are used interchangeably to denote people aged 65 years and older.

DEMOGRAPHICS OF AGING IN THE UNITED STATES

The older population, aged 65 years and above, numbered 41.4 million in 2011, representing 13% of the total US population (Administration on Aging [AoA], 2012a). The percentage of older Americans has more than tripled from that in 1900 (4.1%), and the number has increased more than 13 times (from 3.1 million to 40.2 million). A child born in 2010 could expect to live 77.9 years compared with about 29 years in 1900 (AoA, 2012a). This phenomenal growth has occurred as a result of reduced mortality rates of children and young adults. However, reduced death rates have occurred in the 65 to 84 age group. By 2050, the older population will more than double to 88.5 million, and the over-85 population is projected to increase from 5.8 million in 2010 to 19 million (AoA, 2012a). Moreover, it is predicted that there will be as many people over age 65 years as there are people under 20. Of special note, although the current aging population is not as racially or culturally diverse as the younger population, it is projected to substantially increase over the next four decades (Vincent & Velkoff, 2010). The fastest-growing population of older Americans is the 85 years and older group. The older population will grow significantly between 2010 and 2030 as "baby boomers" (those born during America's post-World War II population explosion, beginning in 1946) continue to turn 65 years old (AoA, 2012a). Aging represents a challenge around the world. Rapidly expanding numbers of very old people around the world represent a social phenomenon that is without precedent. It is projected that by 2025 Asia will be home to 58% of the world's 60+ population (American Association of Retired Persons [AARP] International, 2009).

HEALTH CHALLENGES, RISK FACTORS, AND CONCERNS OF ELDERS

Health Status

Morbidity and mortality patterns of the elderly generally follow patterns of the population as a whole, with cardiovascular disease, cancer, and stroke as the leading causes of death. The majority of older persons have at least one chronic condition, and many have multiple conditions. During the years 2009 to 2011, the most frequently occurring conditions of the elderly included hypertension or taking antihypertensive medication (72%); diagnosed arthritis (51%); all types of heart disease (31%); any cancer (24%); and diabetes (20%) (AoA, 2012b). In 2012, 44% of noninstitutionalized elderly assessed their health as excellent or very good, compared with 64% for persons aged 18 to 64 (AoA, 2012b). Elderly persons also have to cope with disabilities and activity limitations. In 2011, 35% of older men and 38% of older women reported having at least one disability, and over one third reported at least one severe disability. The percentage of disabilities increases with age (AoA, 2012b). As the percentage of elderly people 85 years and older grows, so will the severity and number of chronic illnesses and disabling conditions. Because chronic illness is often related to frailty in the elderly, creative, multidisciplinary approaches to chronic illness management will be needed to optimize independence and functional ability.

Access to Health Care

Accessibility and affordability of health care are challenges for the elderly, particularly for rural and poor elders. Many have not adequately planned for the medical expenses that often accompany the chronic illnesses common among older adults. Currently, access to preventive services is often limited for the elderly. With the recent enactment of the Affordable

Care Act (ACA) Medicare, the primary health insurance for older adults will offer greater coverage for health promotion and preventive services that include immunizations, cardiovascular, cancer, and women's health screenings (National Council on Aging [NCOA], 2012). Medicare coverage is often poorly understood, sometimes leaving elders paying for services that are covered by Medicare. Medicare has many necessary health-related costs, such as prescription drugs and dental care that are not covered by Parts A or B. The elderly are among the greatest consumers of prescription drugs, many times paying for them out of pocket. With the passage of the Medicare Prescription Improvement and Modernization Act of 2003 (P.L. 108-173), eligible persons aged 65 and older now have access to a variety of prescription drug plans. While there are numerous Medicare supplemental insurance plans available for purchase, many Medicare beneficiaries are unable to afford the cost of the premiums. While state Medicaid programs provide coverage for some low-income older people, stringent eligibility requirements leave many without access to Medicaid health insurance. Although older adults have health needs that require a range of services on a continuum, not all services on the continuum are available to older adults in a variety of settings, leading to potential fragmentation of care.

Preventive services for the elderly are often neglected, because many providers do not see any point in prevention during the last years on the age continuum. A related issue is the recruitment and training of health professionals to provide medical and health care for seniors. Until the mid-1970s, medical schools placed little emphasis on geriatrics (Gelfand, 2006). However, professional nursing has been at the forefront in educating advance practice nurses in gerontology and adult nursing, as well as incorporating courses on aging in nursing curricula.

Alternative forms of health care, such as acupuncture and herbal medicine, may not be covered by insurance plans. Medicare Managed Care (Medicare Advantage Plans) is now available to older people, as is Medicare supplemental insurance, which provides coverage for certain services that are not covered by Medicare. Elderly populations often need guidance in selecting Medicare supplement plans that can best meet their needs. The nurse who is educated on guidelines and benefits of Medicare and Medicaid programs and the new ACA will be instrumental in helping older patients seek services critical to their overall health.

Transportation is another issue that impacts access to health care by the elderly, and rural elderly are hit hardest by lack of transportation. Elderly people often rely on friends; family members; lay taxi drivers (people who use private cars and often charge high fees); church volunteers; public transportation; and other forms of community-sponsored transportation to access health services. Nurses can play a key role during debates on Medicare and Social Security reform by promoting health care coverage not only to prevent illness, but also to keep older Americans from losing their savings as they try to pay for health care and, consequently, fall into poverty or sink deeper, if already poor.

Elder Abuse

As functional status and sensory acuity begin to decline, the elderly become vulnerable to an assortment of abusive and neglectful situations. Elder abuse is an umbrella term referring to any knowing, intentional, or negligent act by a caregiver, intimate partner, or any other person that causes harm or a serious risk of harm to a vulnerable population. According to the National Aging Information Center (NAIC, 1998), there are three basic categories of abuse: domestic, institutional, and self-neglect. Domestic elder abuse refers to the maltreatment of an older person residing in his or her own home or the home of a caregiver. Institutional abuse occurs in residential facilities. Self-neglect refers to neglect inflicted when the safety or health of older people is threatened by their living alone. Elder abuse takes on many forms and includes physical abuse, neglect by caregiver, financial exploitation, sexual abuse, self-neglect, emotional/psychological abuse, and abandonment (AoA, 2012c).

In a 2004 survey of State Adult Protective Services agencies, the National Center on Elder Abuse found a 15.6% increase in substantiated elder abuse cases from 2000 to 2004. In 20 of the states, 43% of the victims were age 80 or older (National Center on Elder Abuse [NCEA], n.d.). However, because elder abuse and neglect are largely hidden under the shroud of family secrecy, it is grossly underreported.

Mistreated elders are often frail, dependent on others to meet their most basic needs, over age 70, and women (NCEA, 2012). Elders most vulnerable to abuse and neglect are those with dementia and/or disabilities. Typically, family members, not strangers, inflict abuse on elders. Elders who were abusive parents themselves are at higher risk of abuse. Elder abuse and neglect encompass a variety of events that harm older people, including trauma; swindling and fraud; unattended medical problems; poor hygiene; dehydration; malnourishment; battering; verbal abuse; forced confinement; and other types of mistreatment at the hands of family members, neighbors, and caregivers. Elder abuse results in a wide range of negative health impacts, including the increased likelihood of injury and chronic health conditions, both of which are significant drivers of health care expenditures. Higher morbidity and mortality rates are experienced by older victims of abuse than older people who are not abused (AoA, 2012c). Moreover, older victims of sexual and intimate partner violence suffer from even more pronounced negative physical and emotional health outcomes (AoA, 2012c). Resolving abusive situations may require involvement of protective agencies as well as law enforcement. Community nurses need to be familiar with state abuse reporting laws and how to work with state adult protective services agencies.

Community Safety and Fear of Violence

Many community-dwelling elders are virtually prisoners in their homes because they fear becoming victims of muggings, break-ins, rapes, robberies, and scams. Rates of crime perpetrated against the elderly are different from those perpetrated against younger people. People older than 65 years are more likely to be victims of crime in or near their own homes because elderly people often lack access to transportation and do not travel great distances. The elderly are more vulnerable to crime. Owing to declining physical strength to protect themselves, elderly people, especially women living alone, are easy prey for criminal victimization. Therefore, few venture outside, and many take extraordinary measures to barricade themselves into their homes. This fear is compounded for the elderly poor who live in high-crime neighborhoods. The impact of criminal victimization is more devastating for the elderly than for younger adults. A low or fixed income makes it difficult for many older people to recoup from a robbery. These elderly often live in aging neighborhoods that are undergoing change and economic decline (Gelfand, 2006). Fear for their safety can be a deterrent to elderly people engaging in walking as a form of exercise. This fear can also cause social isolation. Community health nurses can facilitate neighborhood safety campaigns, such as crime watch programs.

Mental Health and Mental Wellness Challenges

Mental health is an important aspect of healthy aging. Ostir, Ottenbacher, and Markides (2004) found a link between positive emotions and frailty. They concluded that a positive outlook on life can help protect against physical and functional decline. Ostir, Berges, Ottenbaccher, Clow, and Ottenbacher (2008) further demonstrated that positive emotion is associated with gains in functional status after stroke. Mental health issues faced by the elderly include social isolation and loneliness, depression, suicide, and alcohol addiction. Tremendous loss and role transition are associated with old age, including retirement, death of friends and loved ones, loss of vitality and energy due to illness or disability, and, in many cases, less contact with children and grandchildren who may live in a different city or state. Social isolation is associated with the very old (aged 85 and older), those in frail health, and the elderly living alone.

Depression is a common problem many elders encounter as they experience health and psychosocial changes. Estimates of depression in older adults living in the community range from less than 1% to 5%, but the estimates rise to 13% for those receiving home health care and 11.5% for elderly hospital patients (National Institute of Mental Health [NIMH], 2008). Older adults are disproportionately likely to die by suicide. In 2004, people age 65 and older accounted for 16% of suicide deaths although they comprised only 12% of the population. Non-Hispanic white men age 85 and older were most likely to die by suicide (NIMH, 2008). Community health nurses and other health care providers need to be aware of the signs and symptoms of elderly depression and suicidal tendencies. A number of depression scales are available for assessing levels of depression in elderly clients. Anxiety symptoms (feeling fearful, tense/keyed-up, or shaky/nervous) have been found to be common among depressed and nondepressed older persons (Mehta et al., 2003). Additionally, anxiety has been observed to be a significant risk factor for the progression of disability in older women (Brenes et al., 2005).

Accidents

Falls are the most common accidents experienced by people over age 70. It is estimated that about two thirds of falls among the elderly are preventable. Whereas a fall in a younger person may not be problematic, a fall by an older person can have devastating results. Common risk factors for falls include use of medications or alcohol, poor physical condition, changes in visual acuity, inner ear disturbance, foot problems, gait and balance disorders, and hazards in the home and community. The presence of osteoporosis increases the likelihood of a broken bone when a fall occurs, particularly in women.

Several risk assessment tools for falls have been developed and are widely available. Scores can be calculated and reviewed with elders to plan fall-prevention strategies. Older adults are also at risk for accidental injury related to driving, fires, overmedication, and hypo- or hyperthermia. Decreased sensory acuity, impaired balance, decreased muscle strength, and decreased reaction time can diminish the ability of elderly people to interpret their environment. Community health nurses are in an excellent position to facilitate communitywide, as well as individual, injury prevention programs that target the elderly.

Disasters and the Elderly

Natural or human-made disasters, such as hurricanes and bioterrorism, can have a devastating effect on elderly populations. The terrorist acts that occurred on September 11, 2001, and the multiple large-scale weather disasters, such as Hurricane Katrina, that have occurred during the past decade have heightened awareness of the special needs of elderly populations. Roughly 71% of the Hurricane Katrina deaths in Louisiana were among persons older than 60. Older persons are likely to be disproportionately vulnerable during disasters because they are more likely to have chronic illnesses; functional limitations; and sensory, physical, and cognitive disabilities than are younger persons (AARP, 2006). Many elderly live alone and on limited incomes, making it nearly impossible to recover from a disaster without special assistance. The elderly are often slow to request help and are unlikely to follow through on a request. Additionally, they may have high nutritional needs, forget to take medicines, and become victims of fraudulent contractors. Recognizing the special needs of elderly populations during a disaster, the U.S. Congress passed the Older American Act, authorizing the Administration on Aging (AoA) to provide assistance for the elderly through state agencies.

HEALTHY PEOPLE 2020 AND OLDER ADULTS

Healthy People 2020 provides science-based, 10-year national objectives for promoting health and preventing disease. Healthy People 2020 goals and objectives are due to be released in final form in 2010. When planning health education and health promotion programs for community elders, community nurses should incorporate priority areas and specific objectives addressed in Healthy People 2020. To stay informed, individuals can subscribe to Healthy People Listserv (http://healthypeople.gov/2020/).

Health Promotion and Health Protection Strategies for Community Elders

Health promotion and health protection are two elements of primary prevention. Health promotion denotes emphasis on helping people change their lifestyles and move toward a state of optimal health, whereas health protection focuses on protecting people from disease and injury by providing immunizations and reducing exposure to carcinogens, toxins, and environmental health hazards. The concept of health for the elderly must be revisited in planning health promotion interventions. Filner and Williams (1979) define health for the elderly as the ability to live and function effectively in society and to exercise self-reliance and autonomy to the maximum extent feasible, but not necessarily as freedom from disease. Messecar (2002) found that older people themselves define health as going and doing something meaningful, which consists of four components: (1) something worthwhile and desirable to do; (2) balance between abilities and challenges; (3) appropriate external resources; and (4) personal attitudinal characteristics. More than any other age group, older Americans are actively seeking health information and are willing to make changes to maintain their health and independence. Health promotion efforts should focus on modifiable risk behaviors, matched to the leading health problems by age (U.S. Department of Commerce, 2002). Hahn (2003) interviewed older ethnic women attending a senior center and found that they defined *healthy* as being able to perform meaningful activities, which in turn keep them healthy. It is evident from these views of health that health care goals for elderly persons must focus on improving functional ability, maintaining independence, and helping them find meaningful activities in life. To maximize health promotion for community elders, a multifaceted approach is needed. Interventions should target individuals and families as well as groups and communities.

Individual- or Family-Focused Interventions

Individual- or family-focused health promotion/health protection interventions are designed to increase the individual's or family's knowledge, skills, and competence to make health decisions that maximize health-promoting and health-protecting behaviors. The goal is empowerment of the elderly and their families to make rational health decisions. Some categories of health promotion and health protection intervention that target the individual, caregivers, and/or family are:

- Health screenings
- Lifestyle modification
- Health education (one-to-one or group)
- Counseling
- Support groups
- Primary health care
- Immunizations

- Home safety
- In-home care (home health, personal care, or household assistance)
- Home-delivered meals
- Social support (telephone reassurance and home visiting)
- Case management
- Home maintenance help

Community-Focused Interventions

Community-focused interventions are activities and programs that are directed toward community elders as a whole or various elderly subgroups in a community. The goal of community-focused interventions is to improve community capacity and availability of the appropriate mix of health and social services required to prolong independence and functional status of community elders. Interventions at the community level primarily involve advocacy, political action, and participation in policy making that affects community elders. Examples of community-focused interventions are:

- Communitywide health educational campaigns that emphasize older people
- Holding campaigns in May, which is designated as "Older American Month"
- Community coalitions to address specific elderly issues, such as development of local information centers, telephone hotlines, or internet sites
- Political involvement to advocate for the needs of the elderly, such as preserving or expanding Medicare coverage for in-home services
- Collaboration with universities, churches, senior centers, senior housing projects, and other established community organizations to provide comprehensive services to subgroups of elders
- Crime prevention activities
- Participation in community-based health fairs

PARTNERSHIPS WITH COMMUNITY ELDERS

Elderly populations, in general, are open to new health practices and respond to a variety of approaches that have the potential to improve their health. To plan effective health programs, community health nurses should validate proposed goals and strategies with the targeted elderly group. Involving elders in planning health promotion and disease prevention activities is essential because older people are sensitive to potential loss of independence, and involving them increases a sense of independence. Action steps for working with older adults in the community include:

- Plan programs where elders usually congregate, such as churches, senior centers, and retirement centers.
- Incorporate outreach activities into all programs.
- Be prepared to offer transportation to group activities.
- Anticipate needs of those with poor vision (e.g., use large print, limit handouts, use a quiet room or loudspeakers).
- Maintain a slow pace for activities and allow adequate time for responses.
- Allow plenty of time for elders to share life experiences.
- Keep teaching sessions relatively short.
- Incorporate multiple repetitions and reinforcement of information.
- Structure health education activities so the elderly feel comfortable asking questions or challenging information that is new or doubtful to them.

- Encourage the involvement of families, friends, and significant others.
- Advocate for improvements in community resources and policies that affect the elderly.
- The following sections discuss selected health promotion and health protection needs of community elders.

Health Services

People over age 65 need regular primary health care services to maintain health and prevent disabling chronic illness and life-threatening conditions. Health promotion services that can form the basis for a community nursing intervention include:

- Immunizations (influenza, diphtheria, tetanus, pertussis (Td/Tdap), zoster, pneumococcal vaccine)
- Screening for chronic illnesses, such as cancers, cardiovascular disease, diabetes and abuse
- Management and control of existing chronic illnesses (health education, case management, and medication management)
- Knowledge of coverage and reimbursement practices (including alternative medicine) of Medicare/Medicare Managed Care, Medicare supplemental insurance, and specific state health insurance programs
- Caregiver support groups and services
- Community outreach and advocacy efforts to ensure linkage of elderly people to needed resources, such as health advocates, health coaches, community gatekeepers
- Referral to existing state pharmacy assistance programs and advocacy to establish such programs where they are needed
- Education and outreach related to the Medicare Prescription Drug, Improvement and Modernization Act of 2003
- Education on medication management (scheduling, adherence, calendars, and so forth)
- Continuous source of primary care
- One-stop shopping for health care
- Connection to chronic illness support groups

Nutrition

Adequate nutrition is important for older adults to maintain health, prevent disease, and slow down progression of existing chronic illnesses. To help the elderly improve or maintain nutritional status, it may be helpful to perform a nutritional assessment and build on existing strengths. An excellent tool that is readily available is the Nutrition Screening Checklist developed by the American Academy of Family Physicians, American Dietetic Association, and the National Council on Aging (Nutrition Screening Initiative, 1992).

Consider a nutritional health partnership program called Eating Healthy, Deliciously! Plan a class or a series of nutrition classes that focuses on basic nutrition as well as risk management nutrition (less salt, less fat, less sugar, more fiber, and so on). If special diet needs are to be covered, consider a series of classes and stratify the group according to specific dietary needs. Nutrition classes are more effective if they are highly interactive—incorporate recipe tasting and recipe sharing, build on existing positive habits, and include ethnic food preferences. Use of colorful, large-print posters and videos is appropriate. Reinforcing handouts are also helpful. Remember, many elderly people like to talk and share their experiences! Provide rewards for class attendance, such as canned goods, paper towels, macaroni, and other nonperishable, healthy food items. Enlist support of grocery stores for gifts. A major challenge is to get older people to attend these classes. Consider asking someone from the community or peer group to help with marketing and outreach.

Exercise and Fitness

The benefits of exercise are well established across the life span. Exercise activity for elders must be suitable to health and functional status. Brach, Simonsick, Kritchevsky, and Newman (2004) found that older adults who participate in 20 to 30 minutes of moderate-intensity exercise on most days of the week have better physical function than older persons who are active throughout the day or who are inactive. In addition, Elsawy and Higgins (2010) recommend older adults engage in strengthening activities that involve all major muscle groups at least two days per week.

The case study in Box 20.1 offers a program idea for increasing exercise fitness.

Fall Prevention

As described earlier in the chapter, falls among the elderly are a major concern. You may want to team up with occupational therapists and physical therapists to conduct a fall-prevention class or classes at a location where elderly people normally congregate (of course, you probably will not impact the elderly needing this class the most; they are at home because of fear of falling if they go out). Some can administer a fall assessment questionnaire, some can perform balance testing, some can demonstrate ways to prevent falls, and still others can provide individualized counseling regarding fall hazards. This collaborative, multidisciplinary project can have a tremendous impact on a problem that sometimes costs the elderly their independence or even causes death. You will need to market the project and obtain space for all screening, balance testing, demonstrations, and counseling. Consider having waiver and consent forms for balance testing in the event of an accidental fall.

Community Safety

To reduce fear of violence that often haunts older people, community nurses need to work with local law enforcement agencies to develop community programs. Prototype programs include Neighborhood Crime Watch Programs, Citizens on Patrol, and other civic organization safety programs. Elders need education regarding physical and psychological self-defense programs. Population-based media campaigns should concentrate on making elders aware of their vulnerability to specific types of crimes in the community, including frequency and time of day of occurrence. Additionally, direct deposit of monthly checks should be encouraged to decrease vulnerability to violence.

Box 20.1 Case Study: Idea for Increasing Exercise Fitness

While conducting a blood pressure screening clinic at a senior nutrition center, a nurse observed that the residents often arrived at the site around 8 AM. Their time was spent sitting until lunch was served at noon. A few played table games such as cards or dominoes, but there was little physical activity. While checking blood pressures, the nurse asked about physical activity and determined that most of them did not feel safe walking in their neighborhood, nor did they know of other forms of exercise. After validating the need for low-impact, chair-type exercise, a program was developed, and several of the participants were trained as exercise leaders. The program was titled "Sitting Down, but Kicking High: Exercise for Seniors." Under the leadership of lay exercise leaders, the program was eventually incorporated into the daily activity schedule.

Driving Safety

As the percentage of older adults in America increases, so does the number of older drivers. It is recommended that older drivers relearn to drive to accommodate neuromuscular and sensory changes that occur with aging. Older drivers should be encouraged to periodically re-evaluate driving ability, including vision and hearing checkups, and evaluation of other physical changes that might affect driving. Encourage elders to ask family and friends if there are concerns about their driving ability. The American Association of Retired Persons (AARP) sponsors driver safety programs to help older motorists improve their driving skills, prevent car crashes, avoid traffic violations, and determine when to stop driving (AARP, 2009). Older drivers should be referred to these resources or others that exist in the local community.

SIGNIFICANT LEGISLATION FOR OLDER AMERICANS

Finally, some important pieces of legislation merit discussion. Two important pieces of legislation that impact the lives of older Americans are the Social Security Act of 1935 and the Older Americans Act (OAA) of 1965. The Social Security Act mandated many programs to serve the elderly, including income assistance and health care. The main provisions included establishing a system of old-age benefits and enabling states to make provisions for blind people, aged people, and dependent and crippled children. The act established a Social Security Board and mechanisms for raising money for retirement income and welfare benefits. One of the most significant amendments came in 1965 and established Medicare and Medicaid health insurance programs. The OAA gave national attention to the needs of the elderly and authorized the AoA within the Department of Health and Human Services. It funded research and training in gerontology and facilitated local, state, and national programs to improve the quality of life of the elderly. Over the years, it has established many services for senior citizens, including area agencies on aging, multipurpose senior centers, nutrition services, volunteer programs, health education, transportation services, in-home health care, and preventive health activities.

Other legislation that helped to improve the quality of life for the elderly includes the Age Discrimination Act of 1974, which prevented age discrimination in employment and prevented forced retirement; the Research on Aging Act of 1974, which created the National Institute of Aging in the National Institutes of Health; and the American Disabilities Act of 1990, which ensured the rights of Americans with disabilities. In 2003, the Medicare Prescription Drug Improvement and Modernization Act was passed requiring the Social Security Administration to implement a plan to make prescription drugs more affordable for Medicare beneficiaries who qualify for the program. Most recently, in March 2010, President Obama signed into law the ACA; this legislation aims to improve Medicare coverage for prevention services and prescription drugs (Mason, Leavitt, & Chaffee, 2012).

Summary

Promoting healthy partnerships with community elders is an exciting venture. A comprehensive paradigm of health for the elderly, including social and environmental health, is needed. The aging population is creating tremendous opportunities for community health nurses to provide innovative, evidence-based health promotion services for the elderly population. The focus of health care for this group will continue to shift from acute medical care to self-care, chronic illness management, and services that promote independence. Additionally, health promotion strategies will emphasize quality-of-life issues as more of the elderly are expected to experience a high level of functioning well into their 80s and 90s. Community health nurses have an opportunity to develop innovative approaches to improving quality of life for elders through advocacy and service delivery.

Critical Thinking Questions

1. What impact does health promotion in younger years have on health status and functioning in older years?

2. If frail elders residing in their homes are provided "lay case management" (such as a health advocate or health coach who calls or visits in-home periodically, supervised by professional nurses), will they experience longer independent living, better health functioning, fewer falls, and fewer hospitalizations than frail elderly who do not get such support?

3. What is the appropriate mix of health and social services that can be provided through senior centers? Are such centers cost-effective?

4. Assume that you have been asked to assess the needs of the elderly population in your community. Outline the specific data that you would collect. Describe how you would collect the data.

5. Visit a senior center and ask a sample of the participants the following question: "What does being healthy mean to you?" Compare the answers with the World Health Organization's definition of health.

6. Conduct an internet search of innovative, evidence-based health promotion programs for elderly noninstitutionalized populations. Discuss how such programs could be implemented in the local community.

REFERENCES

Administration on Aging. (2012a). *AoA programs.* Retrieved July 29, 2013, from http://www.aoa.gov/AoARoot/Aging_Statistics/Profile/2012/docs/2012profile.pdf

Administration on Aging. (2012b). *A profile of older Americans: 2012.* Retrieved July 29, 2013, from http://www.aoa.gov/AoARoot/Aging_Statistics/Profile/index.aspx

Administration on Aging. (2012c). *What is elder abuse?* Retrieved August 13, 2012, from http://www.aoa.gov/AoA_programs/Elder_Rights/EA_Prevention/whatIsEA.aspx

American Association of Retired Persons. (2006). *We can do better: Lessons learned for protecting older persons in disasters.* Retrieved February 14, 2009, from http://assets.aarp.org/rgcenter/il/better.pdf

American Association of Retired Persons. (2009). *Driver safety.* Retrieved February 10, 2009, from http://www.aarp.org/home-garden/transportation/driver_safety/

American Association of Retired Persons International. (2009). *Growing old and less secure: Executive summary.* Retrieved February 13, 2009, from http://www.aarpinternational.org

Brach, J. S., Simonsick, E. M., Kritchevsky, S., & Newman, A. B. (2004). The association between physical function and lifestyle activity and exercise in the health, aging, and body composition study. *Journal of the American Geriatrics Society, 52*(4), 502–509.

Brenes, G. A., Fried, L. P., Guralnik, J. M., Penninx, B. W. J., Simonsick, E. M., Simpson, C., & Williamson, J. D. (2005). The influence of anxiety on the progression of disability. *Journal of the American Geriatrics Society, 53*(1), 34–39. http://www.cdc.gov/mmwr/preview/mmwrhtml/rr6002a1.htm

Elsawy, B., & Higgins, K. (2010). Physical activity guidelines for older adults. *American Family Physician, 81*(1), 55–58.

Filner, B., & Williams, T. (1979). Health promotion for the elderly: Reducing functional dependency. In *Healthy People 2000.* Washington, DC: U.S. Government Printing Office.

Gelfand, D. E. (2006). *The aging network: Programs and services* (6th ed.). New York: Springer.

Hahn, K. (2003). Older ethnic women in faith communities: Culturally appropriate program planning. *Journal of Gerontological Nursing, 29*(7), 5–12.

Mason, D. J., Leavitt, J. K., & Chaffee, M. W. (2012). *Policy and politics in nursing and health care* (6th ed.). St. Louis, MO: Elsevier Saunders.

Mehta, K. M., Simonsick, E. M., Penninx, B. W. J., Schulz, R., Rubin, S. M., Satterfield, S., & Yaffe, K. (2003). Prevalence and correlates of anxiety symptoms in well-functioning older adults: Findings from the health aging and body composition study. *Journal of the American Geriatrics Society, 51*(4), 499–504.

Messecar, D. C. (2002). Older people perceived health as going and doing something meaningful. *Evidence-Based Nursing, 5*(3), 96.

National Aging Information Center. (1998). *Elder abuse prevention.* Washington, DC: U.S. Government Printing Office.

National Center on Elder Abuse. (2012). *How at risk for abuse are people with dementia.* Retrieved August 29, 2012, from http://www.ncea.aoa.gov/Library/Review/Brief/index.aspx

National Center on Elder Abuse. (n.d.). *The scope of elder abuse.* Retrieved January 19, 2012, from http://www.ncea.aoa.gov/

National Council on Aging. (2012). *Straight talk for seniors.* Retrieved August 5, 2013, from http://www.ncoa.org/public-policy-action/health-care-reform/straight-talk-for-seniors-on.html

National Institute of Mental Health. (2008). *Older adults: Depression and suicide facts.* Retrieved February 13, 2009, from http://www.nimh.nih.gov

Nutrition Screening Initiative. (1992). *Nutrition screening checklist.* A cooperative effort of the American Dietetic Association, American Academy of Family Physicians, and the National Council on Aging. Retrieved from http://www.cdaaa.org/images/Nutritional_Checklist.pdf

Ostir, G. V., Berges, I., Ottenbaccher, M. E., Clow, A., & Ottenbacher, K. J. (2008). Associations between positive emotion and recovery of functional status following stroke. *Psychosomatic Medicine, 70*(4), 404–409.

Ostir, G. V., Ottenbacher, K. J., & Markides, K. S. (2004). Onset of frailty in older adults and the protective role of positive affect. *Psychology of Aging, 19*(3), 402–408.

U.S. Department of Commerce. (2002). *An aging world.* United Nations Department of Public Information, DP/2264, March.

Vincent, G., & Velkoff, V. (2010). *The next four decades: The older population in the U.S. 2010–2050.* Retrieved August 31, 2013, from http://www.aoa.gov/AoARoot/Aging_Statistics/future_growth/DOCS/p25-1138.pdf

CHAPTER 21

Promoting Healthy Partnerships With Rural Communities

David Hartley

LEARNING OBJECTIVES

After studying this chapter, you should be able to:

1. Identify health behaviors and health status issues that affect rural populations.

2. Discuss selected social and geographic factors that impact health status and health behavior of rural residents.

3. Describe environmental health promotion strategies that are appropriate for rural populations.

4. Be familiar with the Rural Assistance Center online resources, and with the most common federal programs available to address rural health issues.

Introduction

Thinking about developing partnerships in rural communities should include a consideration of how rural communities, rural people, and rural health issues may differ from their urban counterparts. It is tempting to resort to stereotypes that assume that rural people are engaged in agriculture, that they are self-reliant, conservative, religious, and probably have less education than urban populations. While most of these stereotypes have some basis in historical reality, it would be wise to set them aside and be open to discovering the facts, the problems, the needs, and the strengths that pertain to each rural community. Some of the rural specific issues are true of many rural communities, but probably none are true of all. So we begin by looking at some common rural health issues.

Rural health has different meanings in different parts of the world. In developing countries, it often refers to basic public health services such as clean water, immunizations, and prevention of HIV. In Australia, New Zealand, and to some extent Canada and the United States, it often refers to native or aboriginal populations. In much of the United States, it is commonly used to describe issues that affect timely access to appropriate, effective, affordable services for persons who live in areas of low population density, often at a distance from specialty and tertiary care that results in a greater role for primary care as compared with urban areas. One creative approach to rural health is the concept of "clinical peripherality," which encompasses not only low population density and remoteness from tertiary and specialty care, but remoteness from the administrative offices where decisions are made that might affect quality, cost, or access to care (Swan, Selvaraj, & Godden, 2008).

When the U.S. Office of Technology Assessment published the first comprehensive look at rural health in the United States in 1990, the question "What is rural health?" though not explicitly asked, seemed to be answered by addressing the availability of primary and acute health care services in rural America. Emphasis was placed on listing federal and to some extent state programs to address chronic shortages of personnel, to support small rural hospitals, and to support underserved populations. While rural health continues to be concerned about these issues, with the publication by the Institute of Medicine of *Quality Through Collaboration: The Future of Rural Health* in 2005, there is evidence of a shift toward a population health approach that places less emphasis on categories of services and workforce, and more emphasis on healthy communities. Specifically:

> All rural Americans should have access to the full spectrum of high quality, appropriate care, regardless of where they live . . .

> - Rural communities should focus greater attention on improving population health in addition to meeting personal health care needs . . .
> - A core set of health care services (primary care, dental care, basic mental health care, and emergency medical services) should be available within rural communities . . .
> - The spectrum of services available in rural communities should be based on the population health needs of the local community.

Institute of Medicine (2005, pp. 25–26)

This of course leaves it up to the communities, the policy makers, and the providers of care to determine what constitutes a community and what constitutes a rural community. So let us begin with a brief look at what we mean by "rural."

Newcomers to the field of rural health are often frustrated by the seemingly vast array of definitions of "rural," and cannot understand why we can't just decide on a single definition and stick with it. First, let's look at some common definitions, then let's consider why there are so many.

The most commonly used definitions of rural come from two federal agencies: the United States Bureau of the Census and the White House Office of Management and Budget (OMB). In both cases, the agency has begun by defining what is urban, leaving the definition of rural either explicitly or implicitly as "everything else." The census bureau begins by identifying *urbanized areas* as consisting of densely settled "places," often built up from census blocks that meet minimum population density requirements. When these census blocks are combined with adjacent blocks so as to encompass a population of at least 50,000 people, that is called an "urbanized area." The census bureau also identifies "urban clusters" as places that meet the population density threshold and have at least 2,500 people, but are not adjacent to an urbanized area. Many small rural towns are considered urban clusters by this definition, and, as a result, few federal programs that are intended to assist rural populations rely on this definition.

The OMB definition has been widely used for health planning and policy, because it is based on whole counties, and most of our public health data are available at the county level. The OMB approach is primarily concerned with identifying metropolitan areas (sometimes referred to as metropolitan statistical areas), which consist of one or more "urban core" counties and the surrounding counties that are economically tied to the core. The combined population of the core and surrounding counties must be 50,000 or more, regardless of the size of any of the cities. When using the OMB approach, areas not part of one of these "metropolitan areas" are considered "nonmetro," or rural.

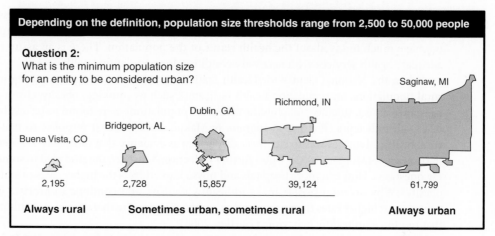

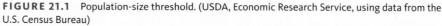

FIGURE 21.1   Population-size threshold. (USDA, Economic Research Service, using data from the U.S. Census Bureau)

Taking a population health perspective, whether at the local, state, or national level, neither of these definitions is adequate. As seen in Figure 21.1, the census bureau definition identifies many small communities as urban. Moreover, the kinds of health status information that help state and federal agencies target resources where they are most needed is often only available for whole counties. On the other hand, there are many whole counties in the United States that are considered "metro" by the OMB definition, yet have vast rural areas within their borders. For example, St. Louis County in northern Minnesota includes Duluth, a city of nearly 100,000, yet extends to the Canadian border, and includes part of the Boundary Waters Wilderness area.

The shortcomings of certain definitions are only one reason why there are so many other definitions. At a minimum, most programs and most researchers have acknowledged that the geography of the United States is not dichotomous. Dividing populations into rural and urban denies the complexity and richness of the American experience. One approach to that complexity has been to develop a continuum from large urban core to rural counties that are adjacent to urban counties, and thence to nonadjacent counties of decreasing population along the continuum. The Educational Research Service within the U.S. Department of Agriculture (USDA) has taken this approach with its "rural–urban continuum" and "urban influence" codes.

There are several useful references that explain these distinctions in greater detail. For the health care provider or health educator who simply wants to know if she can qualify for a recruitment incentive or grant that is restricted to rural areas, an excellent resource can be found at the Rural Assistance Center, also known as RAC online. In addition to rural definitions, this site will generate a custom report for any zip code, indicating whether or not it is rural according to various definitions, and for what federal programs the area is eligible (http://www.raconline.org/funding/rural.php).

GEOGRAPHIC AND SOCIAL FACTORS THAT IMPACT HEALTH IN RURAL AREAS

Those who have made a study of rural health over the past 20 years most often have been concerned with access to services. The traditional approach has been to gather data on services that can be easily quantified, such as the number of primary care physicians, the number of hospital beds, or the number of dentists. Ratios of services to population are then calculated, and the rural ratio is compared with the urban ratio. In many cases, this process leads to the conclusion that rural areas are "underserved." Note, however, that this approach does not have much to say about the health status of the population. There is an assumption that adequate health services are a necessary condition for population health.

When the National Center for Health Statistics published a study comparing urban and rural populations on population health indicators such as smoking, obesity, chronic disease, substance abuse, suicide, and child health, rural populations were found to be less healthy on nearly all indicators (Eberhardt, Ingram, & Makuc, 2001). A first response to that study by rural health advocates was to cite these disparities as evidence that more services were needed in rural areas (Morgan, 2002). Upon further reflection, however, the study led to some disturbing questions. How can more hospitals and physicians address the higher rates of smoking and obesity? Why do rural people make unhealthy choices, and continue to practice unhealthy behaviors at higher rates than urban and suburban people? Are there social and cultural factors that reinforce unhealthy behavior? (Hartley, 2004).

Population health has been defined as "an approach [that] focuses on interrelated conditions and factors that influence the health of populations over the life course, identifies systematic variations in their patterns of occurrence, and applies the resulting knowledge to develop and implement policies and actions to improve the health and well being of those populations" (Kindig & Stoddart, 2003, p. 380). A classic premise of community health is that the determinants of population health and particularly of health behaviors are embedded in relationships that tie individuals to their family and friends, their neighborhoods, and their communities (Eng, Salmon, & Mullan, 1992). These approaches to population health and community health lead to more questions. How do rural communities differ from urban and suburban communities? What is different about those "ties that bind" in rural areas? Is there such a thing as "rural culture?"

A few recent studies make it clear that much of rural America is demographically different from urban America. In age, education, income, and health insurance status, rural is generally worse off. But even in these basic demographics, there is much diversity among rural regions.

As shown in Figure 21.2, the great plains in the heart of the country have a greater portion of the population over 65. That means more people on Medicare, and fewer people in the workforce, among other things. A revealing perspective on demographic diversity was offered by Christopher Murray et al. (2006) in their "Eight Americas" study. By grouping the US population into eight sub-populations based on race, geographic location, population density, income, and cumulative homicide rate, they identified several very different rural Americas. These include the "Northland" which is low-income, northern plains with low population density; Low-income whites in Appalachia and the Mississippi valley; Western Native American; and Southern low-income rural black. Some of their other "Americas" include rural populations, but these four are illustrative of both the diversity of rural America and the disparities associated with that diversity. For example, America 2, northern plains low-income rural whites, had among the highest life expectancy, while America 7, southern low-income rural blacks, had among the lowest. These differences vary between males and females, but amount to as much as 20 years.

Perhaps the most telling demographic marker as a determinant of health and health behavior is illustrated by Figure 21.3, which shows those counties that have been designated as experiencing "persistent poverty." These counties have been found to have 20% or more of the population living below the federal poverty level for three successive census periods (30 years). Whether delivering health services, engaging in health education and health promotion, prenatal care, dental care, or mental health care, life in these areas is qualitatively different from other parts of the country. When federal agencies such as the Health Resources and Services Administration target their programs to special populations, these areas are often included, for good reason. Persistent poverty has long been associated with poor health, as indicated by the

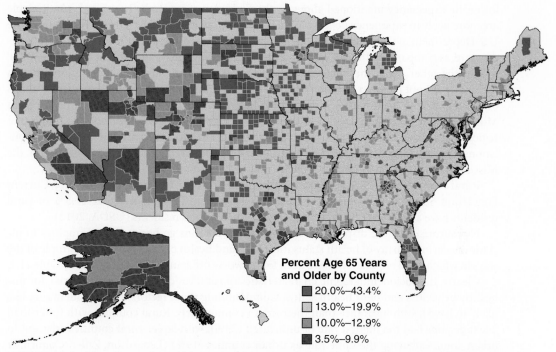

FIGURE 21.2   The aging rural population. United States Census Bureau, Census of Population and Housing, 2010. Accessed online at the Rural Assistance Center. Retrieved from http://www.raconline.org/maps/mapfiles/elderly.jpg

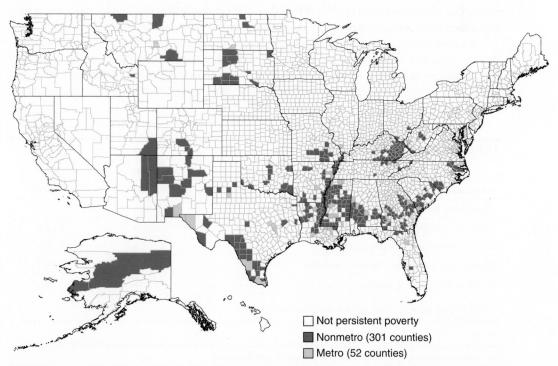

FIGURE 21.3   Persistent poverty counties. These counties had poverty rates of at least 20 percent in each U.S. Census 1980, 1990, and 2000, and American Community Survey 5-year estimates, 2007–11. (Economic Research Service, USDA. Retrieved November 12, 2013, from http://www.ers.usda.gov/topics/rural-economy-population/rural-poverty-well-being/geography-of-poverty.aspx)

lower life expectancy mentioned above in the Eight Americas study. In general, rural people are more likely to experience poverty in their lifetimes, as suggested by a recent report from the U.S. Department of Commerce, noting that 17.7% of rural residents live below the federal poverty line, as compared with 14.8% of urban residents (DeNavas-Walt, Proctor, & Smith, 2012).

On the other hand, the longevity of Murray's America 2 illustrates that regional health disparities are not merely a function of poverty. In their investigation of life expectancy trends over time, Wang, Schumacher, Levitz, Mokdad, and Murray (2013) found rural areas in Minnesota and the Dakotas with low incomes but high life expectancy. They also found that regions with lower life expectancy have persisted from 1985 to 2010, with the same rural populations showing the greatest disparity and actual declines in female longevity in the South, the Mississippi basin, West Virginia, Kentucky, and Indian Country.

Rural counties lag behind in educational attainment, too. Using data from the 2006 Current Population Survey, the Economic Research Service at USDA reports that 17.5% of rural residents have a college degree compared with 30% of urban residents (USDA, 2012).

Not surprisingly, the disparities facing rural populations go beyond demographics to include an alarming array of health status indicators and health behaviors. A small sample of the ways in which rural populations have been found worse off than urban is depicted in Table 21.1.

Clearly, the sociodemographic characteristics of rural residents place them at risk for unhealthy behaviors and poor health status. Compounding those factors, rural residents are less likely to have health insurance than their urban counterparts. Rural counties with fewer than 2,500 persons had the highest rate of uninsured (23%), with larger rural counties adjacent to urban counties having the same rate as urban counties (19%) (Lenardson, Ziller, Coburn, & Anderson, 2009). The Affordable Care Act of 2009 was designed to reduce these numbers, in part, through the expansion of Medicaid eligibility to uninsured individuals up to 133% of the federal poverty level. Unfortunately for rural low-income populations, the Supreme Court ruling that allowed states to opt out of the Medicaid expansion has resulted in many states with significant rural uninsured populations choosing not to expand Medicaid.

In addition, rural communities' lack of public transportation means that those who cannot drive a car, either because they are too young, too old, disabled, or too poor to own one, may not be able to access the few services and programs that serve rural populations, and may not be able to travel to larger communities where more programs and services are available.

TABLE 21.1 Urban–Rural Disparities

	Urban	Rural
Adults who smoke	18%	29%[*]
Adolescents who had five or more drinks in one episode	10%	15%[†]
Adults overweight or obese	60.6%	64.4%[‡]
Self-rated mental health poor or fair	6%	8%[**]
Male suicide deaths per 100,000 population	17	27[††]
Total tooth loss among adults age 65 and over	21%	31%[‡‡]

[*]USCDC, National Center for Health Statistics Health, United States, 2012

[†]Lambert, D., Gale, J., & Hartley, D. (2008). Substance abuse by youth and young adults in rural America. *Journal of Rural Health, 24* (3), 221–228.

[‡]Bennett, K. J., Olatosi, B., & Probst, J. C. (2008). *Health disparities: A rural-urban chartbook.* South Carolina Rural Health Research Center. Retrieved January 4, 2010, from http://rhr.sph.sc.edu/report_by_topic.html#1–09

[**]Ziller, E. C., Anderson, N. J., & Coburn, A. F. (2010). Access to rural mental health services: Service use and out-of-pocket costs. *Journal of Rural Health, 26* (3), 214–224.

[††]Advancing Suicide Prevention. (2005). *Suicide the second-leading cause of death in States with primarily rural populations.* Retrieved December 20, 2009, from http://www.advancingsp.org/Press_Release_8_11_05.pdf

[‡‡]USCDC Health Data Interactive for 2009 retrieved online October 2013.

Indeed, lack of transportation compounds many urban–rural disparities, and is often found to be a factor in designing rural programs or interventions. According to the Economic Research Service of the USDA:

> More than 1.6 million rural households do not have cars, with the proportion of carless households highest in the South, Appalachia, the Southwest, and Alaska. Highly carless rural communities are characterized by persistent poverty and have high concentrations of Black, Hispanic, or Native American residents. Nationwide, over 90 percent of individuals on public assistance do not have a car.
>
> (USDA, 2005)

It is a sad fact that, even in those rural communities where most residents have access to transportation, have a high school education, have health insurance or access to a community health center, and, in short, have relatively fewer of these sociodemographic–geographic issues, we often observe higher rates of smoking, poor nutrition, lack of exercise, and the health problems that follow from these behaviors. That observation has led to the question "Why does rural residence (culture, community, and environment) reinforce negative health behaviors?" (Hartley, 2004). There are no widely accepted answers to this question. A frank discussion of the issue can lead to stereotypes of rural culture and rural people that are simplistic, and do not lead to a solution. Often, rural communities are high in social capital, but may also be low in tolerance for diverse opinions or behaviors, leading to social pressure to conform. Changes in diet may be particularly difficult under such pressure. One rural resident, responding to this question in a personal conversation, noted that if someone in her town started jogging every morning, it would lead others to think that she thought she was better than others in the town. In another such conversation, a rural resident commented on going to high school in a small town, where there are only 25 kids in each grade, and one must conform if one wants to have a social life. Here, too, if smoking and drinking are the norm, it is difficult to resist.

On the positive side, a rural community can come together to address a public health issue, once they accept it as something affecting their whole community, and is something that they can do something about. A great example of this phenomenon is the case of Albert Lea, Minnesota, population about 18,000. With help from AARP and the United Health Foundation, the town launched the Vitality Project, with the goal of helping citizens live longer, healthier lives. The project's strategies are simple: eat more fruits and vegetables, walk instead of drive, and stay productive and social well into old age. Some of the strategies have included sidewalk and trail construction, working with restaurants to add healthier menu options and with grocery stores to feature healthy foods. Schools eliminated sugary treats and started a "walking school bus" program that allows kids to walk to school in groups with adult supervision (Buettner, 2010). According to one report, "the key for Albert Lea was getting the community behind a goal that was not just about weight loss, but also about fostering family relationships, a sense of purpose and healthy living habits" (*USA Today*, 2009).

HEALTH PROMOTION ISSUES THAT RELATE TO RURAL POPULATIONS

Rural populations face all of the same preventable illnesses that are faced by urban populations. To a large extent, prevention of the major contributors to preventable deaths is addressed by public health systems and by primary care practices. There are practitioners in both sectors who can be effective partners in health promotion. However, in rural areas, there are typically fewer primary care practitioners than in urban areas, and they tend to be very busy. Moreover, many rural areas have no local public health department, or one that offers a limited number of services. Prevention initiatives are often undertaken by partnerships involving healthy communities coalitions, hospitals, primary health clinics, schools, social services, law enforcement, and local businesses. While state health departments and the U.S. Centers for Disease Control offer many useful tools for prevention, it is these local partners who must ultimately decide what will work for their communities.

An excellent resource for assessing rural community needs and issues, developing coalitions and local leaders, and targeting specific health issues is *Rural Populations and Health: Determinants, Disparities, and Solutions* (Crosby, Wendel, Vanderpool, & Casey, 2012). In addition to providing more detail on many of the issues discussed in this chapter, the authors offer specific strategies for building coalitions and building capacity in rural communities, with detailed examples addressing smoking prevention, oral health, physical activity, farm-related injuries, mental health, cancer prevention, and adolescent health.

Two issues that challenge these prevention partnerships and coalitions in rural communities are substance abuse and obesity. Both of these threats to the health of the public have been shown to affect rural populations disproportionately. Higher rates of obesity and substance abuse are particularly troubling when observed among rural youth, and in both cases, prevention initiatives that seek to modify not only unhealthy behaviors but also unhealthy environments are proving to be effective. The October 2003 issue of the *American Journal of Public Health* addressed the relationship between health and the built environment (physical environment, urban design, land-use planning, urban sprawl, and housing). The articles raised many good questions about the influence of place of residence on health, but the questions were almost exclusively about urban environments. More recently, research has found that there are significant differences between the urban and rural built environment that have implications for prevention, especially for the prevention of childhood obesity (Yousefian, Ziller, Swartz, & Hartley, 2009).

Obesity

Childhood obesity rates in the United States have only recently leveled off, and the immediate and long-term medical and social consequences of childhood obesity are a continuing concern. Over the past four decades, rates consistently increased. According to the 2007–2008 National Health and Nutrition Examination Survey (NHANES), 16.9% of children age 2 to 19 are obese, while nearly 32% of children and adolescents are overweight or obese (Ogden & Carroll, 2010). Childhood obesity rates are highest among low-income populations and also among racial/ethnic minorities. Research has demonstrated that this trend also applies to rural youth, where the prevalence of obesity and overweight has been shown to be higher than state and national averages and also higher than rates among youth in urban areas (Joens-Matre et al., 2008). A recent national study found that rural children are about 25% more likely to be overweight than their metropolitan counterparts (Lutfiyya, Lipsky, Wisdom-Behounek, & Inpanbutr-Martinkus, 2007). Rates of physical activity have also been found to be lower in rural areas among adults and among rural children when compared with urban and suburban populations (Patterson, Moore, Probst, & Shinogle, 2004).

Attention has been cast on the role that active living plays in obesity prevention among youth in urban and, more recently, in rural areas. The concept of active living incorporates an ecological, population-based approach to physical activity by recognizing that individual behavior, social environments, physical environments, and policies all contribute to behavior change. Active living targets entire communities to promote accessible and safe opportunities for residents to engage in physical activity during transportation, occupation, recreation, and at home (Sallis et al., 2006). Often with funding from the Robert Wood Johnson Foundation (RWJF), communities have assessed how "activity friendly" they are. This assessment process has typically involved a process of walking the sidewalks of a neighborhood with a checklist or other formal assessment tool in hand, observing the condition of the housing, sidewalks, crosswalks, intersections, recreational facilities, school areas, etc. Until very recently, the tools available for these assessments were developed for, and field tested in, urban and suburban neighborhoods. (See, for example, the SPACES instrument [Pikora et al., 2006], the Irvine-Minnesota Inventory [Boarnet et al., 2011], the Active Neighborhood Checklist [Hoehner, 2011], and the Community Park Audit Tool [Kaczynski, Stanis, & Besenyi, 2012].)

Active Living Research and Healthy Eating Research are national programs funded by RWJF, providing research to address childhood obesity. In recent years, these programs have funded a small number of projects to begin exploring the needs of rural communities in this effort. Collaboration among three of their grantees has produced a set of instruments that is designed specifically for use in rural communities (Yousefian et al., 2009, 2010). Known as the Rural Active Living Assessment (RALA) tools, these instruments are especially useful for local community leaders seeking to build partnerships and to involve community members in identifying needs and designing and implementing interventions. A "codebook" has been developed that not only explains how to use the tools, but suggests ways that community members can become involved in assessing their communities' needs. Unlike the urban-based instruments mentioned above, the RALA tools treat the entire rural community as a "neighborhood," and include an inventory of resources that serve the entire town, as well as an inventory of local programs and policies that affect access to physical activity, such as late school buses, "safe routes to school," and public transportation. A Webinar (web-based seminar) presenting the RALA tools was sponsored by the Active Living Research national program office in June 2009, and was attended by approximately 400 interested people, suggesting that there is a significant need for and an interest in addressing physical activity in rural areas. The tools and codebook continue to be modified and improved as more rural communities use them. They are currently being used to assess virtually every town in the state of Maine. They are available from the Active Living Research website (http://www .activelivingresearch.org/node/11947). A complementary tool for assessing the perceived active living environment in rural communities is the Rural Active Living Perceived Environment Support Scale (RALPESS) (Umstattd et al., 2012). This tool is also available from the ALR site.

Substance Abuse

A second major issue that affects rural youth disproportionately is substance abuse. In most rural communities, the substance most used and abused by young people is alcohol. Recent studies have found that rural teens are more likely to use alcohol, to engage in binge drinking, and to drive while intoxicated than urban teens. Young adults living in rural areas are another population at high risk, with higher rates of binge drinking, methamphetamine, and prescription drug abuse than their urban counterparts (Lambert, Gale, & Hartley, 2008; Van Gundy, 2006). We have traditionally focused our prevention efforts on teens in the schools, with programs such as Drug Abuse Resistance Education (DARE), which seek to build self-worth and autonomy in young people to empower them to make wise personal choices. In recent years, however, many states and communities have recognized that "Holding youth solely responsible for underage drinking is like blaming fish for dying in a polluted stream" (attributed to Laurie Lieber, Marin Institute, San Rafael, CA). This realization has led to environmental or ecological approaches to prevention that seek to "purify the water in the stream." One such effort occurred in Piscataquis County, Maine, in 2006.

A statewide survey filled out by students and administered by their school systems on a biennial basis in Maine had shown that several attitudes were highly correlated with youth binge drinking. Examples of questions on the survey (Maine Youth Drug and Alcohol Use Survey, 2009) that reveal these attitudes are as follows:

- My parents think it is not wrong or only a little wrong for me to drink.
- My parents wouldn't catch me if I drank without permission.
- It would be easy to get alcohol if I wanted to.
- A kid in my neighborhood who drinks won't be caught by police.

With help from the Maine Office of Substance Abuse, county educators, law enforcement and public health leaders determined that if they could change these attitudes, they could begin to address youth drinking. Their three-pronged approach included addressing *norms* (what is acceptable in the community), *availability*, and *enforcement*. Enforcement was a critical part of this plan, since it would include not only reducing teens' access to booze, but also communicating the community's standards for acceptable behavior, and could be designed to focus on preventing high-risk behavior such as binge drinking at outdoor keg parties. When law enforcement "busted" a keg party, there was a zero-tolerance rule. Every teen present was escorted home by a peace officer, who then talked to the parents and impressed upon them that this behavior was not acceptable in this community. This strategy helped to engage parents as critical partners, empower them to address the problem, and begin the process of changing community norms. For the strategy to be most effective, it had to begin with a well-publicized written policy from the Sheriff's Department, endorsed by the schools. To assure the zero-tolerance rule (all treated the same), the Sheriff's Department developed a "call-out" system so that extra officers could be brought in to assist when breaking up a drinking party. Officers received special training in "community policing" to make their interventions effective.

Access was also addressed by issuing citations to adults who furnished alcohol to minors. In the year following the implementation of the three-part strategy, citations to adults increased slightly, from three to nine citations, but citations to minors increased from 39 to 138. More importantly, the next year that the survey was administered, attitudes had changed. Perceptions that it was easy to get alcohol had decreased from 76% to 66%, and the perception that adults in the community think teen drinking is wrong went from 61% to 68%. Most importantly, teens who admitted drinking in the last 30 days went from 44% to 36%. While these effects may not be dramatic, trends were going in the right direction, while, throughout the rest of Maine, many of these trends were going in the opposite direction.

Summary

This chapter focused on rural health, its definitions and issues surrounding attempts to measure and affect it. Geographic and social factors unique to rural populations were discussed, as were major health disparities between rural and urban areas. Examples of successful programs for obesity and substance abuse, two major health issues of rural populations, were described.

Critical Thinking Questions

1. From what you know of rural communities, comment on what factors might contribute to the urban–rural differences in health behaviors. Think about the implications of such cultural factors for environmental prevention initiatives addressing substance abuse, obesity, smoking, or other major public health issues. Any statements about rural beliefs or perceptions must be backed by your own personal experience or by references—no stereotypes!

2. Consider the following statement: "Urban–rural differences in health status indicators, including neonatal outcomes, mortality rates, and health risk factors, are not true disparities, because they result from racial and socioeconomic disparities. Rural persistent poverty counties and rural African American and Hispanic populations account for most urban–rural differences." Look for evidence in favor of or against this proposition using data from the Community Health Status Indicators website: http://www.communityhealth .hhs.gov/. Use data chosen from the following counties in making your argument:
   In Mississippi: Bolivar county (rural—delta), Hinds (urban), Rankin (suburban), and

Jackson County (urban—gulf coast). For the Hispanic population, in West Texas, look at Presidio County (rural) and El Paso County (urban). For rural persistent poverty, take a look at McDowell (rural) and Kanawha County (urban) in West Virginia. Look especially at the demographics, measures of birth and death, and the risk factors for premature death. Also, pay attention to the comparison with peer counties as well as the comparison with the US average for each of the indicators. Think about urban–rural differences within a state, as well as how rural counties compare with the US average, which is based on a population that is 80% urban. It may be helpful to prepare a table of the indicators you find most compelling.

3. How would an intervention to prevent smoking in Bolivar County, Mississippi differ from an intervention to prevent smoking in Freeborn County, Minnesota (where the Albert Lea Vitality Project took place)?

REFERENCES

Boarnet, M., Forsyth, A., Day, K., & Oakes, M. (2011, November). The street level built environment and physical activity and walking: Results of a predictive validity study for the Irvine Minnesota Inventory. *Environment and Behavior, 43*(6), 735–775.

Buettner, D. (2010). The Minnesota miracle. *AARP the Magazine, 53*(1B), 42ff.

Crosby, R. A., Wendel, M. L., Vanderpool, R. C., & Casey, B. R. (2012). *Rural populations and health: Determinants, disparities and solutions.* San Francisco, CA: Jossey-Bass.

Day, K., Boarnet, M., Alfonzo, M., & Forsyth, A. (2006, February). The Irvine Minnesota Inventory to measure built environments: Development. *American Journal of Preventive Medicine, 30*(2), 144–152.

DeNavas-Walt, C., Proctor, B. D., & Smith, J. C. (2013). *Income, poverty, and health insurance coverage in the United States: 2012* (U.S. Census Bureau, Current Population Reports, P60–245). Washington, DC: U.S. Government Printing Office.

Eberhardt, M. S., Ingram, D. D., & Makuc, D. M. (2001). *Health United States, 2001 urban and rural health chartbook.* Hyattsville, MD: National Center for Health Statistics.

Eng, E., Salmon, M., & Mullan, F. (1992). Community empowerment: The critical base for primary health care. *Family and Community Health, 15*, 1–12.

Hartley, D. (2004). Rural health disparities, population health and rural culture. *American Journal of Public Health, 94*(10), 1675–1678.

Hoehner, C. M., Ivy, A., Ramirez, L. K., Handy, S. & Brownson, R. C. (2007). Active neighborhood checklist: A user-friendly and reliable tool for assessing activity friendliness. *American Journal of Health Promotion, 21*(6), 534–537.

Institute of Medicine. (2005). *Quality through collaboration: The future of rural health.* Washington, DC: National Academies Press.

Joens-Matre, R., Welk, G. J., Calabro, M. A., Russell, D. W., Nicklay, E., & Hensley, L. D. (2008). Rural urban differences in physical activity, physical fitness, and overweight prevalence of children. *The Australian Journal of Rural Health, 24*(1), 49–54.

Kaczynski, A. T., Stanis, S. A., & Besenyi, G. M. (2012, March). Development and testing of a community stakeholder park audit tool. *American Journal of Preventive Medicine, 42*(3):242–249.

Kindig, D., & Stoddart, G. L. (2003). What is population health? *American Journal of Public Health, 93*, 380–383.

Lambert, D., Gale, J., & Hartley, D. (2008). Substance abuse by youth and young adults in rural America. *Journal of Rural Health, 24*(3), 221–228.

Lenardson, J. D., Ziller, E., Coburn, A., & Anderson, N. (2009). *Profile of rural health insurance coverage: A chartbook.* Portland, ME: Maine Rural Health Research Center, Muskie School of Public Service, University of Southern Maine. Retrieved from http://muskie.usm.maine.edu/Publications/rural/Rural-Health-Insurance-Chartbook-2009.pdf

Lutfiyya, M. N., Lipsky, M. S., Wisdom-Behounek, J., & Inpanbutr-Martinkus, M. (2007). Is rural residency a risk factor for overweight and obesity for U.S. children? *Obesity, 15*(9), 2348–2356.

Maine Youth Drug and Alcohol Use Survey. (2009). *Maine office of substance abuse.* Retrieved from http://www.maine.gov/dhhs/osa/data/mydaus/mydaus2008.htm

Morgan, A. (2002). A national call to action: CDC's 2001 urban and rural health chartbook. *The Journal of Rural Health, 18*, 382–383.

Murray C., Kulkarni S., Michaud C., Tomijima N., Bulzacchelli, M. T., Iandiorio, T. J., & Ezzati, M. (2006). *Eight Americas: Investigating mortality disparities across races, counties, and race-counties in the United States. PLoS Med, 3*, 1513–1524.

Ogden, C. L., & Carroll, M. D. (2010). *Prevalence of obesity among children and adolescents: United States trends 1963–1965 through 2007–2008.* Hyattsville, MD: National Center for Health Statistics, USCDC, Health e-stats.

Patterson, P. D., Moore, C. G., Probst, J. C., & Shinogle, J. A. (2004). Obesity and physical activity in rural America. *The Journal of Rural Health*, *20*(2), 151–159.

Pikora, T., Giles-Corti, B., Knuiman, M. W., Bull, F. C., Jamrozik, K., & Donovan, R. J. (2006). Neighbourhood environmental factors correlated with walking near home: Using SPACES. *Medicine and Science in Sports and Exercise*, *38*(4), 708–714.

Sallis, J. F., Cervero, R. B., Ascher, W., Henderson, K. A., Kraft, M. K., & Kerr, J. (2006). An ecological approach to creating active living communities. *Annual Review of Public Health*, *27*, 297–322.

Swan, G. M., Selvaraj, S., & Godden, D. (2008). Clinical peripherality: Development of a peripherality index for rural health services. *BMC Health Services Research*, *8*, 23. Retrieved from http://www.ncbi.nlm.nih.gov/pmc/articles/PMC2246121

Umstattd, M. R., Baller, S. L., Hennessy, E., Hartley, D., Economos, C. D., Hyatt, R. R., . . . Hallam, J. S. (2012). Development of the rural active living perceived environment support scale (RALPESS). *Journal of Physical Activity and Health*, *9*(5), 724–730.

USA Today. (2009, October 14). *Minnesota town gets healthy together*. Retrieved from December 28, 2009, from http://www.usatoday.com/news/health/2009-10-14-minnesota-health_N.htm

USDA. (2005). *Rural transportation at a glance* (Agriculture Information Bulletin No. 795).

USDA. (2012). *State fact sheet, United States 2012*. Retrieved from http://www.ers.usda.gov/data-products/state-fact-sheets/state-data.aspx?StateFIPS=00#P8e312a7eef274b14b286496040ab15e8_2_39iT0

Van Gundy, K. (2006). *Substance abuse in rural and small town America. Reports on Rural America* (Vol. *1*, No. 2). Durham: Carsey Institute, University of New Hampshire.

Wang, H., Schumacher, A. E., Levitz, C. E., Mokdad, A. H., & Murray, C. J. (2013). Left behind: Widening disparities for males and females in US county life expectancy, 1985–2010. *Population Health Metrics*, *11*, 8

Yousefian, A., Hennessy, E., Umstattd, M. R., Economos, C. D., Hallam, J. S., Hyatt, R. R., & Hartley, D. (2010). Development of the rural active living assessment tools: Measuring rural environments. Preventive Medicine, *50*(Suppl. 1), S86–S92.

Yousefian, A., Ziller, E., Swartz, J., & Hartley, D. (2009). Active living for rural youth: Addressing physical inactivity in rural communities. *Journal of Public Health Management and Practice: Special Issue on Rural Public Health*, *15*(3), 223–231.

A

APPENDIX

A Guide to Nursing Assessment of the Workplace

Ann T. Malecha and Nancy Zamboras

COMPONENTS	QUESTIONS TO ASK
The Company	
Historical development	How, why, and by whom was the company founded?
Organizational chart	What is the formal order of the system, and to whom are the health providers responsible?
Company policies	Is there a policy manual? Are the workers aware of the existence of the manual?
Length of the workweek	How many days a week does the industry operate? Is the industry open year-round?
Length of the work time	Are there several shifts? If yes, describe. How many breaks? Is there paid vacation? If yes, how much? Are there scheduled paid holidays?
Sick leave	Is there a clear policy, and do the workers know it?
Family Medical Leave Act (FMLA)	Are employees paid? Are employees paid during maternity leave?
Employee Benefits	
Insurance programs	What types of insurance programs does the company offer? How much does the company pay? What are the monthly premiums? Who completes the forms?
Health	What type of coverage is offered for spouses, life partners, children, or other dependents? Health Maintenance Organization (HMO)? Preferred Provider Organization (PPO)? What is the average co-pay for an office visit or emergency visit? What are the yearly deductibles?
Dental	Is orthodontic treatment covered?
Prescription medications	What medications are covered?
Vision	What type of vision care is covered (annual exam, glasses, contacts)?

(Continued)

COMPONENTS	QUESTIONS TO ASK
Short- and long-term disability	Does the company pay all or part? Is pregnancy covered?
Flexible spending	What type of spending is covered (e.g., childcare expenses, nonprescription medication)?
Life	What types of life insurance are offered?
Employee assistance program (EAP)	Is the EAP on-site or off-site?
Retirement program	What types of retirement programs are available, and how much funding does the company contribute (e.g., 401K, pension plan)? How many years of employment are required before the employee is vested?
Educational program	Does the company offer continuing education on-site? Does the company financially support off-site continuing education (conferences, certification programs, college courses)?
Employee Relations	
Union representation	If a union is present, is there on-site union representation?
Shared governance	Do shared governance committees exist? How do employees voice their grievances?
The Plant	
General physical setting	What is the overall appearance? Is the environment clean? Comment on heating, air-conditioning, overall lighting, green space, ventilation, compliance with the Americans with Disabilities Act (elevators, ramps, restrooms), etc.
Construction	What is the size and general condition of buildings and grounds?
Parking facilities and public transportation	How far do workers have to walk to get inside? What is the overall appearance of the parking structure: Covered? Lighting? Gated entrance? Security? Escort available to parking after-hours? Open to the public? Does the employee have to pay for parking? If yes, how much? Is vanpooling available? What type of public transportation serves the worksite?
Entrances and exits	How many people use them? How accessible are the entrances? Employee badges required? Security-monitored entrance? During what hours is security available? What are the visitor or contractor policies?
Communication facilities	Are there bulletin boards and newsletters? Common areas where all employees can gather such as inside/outside sitting areas (benches, tables)?
Housekeeping	Is the physical setting maintained adequately? Are public areas (lobbies, hallways, restrooms) clean?
Work Areas	
Space	Are workers isolated or crowded?
Ergonomics	Are work areas ergonomically safe: work stations, desk areas, chairs, lighting, computer monitors and keyboards, and work habits? Does the company conduct periodic ergonomic assessments?

COMPONENTS	QUESTIONS TO ASK
Fall precautions	Is there a chance of workers falling or being injured by falling objects?
Safety signs and markings	Are dangerous areas well marked to protect employees from slips, trips, or falls?
Safety equipment	Do the workers make use of hard hats, safety glasses, face masks, radiation badges, and so forth? Are requirements met for the Occupational Safety and Health Administration (OSHA) standards regarding use and maintenance of personal protective equipment (PPE), as well as specific provisions on the use, design, and performance requirements for various types of PPE (eye, face, head, and respiratory protection)?
Nonwork Areas	
Lockers	If the work is dirty, workers should be able to change clothes. Can workers accidentally carry toxic substances home on their clothes? Does the company supply work clothes?
Break rooms, restrooms, recreation rooms	Do workers have an area for resting and taking a break? Is it shared with the public? How accessible are the restrooms? What are the conditions of these areas? What is the policy for taking a break? Do workers feel free to use the facilities? What is the policy on break time? Can a worker who is not feeling well lie down?
Cafeteria or dining area	What types of dining areas exist for employees? Is water readily available? What kinds of food are available on-site (cafeteria, vending machines, etc.)? Are employees permitted to go off-site for meals?
Communications/technology	What are the policies on: receiving personal telephone calls? Voice mail? Use of mobile/cellular phones? Pagers? Personal e-mail? Other handheld technology?
Other nonwork areas	What is the company's smoking policy? Are there designated areas for smoking? Does the company provide on-site childcare?
The Working Population	
General characteristics	
Demographic description of employee population	What is the total number of employees? Usually, if an industry has 500 or more employees, full-time nursing services are recommended. What are the age, gender, socioeconomic, education, relationship status, and race/ethnic distributions?
Cultural considerations	What languages are spoken at the worksite? Do employees observe religious/ethnic holidays? What level of education is required? What is the percentage of skilled and nonskilled employees? What is the percentage of exempt and nonexempt employees? What percentage of employees are physically or mentally challenged?
Work status	How many employees work full-time or part-time? What is the policy on overtime? What is the policy on job sharing? What are the policies on promotion?

(Continued)

COMPONENTS	QUESTIONS TO ASK
Absenteeism	Who keeps a record on absenteeism? What is the absenteeism policy? How many days per year are employees allowed for absences? What are the five most common reasons for absence? What is the return-to-work policy?
International travel or long-term international assignments	Do employees travel internationally for work? If yes, what type of health care is required before travel or international assignment? Whom do employees contact for health care concerns while living out of the country? Does the worksite receive international visitors?
Physical work demands	What percentage of workers engage in physically demanding work or sedentary work?
Outdoor work	Do employees work outside? In what seasons? What health promotion interventions are addressed for outdoor work?
The Industrial Setting and Operations	
Nature of the operations	What does the company produce and how? Ask for a brief description of each stage of operations so that the nurse can compare the needs and abilities of the worker with the needs of the job.
Safety committee	Is there a designated safety committee? If yes, who serves on the committee, and when does the committee meet? If no committee, who oversees safety and fire issues for the worksite? Who is responsible for training of first responders? Are there specific situations or substances in the plant that pose a potential for danger and/or fire? How often are there organized fire drills? Are workers aware of what to do in other emergencies (tornado, earthquake, bomb threat, serious injury, death, etc.)?
Raw materials used	What are they and how dangerous are they? How are they stored? Check the Code of Federal Regulations and the Federal Register for guidelines on storage.
Waste products produced	What is the system for waste disposal? Are pollution-control devices in place and functioning?
Equipment used	What types of equipment are used: fans, blowers, fast-moving, wet, or dry? Is the equipment portable or fixed? Heavy or light? Ask to have each piece of large equipment marked on a scale map. What type of training do workers receive to operate equipment?
Nature of the final product	Can the workers take pride in the final product or do they make only parts?
Exposure to hazardous materials	To which hazardous materials are the workers exposed? Where are the material safety data sheets (MSDS) kept? How often do workers receive training on the MSDS? Are workers exposed to animals and/or animal products?
The Health Program	
Policies and procedures	What type of policies and procedures exist? Are they up to date and written clearly?

COMPONENTS	QUESTIONS TO ASK
Job descriptions for health care providers	Who provides health care to the employees? Are there job descriptions? Is health care delivered at the worksite? Off-site? Is there a medical director for the company? If yes, what are the responsibilities of the medical director (oversees standing orders, first aid/emergency policies)?
Preplacement physicals	Are they required? What types of physicals are offered? Who pays for the physical exams? Who performs the physical exams? Location?
Drug and alcohol screening	Are these screenings required? What types of screening: preplacement, DOT, for cause, random? Who pays for the screenings? Location?
First aid and personnel	What type of first-aid care is available? Who is trained to deliver first aid?
Facilities and resources	What types of space and equipment are available for delivering health care? Where is a sick or injured employee taken? Where is emergency equipment kept? Are automated external defibrillators (AEDs) available?
Supplies	What are they? Where are they kept? Who is responsible for maintenance and reordering? What is the annual budget for supplies? Make a list of the available supplies and describe the condition of each item.
Records, reports, and retention of documents	What medical records exist? Who maintains the OSHA log on work-related injuries and illnesses? Who has access to medical records? How long and where are the medical records kept?
Services provided in the past 12 months	
Clinical care provided	Acute and/or chronic care? Describe the five most common presenting complaints. Is medication dispensed at the worksite? If yes, what types? Where is the medication stored? Are immunizations provided? Who provides the clinical care services?
Work-related injuries/illnesses	How many accidents in the past 12 months? What type of accidents? Health outcomes for injured/ill workers? Who is the workers' compensation carrier? Does the industry have a designated case manager to manage return-to-work issues?
Screening provided	What types of screenings are provided?
Referrals	What types of referrals are made? Is there a list of referral health providers, agencies, and community resources?
Health education and health promotion activities	Does the company support health promotion activities? If yes, what type? Do employees have access to physical fitness facilities either on-site or off-site?

Source: Serafini, P. (1976). Nursing assessment in industry: A model. *American Journal of Public Health, 66*(8), 755–760.

Postscript

It has been over 100 years since Lillian Wald coined the term *public health nurse*. It seems fitting that we "wrap up" this edition with an editorial inspired by Ms. Wald's work in New York City at the turn of the last century. As it was included in the third, fourth, fifth, sixth and now the seventh editions of *Community as Partner*, we fervently hope that such an editorial will not be necessary at the beginning of the next millennium.

A Call for Transformation[*]

Standing in the room where Lillian Wald once lived at Henry Street was an inspiring experience. More than 100 attendees at the American Public Health Association's annual meeting in New York came together to hear Clair Coss read her play about the woman who coined the term "public health nurse" and then visit the historic Henry Street Settlement. Each of us reflected on what public health nursing was in those early days: comprehensive health and illness care that embodied social reform and political involvement.

What happened to this once-glorious group that picketed against war, fought for the rights of women and children, aided the immigrant, initiated school health programs, and saw to it that the poor and disenfranchised received a fair wage and access to health care? In 1920, the public health nurse was described as "...one of the very greatest agents in the advancement of health, both individual and public, in this country" (1). These early professionals accomplished the goals of reducing mortality and morbidity so well that they became a threat to those in power. One of the strongest opponents of home visiting was the American Medical Association (AMA), which successfully fought against federally financed public health programs. In 1930, the AMA condemned such programs as "...unsound in policy, wasteful and extravagant, unproductive of results and tending to promote communism...." (2). In addition, health became a medical concern and, as a result, health problems were depoliticized. Those problems rooted in social disarray were reduced to individual, biologic, or situational factors, and the focus became the individual. Even the sacrosanct home visit became limited to the care of a medically diagnosed problem in order to carry out medically prescribed activities. Funding of programs outside the hospital was predicated on stamping out disease (always with medical prescription to back it up). Other funding was aimed at specific problems, so that we had (and still have) immunization clinics; Women, Infants, and Children programs; sexually transmitted disease clinics; and the like. But the community is not a series of fragmented risk groups. It is a collection of people who want and deserve comprehensive nursing care: primary health care given distributively whether the people are sick or well. The district nurses did that in the early part of this century. Where are they now?

Now is the time to end our focus on fragmented programs and to return to our raison d'etre, the improvement of health: not health as an end, but as a means to a full life. Health cannot occur when the means of achieving a living wage are controlled by a small minority; when agencies charged with maintaining and improving a safe environment are influenced by the polluters they are supposed to police; when the whole structure is predicated on health as a commodity to be doled out to the "deserving" (insured) by a group whose primary mission is to cure disease; when violence, from child abuse to war, is tolerated; when age defines

*Source: Anderson, E. T. (1991). Editorial: A call for transformation. *Public Health Nursing, 8*(1), 1–2.

usefulness and is given as a reason to withhold care and treatment; and when a majority of the population is relegated to second-class status because of gender, race, or ethnicity.

Community health nurses can transform our fragmented, disease-oriented "system," not by bemoaning the loss of our glorious past, but by looking into the future, by focusing on a goal and the strategies to achieve it. Health for all through primary health care means that the nurses first ask the people what they want to improve their health and then take the responsibility to work as partners with them to achieve it (empowerment). This means working with others, not just the health team, but community groups, business and education leaders, politicians, engineers, and others to overcome inequities.

Community health nurses in the model of Lillian Wald can make a difference. Let us begin immediately either to change our public health care system (now in "disarray" (3)) or forge out on our own as Ms. Wald did, get our own financing, and deliver district nursing as it should be. We know we can reduce mortality and morbidity as she did; our research has demonstrated this. What we need is a galvanizing force to do so. Our challenge is this: Join with the community to transform an unjust and failing health care system to one that reflects health for all, the legacy of Lillian Wald.

Elizabeth T. Anderson, Dr. P.H., R.N., F.A.A.N.
Galveston, TX

REFERENCES

1. Welch, W. H. (1920). *Papers and addresses* (*Vol. 3*, p. 165). Baltimore, MD: Johns Hopkins University Press.
2. Donahue, M. P. (1985). *Nursing: The finest art* (p. 339). St. Louis, MO: C. V. Mosby.
3. Committee for the Study of the Future of Public Health, Division of Health Care Services, Institute of Medicine. (1988). *The future of public health* (p. 19). Washington, DC: National Academy Press.

Index

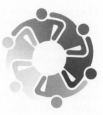

Note: Page numbers followed by f indicate figures; those followed by t indicate tables; and those followed by b indicate boxed material.

CCS0915